D0611478

Erectile Dysfunction

Contents

List of contributors

Michael A Adams
Department of Pharmacology and Toxicology
Queen's University
Kingston, Ontario, Canada K71 3N6

Karl-Erik Andersson
Department of Urology
University of Virginia Health Sciences Center
Box 422
Charlottesville, Virginia 22908, USA

James D Banting
Department of Pharmacology and Toxicology
Queen's University
Kingston, Ontario, Canada K71 3N6

Culley C Carson
Division of Urology
University of North Carolina School of Medicine
427 Burnett-Womack Building, CB #7235
Chapel Hill, North Carolina 27599-7235, USA

Andrea Cestari
Department of Urology
Istituto Scientifico H San Raffaele
Via Luigi Prinetti, 29
I-20127 Milan, Italy

George J Christ
Laboratory of Molecular and Integrative Urology
Room 716S, Forchheimer Building
Albert Einstein College of Medicine
1300 Morris Park Avenue
Bronx,
New York 10461, USA

Ahmed I El-Sakka
Department of Urology
University of California, San Francisco
Box 0738
San Francisco, CA 94143-0738, USA

Giorgio Guazzoni
Department of Urology
Istituto Scientifico H San Raffaele
Via Luigi Prinetti, 29
I-20127 Milan, Italy

Jeremy PW Heaton
Departments of Urology and Pharmacology and Toxicology
Queen's University
Kingston, Ontario, Canada K71 3N6

Enrique Lledo Garcia
Unidad de Urologia
Area de Cirugia
Fundacion Hospital Alcorcon
Alcorcon, Madrid, Spain

Tom F Lue
Department of Urology
University of California, San Francisco
Box 0739
San Francisco, California 94143-0739, USA

Kazushi Manabe
Department of Pharmacology and Toxicology
Queen's University
Kingston, Ontario, Canada K71 3N6

Murray C Maytom
Pfizer Central Research
Ramsgate Road
Sandwich CT13 9NJ, UK

Eric JH Meuleman
Academisch Ziekenhuis Nijmegen
Department of Urology
Postbus 0191
6500 HB Nijmegen, The Netherlands

Ignacio Moncada Iribarren
Unidad Andrologia
Servicio de Urologia
Hospital General Universitario
Gregorio Marañon
Madrid, Spain

Alvaro Morales
Department of Urology
Queen's University
Kingston, Ontario, Canada K7L 2V7

Francesco Montorsi
Institute of Human Anatomy
University of Milan School of Medicine
and Department of Urology
Istituto Scientifico H San Raffaele
Via Luigi Prinetti, 29
I-20127 Milan, Italy

Ian H Osterloh
Pfizer Central Research
Ramsgate Road
Sandwich CT13 9NJ, UK

Harin Padma-Nathan
Department of Urology
University of Southern California School of Medicine
and The Male Clinic
9100 Wilshire Blvd
Suite 350
Beverly Hills, CA 90212, USA

Hartmut Porst
Urological Office,
Never Iungfernsteig 6a
20354 Hamburg, Germany

John P Pryor
Institute of Urology
48 Riding House Street,
London W1P 7PN, UK

David Ralph
Institute of Urology,
48 Riding House Street,
London W1P 7PN, UK

Patrizio Rigatti
Department of Urology
Istituto Scientifico H San Raffaele
Via Luigi Prinetti, 29
I-20127 Milan, Italy

Iñigo Saenz de Tejada
Departamento de Investigacion
Hospital Ramon y Cajal
E-28034 Madrid, Spain

William D Steers
Department of Urology
University of Virginia Health Sciences Center
Box 422
Charlottesville, Virginia 22908, USA

J Lisa Tenover
Division of Geriatric Medicine and Gerontology
Emory University School of Medicine
Wesley Woods Center on Aging
1817 Clifton Road, NE
Atlanta, Georgia 30329, USA

Martyn A Vickers, Jr
Department of Veterans Affairs
Medical and Regional Office Center
1 VA center
Rogus, Maine 04330, USA

Pierre A Wicker
Pfizer Central Research
Ramsgate Road
Sandwich CT13 9NJ, UK

Foreword

It is very timely that this volume coincides with the introduction of the first scientifically proven oral therapy for erectile dysfunction. Strict scientific investigational trials have also begun or will begin in various regions of the world for other oral agents to be used in the treatment of erectile dysfunction. Heretofore, the pharmacological treatment of erectile dysfunction has been limited to intracaversonal injection or intraurethral therapy with a few sporadic reports of mediocre results with topicals. The emerging oral therapeutic agents are more likely to succeed because the development of these pharmaceutical agents has been paired with an understanding of the events occurring in the corpora cavernosa tissue with erection and detumescence at the molecular level. It is imperative that any physician involved in the pharmacological management of erectile dysfunction have a solid foundation in understanding the molecular biology of erection and the scientific rationale for the various therapeutic choices.

This volume is an excellent beginning for achieving that goal. It is edited by Alvaro Morales of Queen's University in Kingston, Ontario; his individual accomplishments in this field and the accomplishments of his department are recognized around the world. Queen's University has been a pioneer in the evaluation of previous oral therapies and the new emerging oral therapies, so it is appropriate that a volume such as this emanates from this institution. Dr Morales has gathered an excellent representative group of participants to contribute to this volume. The chapters allow a reader to understand the basic mechanisms of penile erection and to understand how knowledge in this area has led to the development of new therapies. The reader will also be able to understand the emerging therapies more clearly by mastering the concepts presented in this volume. Pharmacologic management of erectile dysfunction will become more complicated, will require more precise diagnosis to determine the suitable agent(s) for the individual patient's problem, and may involve, in the not too distant future, the use of several different approaches at the molecular level. This is a well conceived volume with many excellent chapters that will help physicians address these issues.

Ronald W Lewis

Preface

Few fields in medicine can match the rapid progress that has been made in our understanding of male erectile function. These changes have been profound, and fundamental. Baseless speculation about the essential vascular mechanisms of erection and the belief in a predominantly emotional etiology have given way to the identification of the molecular events resulting in an erection and to effective pharmacological treatment of their alterations. The current state of the art is a pre-eminent example of what is achievable by systematic and conscientious application of basic research and clinical observation. Many clinicians and basic scientists throughout the world have made enormous contributions to the study of this fundamental physiological process.

It is particularly gratifying to note that the study of sexual function has now achieved a place among the scientific disciplines. Gone for ever are the days of the patronizing dismissal of patients with erectile problems and of unsubstantiated treatments. The task now is to enhance and disseminate the acquired knowledge among health-care professionals. It is equally important to sensitize all levels of society to the personal and interpersonal impact of sexual dysfunction, the successful therapeutic avenues currently available and the promising treatments now emerging. One hopes that the new century will largely eliminate the silent frustration of couples unaware of these opportunities. The advent of effective pharmacotherapy has brought more options and new challenges. *Erectile Dysfunction: Issues in Current Pharmacotherapy* was carefully planned to bring together a practical compilation of relevant topics to address scientifically this ever-increasing selection of treatments. Each chapter is crisp but deals with its topic in depth and with authority. I am profoundly indebted to each and every contributor for their generous dedication and willingness to participate in this endeavour. Their selfless enthusiasm and well-deserved international reputation are gratefully acknowledged. Their expertise in the topic about which they wrote is vast, but has been delivered in a concise and easily understandable manner. I wish to express my thanks also to Mr Robert Peden for his continuous support and guidance from the planning to the editing of this volume and to Mrs Sheila Milonas for superb secretarial support.

Alvaro Morales
Kingston, Canada

1

An update on the physiology of erection

Enrique Lledo Garcia, Ignacio Moncada Iribarren, Iñigo Saenz de Tejada

From the Sumerians to Galen

Male impotence is an ancient entity, as old as human beings. The first written evidence for it comes from the Sumerian tablets; this, however, is a mere historical record of the illness, and not an elaborate text containing possible remedies.

Egyptian papyri offer the first detailed descriptions of erectile impotence. In these documents two types of disease are mentioned (Brenot 1994). Firstly, "natural impotence", where the male is generally unable to have sexual intercourse, and secondly "supernatural impotence", where a spell causes the individual to lose his virility when he meets his partner.

Several centuries later, Hippocrates tried to explain several problems related to sexuality and fecundity (Brenot 1994). This author outlined two concepts that were to remain unchallenged until the Renaissance.

First came the belief that sperm come from the spinal marrow, reaching a particular duct of the penis via the kidneys, ureters and testes. On the other hand, the concepts of impotence and sterility were also identified and exemplified in the descriptions of eunuchs. Even though it is certain that Hippocrates outlined the existence of "some fine nerves that branch to the copulatory organs", he assumed that this innervation originated anatomically in the testes. Therefore, in these individuals, castration would eliminate sexual potency as well as their reproductive capacity.

Hippocrates exemplified his "pathogenic" explanations of impotence in terms of the population of Scythia (Brenot 1994). According to him, these individuals over-indulged in horse-riding, and this was the cause of their high incidence of erectile dysfunction. He even applied "psychoanalytical" concepts to this population, thus explaining what seems to be psychogenic impotence.

Aristotle (fourth century BC) outlined a more "spiritual" vision of sexuality. According to him, semen originates from the masculine soul. Men are superior to women, and this view is confirmed by their procreative capacity, which in women is limited to a much younger age. Aristotle established the fecundity age-limit in men at 71 years.

This author's theories were taken up several centuries later, and remained almost unaltered until the Renaissance. Galen continued the same "spiritual" line of thought as Aristotle. His great doubts referred to the origin of semen and the physical location of conception (Musitelli et al 1996). The absence of accurate anatomical studies frequently helped to sustain misconceptions. Saint Thomas Aquinas and René Descartes conceived the existence of a "masculine semen" and a "feminine semen" that would be mixed during the sexual act to form an embryo. The persistence of the Aristotelian idea of masculine predominance is also found in the few known anatomical descriptions that exist. André Vésale (Vesalius) and Ambroise Paré represented the organs of the feminine internal genitalia with the same shape as the external masculine ones: thus the uterus and the vagina were seen as an internalised penis and the ovaries were called testes (Brenot 1994).

The progressive views of Leonardo da Vinci

Leonardo da Vinci tried to challenge some of Aristotle's concepts (O'Malley and Saunders 1952). One of the most firmly established ideas from Aristotle's time was that the erection was produced by a massive entry of air (*spirit*) into the penis through nerves originating in the respiratory system and the spinal marrow. Leonardo cast doubt on this theory, and suggested alternatives based on anatomical observations. He studied the corpses of hanged men whose erection had persisted after death. He claimed that the penis was filled with blood and not with air in the erectile state, and cited the physical aspect of penile skin and the glans in erection, bearing little resemblance to an air-filled organ, to support his theory. It is, in fact, the first time in history that an explanation of this nature is offered. Subsequently, other anatomists such as Paré and Hunter (sixteenth and eighteenth centuries) confirmed these theories, but at a much later point in time.

The sixteenth to nineteenth centuries: anatomical progress and attempts to explain "venous retention"

Ambroise Paré provided interesting anatomical, clinical and even therapeutic concepts in the sixteenth century (Jardin 1996). After performing numerous dissections, this author outlined the internal structure of the penis as formed by "nerves, veins, arteries, four muscles, two ligaments and a urinary conduit". He claimed that these ligaments were spongy (corpora cavernosa or corpus spongiosum), and that they were linked to vascular and nervous branches, which filled with blood during erection. He introduced the concepts of priapism and erectile dysfunction, going so far as to give remedies and offer diagnostic tests. Paré compiled his observations into the huge corpus of his *Complete Works*, which contains two important volumes on this subject (*Ten Books on Surgery* and *Book of Reproduction*).

From the sixteenth century onwards a cascade of more objective explanations of the mechanisms of erection appeared. In 1573 Varolio published the hypothesis that the blood that enters the penis during erection is retained by means of a contracted venous muscular layer. De Graaf (de Vries 1996) in 1668 suggested that the blood was held specifically in two anatomical spaces of the penis (the corpora cavernosa), though Dionis perfected this theory in 1718 with the idea that the corpus spongiosum also retained blood and helped to prevent its drainage (Brenot 1994).

John Hunter in the eighteenth century is the first anatomist who elaborated a complete explanation of the physiology of erection, based on observations in animal and human corpses (Androutsos 1994). According to this author, the erection is produced by a massive entry of blood into the corpus cavernosum, which is retained there owing to a consequent venous spasm. When these veins are relaxed, the erection concludes. Hunter suggested that both the corpus spongiosum and the glans are also filled with blood to a similar pressure.

Up to this time many authors had still thought that perineal musculature was fundamental in helping to maintain the erection. In the nineteenth century many authors cast doubt on this concept, and an "intracavernous" vision of erection emerged: the need for a primarily cavernous mechanism, not dependent on perineal musculature but on a tissue structure that itself allows initial blood entry and its subsequent retention, is established. This mechanism is mainly outlined by Dionis. In the second half of the nineteenth century Magendie, Bernard and Boeckel reinforced the idea of the primary role of the cavernous bodies in the production and maintenance of erection.

The twentieth century: definitive advances

In the twentieth century anatomical studies were carried out on penile venous anatomy and on the so-called "theory of venous retention". Bondil and Wespès (1992) concluded in 1935 that the main gaps remaining were the exact mechanism involved in retention, as well as the role of the corpus spongiosum.

Anatomical studies aside, few contributions on this subject were made in the second half of the twentieth century. It was only in 1982 that Virag (1982) published the effect of vasoactive intravenous drugs in *The Lancet* for the first time. From then on in-depth research was carried out on the physiological and biochemical mechanisms of erection. In 1983, Brindley (1983) discovered the beneficial action of intracavernous injections of phenoxybenzamine, and in 1986 Ishii et al introduced the use of prostaglandin E_1. The rate of advance of these discoveries has been spectacular in recent times, shedding new light on penile hemodynamics, neuroanatomy, functional anatomy and the pharmacology of erection. Great advances in the understanding of the role of neurotransmitters in the relaxation of smooth cavernous muscle and pharmacological research into erectile mechanisms have also taken place. These discoveries have led to substantial improvements in the diagnosis and treatment of erectile dysfunction.

Functional vascular and neurological penile anatomy

Introduction

Knowledge of penile anatomy is essential in order to understand the physiology of the states of erection and flaccidity (Figure 1). The penis contains the urethra and three erectile bodies: two corpora cavernosa and the corpus spongiosum. Different fascial sheaths can be observed: Buck's fascia wraps the erectile bodies, and is firmly attached to the underlying tunica albuginea. Surrounding this fascia is Colles' fascia or the superficial penile fascia, which joins Scarpa's fascia of the lower abdominal wall and the dartos fascia of the scrotum. Above this fascia is the skin (Tobin and Benjamin 1944).

Two ligamentous attachments, linked to Buck's fascia, suspend the body of the penis proximally from the linea alba to the pubic bone: the suspensory ligament, which extends from the pubic symphysis to Buck's fascia, and the fundiform ligament, which lies distal to the suspensory

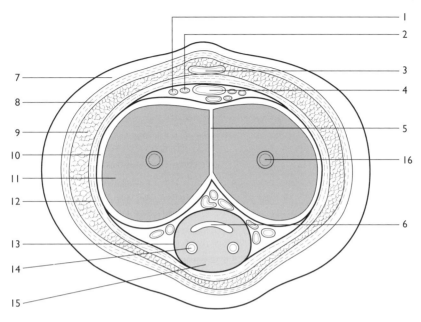

Figure 1
Penile anatomy: (1) Dorsal nerve; (2) dorsal artery; (3) superficial dorsal vein; (4) deep dorsal vein; (5) intercavernosal septum; (6) urethra; (7) skin; (8) dartos; (9) subcutaneous tissue; (10) tunica albuginea; (11) corpora cavernosa; (12) penile fascia; (13) corpus spongiosum albuginea; (14) bulbourethral artery; (15) corpus spongiosum; (16) cavernosal artery.

ligament, arising from the lower part of the linea alba, passing on either side of the penis, and coming together, inferiorly, as part of the scrotal septum. Proximal to the suspensory ligament, the right and left corpora cavernosa diverge, forming a crus, which reaches the ischial tuberosities, on either side. Ischiocavernous muscles cover each of the crura, and may play a role in the final rigid phase of erection.

The urethra is surrounded by the corpus spongiosum throughout the entire ventral groove formed by both corpora cavernosa in the pendulous portion of the penis. Proximally, it forms the bulb, which is attached to the inferior layer of the urogenital diaphragm. Distally, the corpus spongiosum expands, forming the glans penis. The spongiosum is composed of sinusoidal spaces of a larger size than those of the cavernosal bodies and with less smooth muscle.

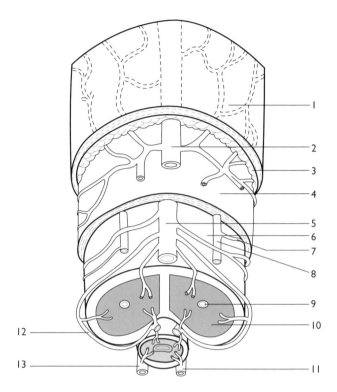

Figure 2
Penile vascular anatomy: (1) dartos; (2) superficial dorsal vein; (3) subcutaneous tissue; (4) penile fascia; (5) deep dorsal vein; (6) tunica albuginea; (7) dorsal artery; (8) penile dorsal artery branch; (9) cavernosal artery; (10) corpus cavernosum; (11) urethral veins; (12) circumflex veins; (13) bulbourethral veins.

The corpora cavernosa are two cylinders, dorsally located in the penis. Geometrically, they are paired tubular structures that connect freely through a common perforated midline septum, and may therefore be considered physiologically as a single blood space (Goldstein et al 1985). Each corpus cavernosum is wrapped in a thick fibrous sheath, the tunica albuginea, forming a white coat. Two layers may be identified in this structure: an outer longitudinal and an inner circular coat. Ventrally, the tunica albuginea forms a groove for the corpus spongiosum. Ventromedially, the tunica is thinner as the outer coat becomes attenuated, leaving only the inner coat. The erectile tissue is composed of multiple lacunar spaces, interconnected and lined by vascular endothelium. The trabeculae are the walls of these spaces, and are formed by smooth muscle (around 45%) and a fibroelastic framework of, mainly, collagen (Goldstein and Padma-Nathan 1990).

Vascular anatomy and neuroanatomy

Arterial and venous vascularization

Penile vascular anatomy is composed of a stratified arterial and venous network (Figure 2) of progressive complexity. The internal pudendal artery, a branch of the hypogastric artery, is mainly responsible for the blood supply to the deep structures of the penis (Figure 3). In the pelvis, it becomes the common penile artery after branching off the perineal artery. Near the bulb of the urethra it gives off four terminal branches before reaching the corpora cavernosa: bulbar, urethral, dorsal and cavernosal arteries (Breza et al 1989). The cavernosal artery pierces the tunica, entering each corpus cavernosum at the hilum of the penis, where the two corpora come together, running near the center of each

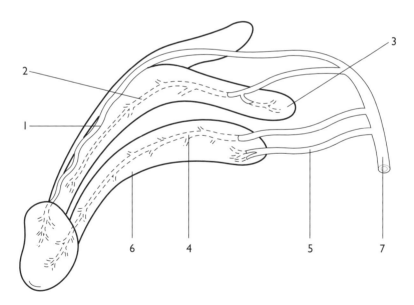

Figure 3
Arterial anatomy of the penis. (1) Dorsal artery; (2) cavernous artery;
(3) corpus cavernosum; (4) urethral artery; (5) bulbar artery;
(6) corpus spongiosum; (7) pudendal artery.

corpus. It gives off numerous terminal branches called helicine arteries. These muscular arteries are corkscrew-shaped and open directly into the lacunar spaces. There are multiple layers of smooth muscle surrounding these resistance arteries, and these act as a sphincter. In flaccidity this muscle is contracted, allowing only small amounts of blood into the lacunar spaces. After the proper stimulus, this muscle relaxes, and the arteries dilate and straighten, increasing blood flow and pressure to the lacunar spaces. The cavernosal arteries supply the bulk of the blood that is delivered to the corpora cavernosa.

The dorsal artery is a terminal branch of the internal pudendal artery. It travels along the dorsal surface of each corpus beneath the Buck's fascia between the deep dorsal vein (medially) and the dorsal nerves (laterally), reaching the glans penis. It gives off circumflex branches that contribute to the blood supply of the urethra; its terminal branches provide blood to the glans and account for glans congestion during erection (Devine and Angermeier 1994). On occasions the dorsal artery perforates the tunica and contributes to the blood supply of the corpora cavernosa.

The urethra is mainly irrigated by the bulbar artery (in its most proximal portion) and the urethral artery, which runs along the corpus spongiosum, providing blood supply to the penile urethra and corpus spongiosum. Sometimes, bulbar and urethral arteries have a common origin in a bulbourethral artery (Breza et al 1989; Devine and Angermeier 1994). Finally, the penile skin and the prepuce are irrigated by branches of the external pudendal artery.

Venous blood drainage from the penis is carried out by three systems: superficial, intermediate and deep (Figure 4).

The superficial system drains venous blood from the skin and subcutaneous tissue above Buck's fascia. These veins drain into the superficial dorsal vein, which usually drains into the left external pudendal branch of the internal saphenous vein.

The intermediate venous system drains blood from the glans, the corpus spongiosum and the two distal thirds of the corpora cavernosa. It lies beneath Buck's fascia and is composed of the deep dorsal vein and the circumflex veins. The deep dorsal vein runs as a single trunk in a groove between both corpora. It enters the pelvis through the suspensory ligament to drain into the periprostatic (Santorini's) plexus.

The deep drainage system is composed of the cavernosal veins and the crural veins.

Corpora cavernosa drainage is by way of venules located at the periphery of the erectile tissue, forming a network under the tunica albuginea. These venules coalesce to form the emissary veins, which pierce the tunica and drain either directly into the deep dorsal vein or by way of the circumflex veins.

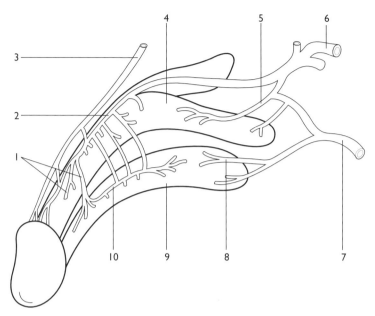

Figure 4
Venous anatomy of the penis. (1) Circumflex veins; (2) deep dorsal vein; (3) superficial dorsal vein; (4) corpus cavernosum; (5) cavernous veins; (6) periprostatic venous plexus; (7) pudendal vein; (8) bulbo-urethral veins; (9) corpus spongiosum; (10) urethral veins.

    Subtunical venules are functionally very important. Their compression and elongation by the expansion of the trabecular structures against the tunica, secondary to the change in penile volume during erection, causes a dramatic increase in the resistance to blood outflow from the corpora. This is known as the corporo-veno-occlusive mechanism, which is triggered by the relaxation of trabecular smooth muscle (Krane et al 1989). This mechanism allows the maintenance of high intracavernosal pressure with low maintenance flow. Once erection has been established, only 1–5 ml of blood are needed to maintain intracavernosal pressures within a physiological range (60 and 100 mmHg) (Saenz de Tejada et al 1991a).

Lymphatic system

The lymphatic drainage of the penis is through the superficial and deep inguinal lymph nodes of the femoral triangle, which, in turn,

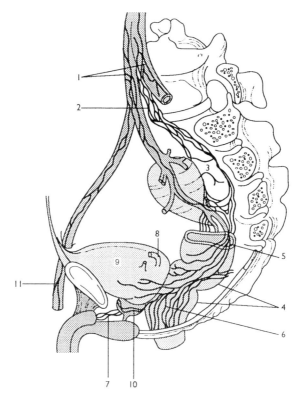

Figure 5
Neuroanatomy: autonomic innervation – hypogastric or pelvic
plexus. (1) Iliac plexus; (2) hypogastric plexus; (3) hypogastric
nerves; (4) pelvic ganglia; (5) pelvic plexus; (6) lower hemorrhoidal
plexus; (7) cavernosal nerves; (8) deferential plexus; (9) bladder
plexus; (10) prostatic plexus; (11) femoral plexus.

drain into the external and common iliac lymph nodes. However, the
lymphatic drainage of the posterior urethra is to the internal iliac
lymph nodes. Drainage from the anterior urethra is also via the
inguinal lymph nodes (Devine and Angermeier 1994).

Functional neuroanatomy

Three groups of peripheral nerves play a role in erectile function:
thoracolumbar sympathetic, lumbosacral parasympathetic and lumbosacral somatic (Figure 5) (De Groat and Steers 1988; Steers 1990).

The thoracolumbar sympathetic center is anatomically located in the intermediolateral gray matter of the tenth thoracic to the second lumbar spinal cord segments. Three main levels of synapsis can be observed: the paravertebral ganglion chain; the hypogastric – forming the superior hypogastric plexus and the pelvic plexus; and postganglionic fibers, which join to form the cavernous nerve, which enters the penis near the posterolateral side of the prostate.

The sacral parasympathetic center is located in the intermediolateral gray matter of the spinal cord from the second to the fourth sacral segments (Lue et al 1984; Steers 1990). The sacral preganglionic nerves constitute the pelvis nerve which reaches the pelvic plexus and from which the cavernous nerve, which innervates the penis, emerges.

The cavernous nerve, containing sympathetic and parasympathetic postganglionic and some preganglionic fibers, provides innervation to each corpus cavernosum. Two branches may be found. One is the lesser cavernous nerve, which supplies the erectile tissue of the corpus spongiosum as well as the penile urethra. The other branch, the greater cavernous nerve, stays beneath the prostatic venous plexus and enters the corpora cavernosa around the cavernous vessels in the hilum of the penis.

The cavernous nerve is one of the elements of the so-called neurovascular bundle. It runs between the posterolateral surface of the prostate and the rectum, and lies above the endopelvic fascia and under Santorini's venous plexus. Posterolateral to the prostate, the bundle gives off fine branches to supply the prostatic capsule. At the prostatic apex the nerve passes very near to the urethral lumen at the 3 and 9 o'clock positions, and enters the penile crura at 1 and 11 o'clock. This is the main nerve responsible for providing signal transmission to the erectile tissue, eliciting relaxation of smooth muscle and, thus, erection. The understanding of this neuroanatomy of erection has stimulated strategies for the preservation of potency in operations such as radical prostatectomy, normally associated with a high rate of postoperative impotence (Walsh and Donker 1982; Lue et al 1984).

The pudendal nerve is responsible for somatic innervation. It is composed of motor efferent fibers innervating the ischiocavernosal and bulbocavernosal muscles, as well as sensory fibers from the penis and perineal skin. Along the way it gives off several branches, such as the perineal nerve, with branches to the posterior part of the scrotum, and the rectal nerve, supplying the inferior rectal area. But the most important of these is the dorsal nerve of the penis, which arises as the last branch of the pudendal nerve. This nerve runs along the dorsal penile shaft lateral to the dorsal artery. Multiple fascicles fan out from the dorsal nerve, supplying proprioceptive and sensory nerve terminals on the surface of the tunica albuginea and sensory terminals in the skin and glans penis. Deep dorsal veins, dorsal arteries and dorsal nerves constitute the neurovascular bundle of the penis, a structure that must be handled very carefully when penile surgery is to be performed, as damage to it may cause anesthesia in the glans and penile shaft as well as necrosis of the glans if there is not enough arterial supply from the urethral arteries (Amarenco and Casanova 1991).

Central nervous system control of erection is very important, both eliciting and inhibiting responses to stimulus as modulator of spinal activity. It could be said that the CNS regulation functions comprise the psychogenic integration of stimulus and the secondary activation, maintenance and inhibition of erection.

It is known that penile erections are elicited by local sensory stimulation of the frenulum, glans penis and penile skin (reflexogenic erections) and by central psychogenic stimuli received by or generated within the brain (psychogenic erections). Reflexogenic and psychogenic erectile mechanisms probably act synergistically in the control of penile erection (Krane et al 1989).

Reflexogenic and psychogenic erections are the result of different forms of stimulus reception and secondary response break-out. Reflexogenic erections are mediated by a spinal reflex pathway in which the afferent limb consists of sensory receptors in the penile skin and the glans, and the dorsal nerve that joins the pudendal nerve to reach the sacral spinal cord. The efferent limb arises in the sacral parasympathetic center and contributes fibers to the pelvic nerve, which enters the erectile tissue as the cavernosal nerve.

However, the pathways for psychogenic erections are less well understood. They are initiated in supraspinal centers by auditory, olfactory, imaginative or visual stimuli. The brain exerts an important modulating influence over spinal reflex pathways after processing this information, activating or inhibiting erections.

Modulation of penile erection occurs in diverse areas of the brain. This is predictable on the basis of the elevated number of stimuli that are known to elicit erectile responses. The thalamic nuclei, the rhinencephalon and the limbic structures are involved in the modulation of psychogenic penile erections.

The medial preoptic–anterior hypothalamic area, the cortico-subcortical region of the limbic system, and the medial preoptic–anterior hypothalamic area integrate messages from diverse regions. Efferent pathways from the medial preoptic–anterior area enter the medial forebrain bundle and then pass caudally into the midbrain tegmental region near the lateral part of the substantia nigra. Caudal to the midbrain the efferent pathway travels in the ventrolateral part of the pons and medulla, reaching the spinal centers via the lateral funiculus of the spinal cord.

The function of higher centers is less clear. It has been postulated that three systems are involved in penile erection: the gyrus rectus, the cingulate gyrus and the hippocampus and hippocampal projections to the septum (De Groat and Steers 1988; Steers 1990).

Physiology of erection

Hemodynamics of erection

The penis accumulates blood under pressure during erection (Saenz de Tejada et al 1991), acting as a capacitor (Figure 6). In the state of

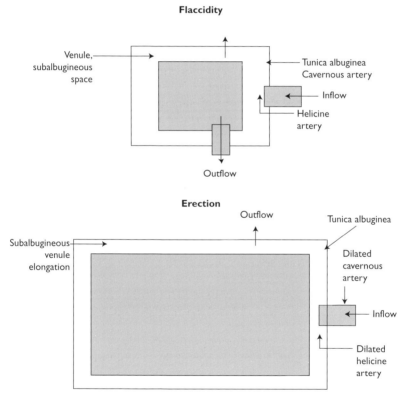

Figure 6

Schematic view of erection/flaccidity mechanisms. Top: flaccidity state, smooth-muscle contraction: lacunar space low flow, low pressure. Bottom: erection state, smooth-muscle relaxation: lacunar space high pressure, veno-occlusive mechanism.

flaccidity the cavernosal and helicine resistance arteries are contracted; thus a state of low flow and low pressure exists in the penis. Peak flow velocity is not detectable or below 15 cm/s under those conditions (Moncada et al 1992). This fact creates a large pressure gradient between the cavernosal artery and the lacunar spaces, which is needed to maintain the flaccid state of the penis. The first event leading to penile erection is dilatation of cavernosal and helicine arteries. In a healthy potent man, a twofold dilatation of the cavernous artery from 0.5 mm to 1 mm in diameter and a peak flow velocity of over 30 cm/s can be detected (Lue and Tanagho 1987). High flow enters the corpora cavernosa during both diastolic and systolic phases. The dilated blood vessels allow transmission of systemic pressure to the corpora. Progressively, the penis begins to show a change in volume and fullness, and the intracavernosal pressure begins to rise.

Dilatation of the lacunar spaces with expansion of the erectile tissue against the tunica albuginea is a consequence of relaxation of the trabecular smooth muscle, which increases the compliance of the tissue. Subtunical venules are elongated and probably compressed against the tunica albuginea because of the change in volume of the penis and the expansion of the erectile tissue. The functional result of this anatomical change of compression of the venules is a large increase in the resistance to the passage of flow through these vessels, which is the functional basis of the corporo-veno-occlusive mechanism (De Groat and Steers 1988).

The contractile physiological activity of the penile muscle is regulated by several factors: adequate levels of agonists (neurotransmitters, hormones and endothelium-derived substances), adequate receptor expression, integrity of the transduction mechanisms, calcium homeostasis, and interaction between contractile proteins, as well as the intercellular communication among the muscular cells (gap junctions) (Christ 1995).

The tone of the trabecular smooth muscle is the main regulating factor of the corporo-veno-occlusive mechanism. When the smooth muscle is contracted, there is low resistance to outflow, allowing for the easy evacuation of the corporeal bodies and so contributing to the maintenance of penile flaccidity. Conversely, following smooth-muscle relaxation, the penis rapidly expands and elongates to its maximal capacity, together with a large increase in outflow resistance: around 100-fold compared to the flaccid state.

When the compliance limit for the fibroelastic elements of the penis has been reached the intracavernosal pressure increases rapidly. When it rises above the diastolic pressure, inflow occurs only in the systolic phase (Fournier et al 1987). The intracavernosal pressure evens out at a pressure nearing that of the cavernosal artery systolic occlusion pressure minus the loss of pressure from corporeal drainage. Arterial pressure rather than arterial flow appears to govern penile rigidity under physiological conditions in which an effective corporo-veno-occlusive mechanism is in place (De Groat and Steers 1988).

Several parameters can be used to express the quality of the erectile response. The most important is penile rigidity (Lavoisier et al 1988), but other factors that depend on the architecture and geometry of the penis are also relevant. A recent study describes the link between penile buckling forces and their underlying constituents (Hatzichristou et al 1995). The major factors associated with penile rigidity in this study were: (1) high values of intracavernosal pressure (pressure was related to rigidity in an exponential fashion); (2) high values of penile aspect ratio (the relationship between penile diameter and length); and (3) high expandability of erectile tissue, implying the ability to achieve maximal volume at low-pressure values during pressure loading.

Regulation of penile smooth-muscle contractility

The hemodynamics of the penis and, therefore, erection are regulated by the smooth muscle of the penis. It constitutes 45% of the total volume of the cavernosal bodies (Wespès et al 1991). The molecular structure of the cytoskeleton and the contractile proteins are important in order to maintain the passive and active characteristics of penile smooth muscle.

Mechanical properties of cavernosal tissue are of two types:

- *Passive*: these depend on the relative proportion between muscular and non-muscular components, particularly collagen, and on the orientation of smooth muscle (Goldstein et al 1985; Steers 1994).
- *Active*: these are most influenced by adequate levels of agonists (neurotransmitters, hormones and endothelium-derived factors), adequate expression of receptors, integrity of transduction mechanisms, calcium homeostasis, and interactions with contractile proteins, as well as intercellular communication between smooth-muscle cells (gap junctions) (Steers 1994).

Ultrastructural examination of a smooth-muscle cell reveals thin, thick and intermediate filamentous structures (Steers 1994). Thin filaments are mainly composed of actin. Thick filaments are formed of myosin. Intermediate filaments contain either desmin or vimentin. Each type of filament has a specific function.

Following phosphorylation of myosin by ATP, attachments form between the globular heads of a light chain of myosin and actin. These attachments confer contractile tone on the smooth muscle (Hai and Murphy 1988). Maintenance of this tone is achieved at the expense of little ATP, owing to the establishment of a latch state of the cross-bridges between actin and myosin. This state of tone demands a high concentration of cytoplasmic free calcium.

An adequate concentration of free calcium is required for the regulation of smooth-muscle tone. Several mechanisms are needed to achieve this (Figure 7):

* influx of extracellular calcium through voltage-regulated channels;

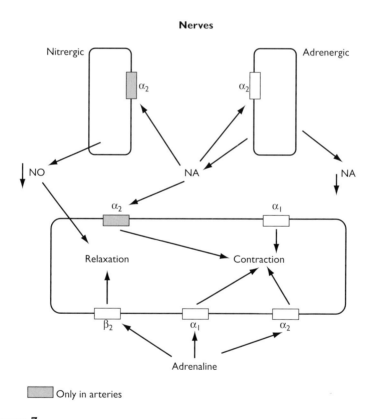

Figure 7
Adrenergic mechanisms of penile smooth muscle (arterial and trabecular). NA: noradrenaline α = alpha-adrenergic receptor; β = beta-adrenergic receptor.

- activation of membrane-bound receptors that allow extracellular calcium to enter the cell through receptor-operated channels; and
- activation of release mechanisms of calcium from sarcoplasmic reticulum.

Relaxation of smooth muscle is achieved by lowering cytosolic calcium. The critical event for this process is the accumulation of the cyclic nucleotides cAMP and cGMP in response to various agonists. Protein kinase G and protein kinase A activate multiple mechanisms that reduce intracellular calcium. In addition to the induction of cGMP formation, nitric oxide has been shown to stimulate Na^+ pump activity. This would induce hyperpolarization, with subsequent closure of voltage-sensitive Ca^{2+} channels.

Other substances accomplish muscle relaxation by way of a cAMP-dependent mechanism, such as prostaglandin E, vasoactive intestinal polypeptide (VIP) and catecholamines.

Smooth-muscle responses are characteristically coordinated through gap junctions (Christ et al 1991). These consist of intercellular channel formations due to homologous cell membrane protein junctions (conexins). These channels act as a common cytoplasmic pathway for the flow of molecules (inositol triphosphate) and calcium ions (Christ et al 1993). The major protein component of gap junctions of penile smooth-muscle cells is conexin 43 (Campos de Carvallo et al 1993).

Regulatory mechanisms of penile smooth-muscle contractility

Several mechanisms are activated to regulate penile smooth-muscle contractility. They can be divided into two groups: (1) neurogenic control (adrenergic, cholinergic and non-adrenergic, non-cholinergic neuroeffector systems) and (2) endothelial control (substances released by the endothelium lining penile arteries and lacunar spaces) (Saenz de Tejada 1992) (Figures 7 and 8).

Neurogenic control

Adrenergic mechanisms:

The detumescence of the erect penis is mediated by adrenergic nerve terminals whose neurotransmitter, noradrenaline, activates adrenergic receptors. Cavernosal and helicine arteries, as well as cavernosal smooth muscle of humans, receive adrenergic innervation (Andersson 1993).

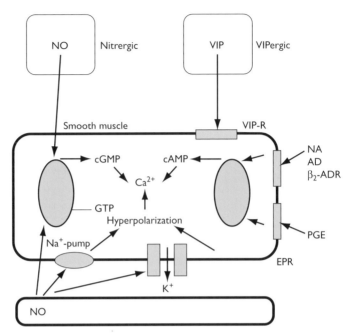

Figure 8

Schematic view of the smooth-muscle relaxation pathways. cGMP, cAMP, hyperpolarization. NA: noradrenaline; AD: adrenaline; β_2-ADR: adrenergic receptor (β_2); PGE-EPR: prostaglandin receptor; VIP-R: VIP receptor; NO: nitric oxide.

There are two types of α adrenergic receptors in penile tissue: α_1 and α_2. α_1-Receptors are the principal mediators of arterial and trabecular smooth contraction with α_2-receptors having a less significant role (Breza et al 1989; Goldstein and Padma-Nathan 1990). α-Adrenergic receptors can be activated not only by local nerve release of noradrenaline, but also by circulating catecholamines, adrenaline or noradrenaline.

Recent pharmacological and functional studies have suggested the presence of more than one α_1-receptor subtype in human corpus cavernosum. In situ hybridization analysis and RNase protection assays of mRNA isolated from whole tissue demonstrated the presence of mRNA transcripts for three α_1-adrenergic receptor subtypes (α_{1d}, α_{1b} and α_{1a}) (Kamm and Stull 1989). The α_{1d} and α_{1a} subtypes are the ones expressed with greater density in the trabecular muscle (Wegner et al 1995).

Cholinergic mechanisms

Acetylcholine is the preganglionic neurotransmitter of parasympathetic nerve input. Even though the parasympathetic sacral center is very important in the initiation of erection, acetylcholine is not the main neurotransmitter mediating dilator neurogenic response; rather it is a non-adrenergic, non-cholinergic (NANC) neurotransmitter, the chemical nature of which has now been defined as nitric oxide.

The modulator effects of acetylcholine facilitate relaxation of trabecular muscle and vasodilatation. Relaxation is brought about by inhibiting the release of noradrenaline by way of prejunctional muscarinic receptors on adjacent adrenergic nerve endings (Saenz de Tejada et al 1988a, 1989). In addition, cholinergic nerves enhance neurogenic NANC relaxation by an as yet unidentified mechanism.

The non-adrenergic, non-cholinergic neuroeffector system

An NANC neuroeffector is the principal neurotransmitter involved in trabecular and arterial smooth-muscle relaxation and erection. VIP (a peptide of 28 amino acids) was initially put forward as the principal NANC neurotransmitter (Lue and Tanagho 1987; Andersson 1993). This is questionable, since NANC action produces an increase of cGMP and the transduction pathway for VIP in penile smooth muscle implicates cAMP. VIP, when it is directly injected in cavernous bodies, is rarely capable of inducing penile erection (Ignarro et al 1990). This peptide is probably a co-neurotransmitter.

Nitric oxide has been identified as the NANC relaxing factor in several experimental studies. The producing enzyme, nitric oxide synthase, has been localized by immunohistochemistry in the peripheral autonomic nerves innervating vascular and non-vascular smooth muscle (Bredt et al 1990). Experimentally, transmural electrical stimulation of nerves within human corpus cavernosum tissue induces nitric oxide production and relaxation (Kim et al 1991; Simonsen et al 1995) which are attenuated by the administration of nitric oxide synthase inhibitors. Such substances (N^G-methyl-L-arginine, N^G-nitro-L-arginine) also produce a decline of the erectile response to stimulation of pelvic nerves in vivo (Holmquist et al 1991; Burnett et al 1992; Trigo-Rocha et al 1993).

In addition, we now know that administration of selective phosphodiesterase inhibitors facilitates penile erection, an effect that would be expected from a physiological response that depends on the nitric oxide/cGMP pathway.

Endothelial control

Endothelium-derived relaxing factor

Vascular endothelium releases a relaxing substance when it is directly affected by biochemical (acetylcholine, bradykinin) or physical (shear stress) stimuli. This substance, named endothelium-derived relaxing factor (EDRF), needs the integrity of the endothelium, and is able to diffuse to the sub-endothelial smooth muscle, causing vasodilatation. This mechanism was first described by Furchgott in 1980 (Furchgott and Zawadski 1980). EDRF was later identified as nitric oxide (Adzadzoi et al 1992). Vasodilator substances can be divided into two groups: those which require the endothelium for their action (endothelium-dependent vasodilators like acetylcholine and bradykinin) (Kimoto et al. 1990; Kim et al 1991), and a second group of vascular smooth-muscle-relaxing vasodilator drugs that act directly on the smooth muscle (endothelium-independent vasodilators).

Having diffused the smooth muscle, endothelium-derived nitric oxide stimulates soluble guanylate cyclase with accumulation of cGMP (Ignarro et al 1990; Vane et al 1990). Endothelium-dependent relaxation of trabecular smooth muscle is blocked by nitric oxide synthase inhibitors (N^G-monomethyl-L-arginine, N^G-nitro-L-arginine), by guanylate cyclase blockers (ODQ) and by nitric oxide scavengers (oxyhemoglobin). However, the activity of EDRF in response to acetylcholine or bradykinin in penile arteries is only partially reversed after administration of an inhibitor of nitric oxide synthase. Therefore, the endothelium-dependent relaxing mechanisms of penile resistance arteries seem to be different from those observed in the trabecular smooth muscle.

Endothelin

Endothelins are a family of three peptides: endothelin-1 (Inoye et al 1989), endothelin-2 and endothelin-3. Endothelin-1 is a potent vasoconstrictor that also has growth factor activity, acting on fibroblasts, smooth muscle and endothelial cells (Furchgott and Zawadski 1980; Blanco et al 1988; Azadzoi et al 1992). This substance could be involved in the maintenance of the flaccidity state of the penis, since it is synthesized by corpus cavernosum endothelium and produces long-lasting contraction of smooth muscle (Holmquist et al 1990; Saenz de Tejada et al 1991b).

Prostanoids

This group of substances includes the prostaglandins PGE_2, PGE_1, $PGF_{2\alpha}$, and prostacyclin (PGI_2) (Jeremy et al 1986; Saenz de Tejada et

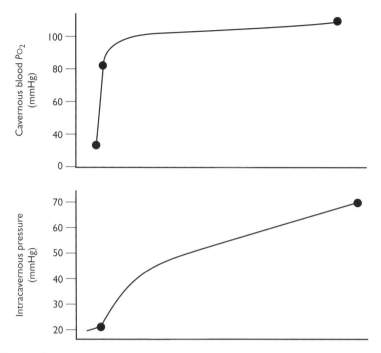

Figure 9
Simultaneous determination of oxygen pressure and cavernous pressure in flaccidity/erection after injection of papaverine–phentolamine. Po_2 goes up after injection, from venous values to arterial values.

al 1988b). PGE is the only endogenous prostaglandin that induces relaxation of the trabecular smooth muscle, while PGE and PGI_2 are potent dilators of penile arteries.

Oxygen tension as a regulator of cavernous vasoactive substances

Molecular oxygen is a regulator of the synthesis of various endogenous vasoactive substances in cavernous tissue, which makes this molecule an important modulator of the erectile activity of the penis (Figure 9). The partial oxygen pressure (Po_2) in the blood of the cavernous body during the flaccid state is similar to that of venous blood (around 35 mmHg), but increases during erection, owing to the increase in arterial blood flow at the onset of erection, the Po_2 reaching approximately 100 mmHg (Kim et al 1993).

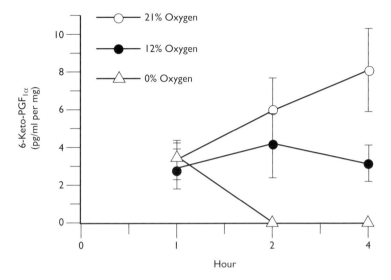

Figure 10
Effect of Po₂ *in prostacyclin (PGI₂) production. Prostacyclin synthesis*
is inhibited when Po₂ *is on venous values.*

Oxygen and L-arginine are substrates for the synthesis of nitric
oxide by the enzyme nitric oxide synthase. Thus oxygen tension
determines substrate availability for the reaction, and is therefore a
potent regulator of nitric oxide synthesis (Kim et al 1993).

In the flaccid penile state, the oxygen concentrations measured in
the cavernous bodies are very low, and the synthesis of nitric oxide is
profoundly inhibited, preventing the relaxation of trabecular smooth
muscle. This inhibition also helps to maintain penile flaccidity by
facilitating the predominance of constrictor tone. In the erectile state
vasodilatation of the arteries and the trabecular smooth muscle occur.
These events allow oxygen concentration to increase to arterial levels, which provides a sufficient substrate for nitric oxide synthesis. It
has been estimated that the minimal pressure of oxygen in the cavernous bodies necessary to achieve full activity of the nitric oxide synthase is between 50 and 60 mmHg. Lower concentrations would
induce a partial synthesis of nitric oxide, with subsequent partial
relaxation of the trabecular muscle.

The oxygen concentration to which the cavernous bodies are
exposed also regulates the synthesis of prostanoids (Daley et al 1996)
(Figure 10). The prostaglandin H synthase (cyclo-oxygenase) is also
an oxygenase and uses oxygen as substrate for the synthesis of

prostanoids. In the case of PGE, the relaxing prostaglandin of the trabecular muscle, physiological variations in the oxygen concentration will also condition its endogenous production: inhibited in flaccidity and stimulated in erection.

The synthesis of the vasoconstrictor, endothelin, is also subject to modulation by the oxygen concentration. Conversely, low oxygen concentrations promote its synthesis, and high levels (Po_2 100 mmHg) inhibit it.

References

Amarenco G, Casanova, JM (1991). Lesion of the nerve of the penis in Peyronie's disease. *Prog Urol* **1**: 906–10.

Andersson KE (1993). Pharmacology of lower urinary tract smooth muscles and penile erectile tissues. *Pharmacol Rev* **45**: 253–309.

Androutsos G (1994). John Hunter, un pionnier de la sexologie au XVIIIe siécle. Poster at 23e Séminaire AIHUS, Paris 1993. In: Brenot PH. *Male Impotence: a historical perspective*. L'Esprit du temps, Paris.

Azadzoi KM, Kim N, Brown ML, et al (1990). Endothelium derived nitric oxide and cyclooxygenase products modulate corpus cavernosum smooth muscle tone. *J Urol* **147**: 220–5.

Blanco R, Saenz de Tejada I, Goldstein I, et al (1988). Cholinergic neurotransmission in human corpus cavernosum. II. Acetylcholine synthesis. *Am J Physiol* 254 (*Heart Circ Physiol* 23): H468.

Bondil P, Wespès E (1992). Anatomie et physiologie de l'erection. *Progrès en Urologie* **2**: 721–857.

Bredt DS, Hwang PM, Snyder SH (1990). Localization of nitric oxide synthase indicating a neural role for nitric oxide. *Nature* **347**: 768.

Brenot PH (1994). *Male Impotence: a historical perspective*. L'Esprit du temps, Paris.

Breza J, Aboseif SR, Orvis BR, et al (1989). Detailed anatomy of penile neurovascular structures: surgical significance. *J Urol* **141**: 437–43.

Brindley GS (1983). Cavernosal alpha-blockage: a new technique for investigating and treating erectile impotence. *Br J Psychiatry* **143**: 332–7.

Burnett AL, Lowenstein CJ, Bredt DS, et al (1992). Nitric oxide: a physiologic mediator of penile erection. *Science* **257**: 401–3.

Campos de Carvalho AC, Roy C, Moreno AP, et al (1993). Gap junctions of connexin43 are found between smooth muscle cells of human corpus cavernosum. *J Urol* **149**: 1568–75.

Christ, GJ (1995). The penis as a vascular organ. The importance of corporal smooth muscle tone in the control of erection. *Urol Clin North Am* **22**: 727–45.

Christ GJ, Moreno AP, Parker ME, et al (1991). Intercellular communication through gap junctions: a potential role in pharmacomechanical coupling and syncytial tissue contraction in vascular smooth muscle isolated from the human corpus cavernosum. *Life Sci* **49**: PL195–200.

Christ GJ, Brink PR, Melman A, et al (1993). The role of gap junctions and ion channels in the modulation of electrical and chemical signals in human corpus cavernosum. *Int J Impot Res* **5**: 77–96.

Daley JT, Brown ML, Watkins MT, et al (1996). Prostanoid production in rabbit corpus cavernosum: I. Regulation by oxygen tension. *J Urol* **155**: 1482–7.

De Groat WC, Steers W (1988). Neuroanatomy and neurophysiology of penile erection. In: *Contemporary Management of Impotence and Infertility*, eds EA Tanagho, TF Lue, R D McClure. Williams & Wilkins, Baltimore.

Devine CJ, Angermeier KW (1994). Anatomy of the penis and male perineum. *AUA Update Series* Vol XII, Lesson. 2.

Fournier GR, Juenemann KP, Lue TF, et al (1987). Mechanisms of venous occlusion during canine penile erection: an anatomic demonstration. *J Urol* **137**: 163–7.

Furchgott RF, Zawadski JV (1980). The obligatory role of endothelial cell in the relaxation of arterial smooth muscle by acetylcholine. *Nature* **288**: 373–6.

Goldstein AMB, Padma-Nathan H (1990). The microarchitecture of the intracavernosal smooth muscle and the cavernosal fibrous skeleton. *J Urol* **144**: 1144–6.

Goldstein AMB, Meehan JP, Morrow JW, et al (1985). The fibrous skeleton of the corpora cavernosa and its probable function in penile erection. *Br J Urol* **57**: 574–8.

Hai CM, Murphy RA (1988). Crossbridge phosphorylation and regulation of the latch state in smooth muscle. *Am J Physiol* **255**: C86–94.

Hatzichristou DG, Saenz de Tejada I, Kupferman S, et al (1995). In vivo assessment of trabecular smooth muscle tone, its application in pharmacocavernosometry, and analysis of intracavernosal pressure determinants. *J Urol* **153**: 1126–35.

Holmquist F, Andersson K-E, Hedlund H (1990). Actions of endothelin on isolated corpus cavernosum from rabbit and man. *Acta Physiol Scand* **139**: 113–22.

Holmquist F, Stief CG, Jonas U, et al (1991). Effects of nitric oxide synthase inhibitor Ng-nitro-L-arginine on the erectile response to cavernosus nerve stimulation in the rabbit. *Acta Physiol Scand* **143**: 299–304.

Ignarro LJ, Bush PA, Buga GM, et al (1990). Nitric oxide and cyclic GMP formation upon electrical field stimulation cause relaxation of corpus cavernosum smooth muscle. *Biochem Biophys Res Commun* **170**: 843–50.

Inoue A, Yanagisawa M, Kimura S, et al. (1989) The human endothelin family: three structurally and pharmacologically distinct isopeptides predicted by three separate genes. *Proc. Natl. Acad. Sci USA* **86**: 2863–7

Ishii N, Watanabe H, Irisawa C, et al (1986). Therapeutic trial with prostaglandin E1 for organic impotence. In: *Proceedings of the Fifth Conference on Vasculogenic Impotence and Corpus Cavernosum Revascularization*. Second World Meeting on Impotence, Prague, International Society for Impotence Research (ISIR), 11.2.

Jardin A (1996). The history of urology in France. In: *De Historia Urologiae Europaeae*, ed. JJ Mattelaer, Historical Committee, European Association of Urology, Vol. 3, pp. 11–34.

Jeremy JY, Morgan RJ, Mikjalidis DP (1986). Prostacyclin synthesis by the corpora cavernosa of the human penis: evidence for muscarinic control and pathological implications. *Prostaglandins Leukot Med* **23**: 211–16.

Kamm K, Stull J (1989). Regulation of smooth muscle contractile elements by second messengers. *Annu Rev Physiol* **51**: 299–313.

Kim N, Azadzoi KM, Goldstein I, et al (1991). A nitric oxide-like factor mediates non-adrenergic non-cholinergic neurogenic relaxation of penile corpus cavernosum smooth muscle. *J Clin Invest* **88**: 112–18.

Kim N, Vardi Y, Padma-Nathan H, et al (1993). Oxygen tension regulates the nitric oxide pathway: physiological role in penile erection. *J Clin Invest* **91**: 437–42.

Kimoto Y, Kessler R, Constantinou CE (1990). Endothelium dependent relaxation of human corpus cavernosum by bradykinin. *J Urol* **144**: 1015–17.

Krane RJ, Goldstein I, Saenz de Tejada I (1989). Impotence. *N Engl J Med* **321**: 1648–59.

Lavoisier P, Proulx J, Courtois F, et al (1988). Relationship between perineal muscle contractions, penile tumescence, and penile rigidity during nocturnal erections. *J Urol* **139**: 176–9.

Lue TF, Tanagho EA (1987). Physiology of erection and pharmacological management of impotence. *J Urol* **137**: 829–36.

Lue TF, Takamura T, Schmidt RA, et al (1984). Neuroanatomy of penile erection: its relevance to iatrogenic impotence. *J Urol* **131**: 273–80.

Moncada I, Concejo J, Escribano G, et al (1992). Eco-Doppler Duplex asociado a inyección intracavernosa de prostaglandina E1 en el diagnóstico de la impotencia. *Arch Esp Urol* **45**: 45–51.

Musitelli S, Jallous H, De Bastiani T, et al (1996). The structure and the function of the testicles from Aristotle to the *textus examinatus* of Claudius Aubry (1868). In *De Historia Urologiae Europaeae*, ed. JJ Mattelaer, Historical Committee, European Association of Urology, Vol. 1, pp. 132–43.

O'Malley CD, Saunders JB (1952). *Leonardo da Vinci on the Human Body*. Schumann, New York.

Saenz de Tejada I (1992). Mechanisms for the regulation of penile smooth muscle contractility. In: *World Book of Impotence*, ed. T Lue. Smith-Gordon, London.

Saenz de Tejada I, Blanco R, Goldstein I, et al (1988a). Cholinergic neurotransmission in human corpus cavernosum. I. Responses of isolated tissue. *Am J Physiol* **254**: H459–67.

Saenz de Tejada I, Carson MP, Taylor L, et al (1988b). Prostaglandin production by human corpus cavernosum endothelial cells (HCC EC) in culture. *J Urol* **139**: 252A (abstract 358).

Saenz de Tejada I, Kim N, Lagan I, et al (1989). Regulation of adrenergic activity in penile corpus cavernosum. *J Urol* **142**: 1117–21.

Saenz de Tejada I, Moroukian P, Tessier J, et al (1991a). Trabecular smooth muscle modulates the capacitor function of the penis. Studies on a rabbit model. *Am J Physiol* **260**: H190–5.

Saenz de Tejada I, Carson MP, de las Morenas A, et al (1991b). Endothelin: localization, synthesis, activity and receptor types in human penile corpus cavernosum. *Am J Physiol* **261**: H1078–85.

Simonsen U, Prieto D, Saenz de Tejada, et al (1995). Involvement of nitric oxide in the non-adrenergic non-cholinergic neurotransmission of horse deep penile arteries: role of charybdotoxin-sensitive K⁺-channels. *Br J Pharmacol* **116**: 2582–90.

Steers WD (1990). Neural control of penile erection. *Semin Urol* **8**: 866–79.

Steers WD (1994). Smooth muscle physiology. *AUA Update Series* Lesson 30.

Tobin CE, Benjamin JA (1944). Anatomical study and clinical consideration of the fasciae limiting urinary extravasation from the penile urethra. *Surg Gynecol Obstet* **79**: 195–204.

Trigo-Rocha F, Aronson WJ, Hohenfellner M, et al (1993). Nitric oxide and cyclic guanosine monophosphate: mediators of pelvic nerve-stimulated erection in dogs. *Am J Physiol* **264**: H419–22.

Vane JR, Anggard EE, Botting RM (1990). Regulatory functions of the vascular endothelium. *N Engl J Med* **323**: 27–36.

Virag R (1982). Intracavernous injection of papaverine for erectile failure. *Lancet* **ii**: 938.

de Vries JDM (1996). The history of urology in the Netherlands. In: *De Historia Urologiae Europaeae*, ed. JJ Mattelaer, Historical Committee, European Association of Urology, Vol. 3, pp. 65–110.

Walsh PC, Donker PJ (1982). Impotence following radical prostatectomy: insight into etiology and prevention. *J Urol* **128**: 492–7.

Wegner HEH, Andresen R, Knispel HH, et al (1995). Evaluation of penile arteries with color-coded duplex sonography: prevalence and possible therapeutic implications of connections between dorsal and cavernous arteries in impotent men. *J Urol* **153**: 1469–71.

Wespès E, Goes PM, Schiffmann S, et al (1991). Computerized analysis of smooth muscle fibers in potent and impotent patients. *J Urol* **146**: 1015–17.

2

Common features regulating the systemic circulation and the penile vasculature

Michael A Adams, James D Banting, Kazushi Manabe, Jeremy PW Heaton

Introduction

The common factors underlying human erectile dysfunction most commonly relate to alterations either in vascular control mechanisms or in the tissues that they regulate. The generation of a "normal" or physiological erection involves a coordinated pattern of neural pathway activation that initiates a cascade of vascular events in the penile and pre-penile vasculature. Some fundamental principles can be identified to describe this response. The magnitude of the final response is determined by the degree of coordination and temporal integration of a number of activating and inactivating processes at many different levels, including local, neural and humoral factors. In addition, these systems can act both in concert and in opposition to each other (Krane et al 1989; Saenz de Tejada et al 1991; Anderson 1993; Lerner et al 1993). This type of multiplicity and overlap of control systems should be anticipated for any process that is fundamental for a reproductive function critical to the survival of the species (Adams et al 1997). A further important conceptual point is that the most dynamic regulation is available in a control system that can respond effectively and rapidly in both directions from its starting point. Thus, the most effective operating point of a control system would be at the midpoint of the stimulus–response relationship.

Interestingly, this type of regulation is not a particularly prominent part of the regulation of the penile vasculature. In the penis, the primary control systems regulate penile arterial inflow more as a function of a two-state control sequence. Thus, a neural signal induces tumescence (high net vasodilator tone) from a quiescent resting state (high net vasoconstrictor tone and low blood flow) within seconds to minutes, in which the most dynamic period of hemodynamic change occurs (progressive increase in blood flow during active relaxation) in the transition period.

The elements

Early in this decade nitric oxide (NO) was hypothesized to be the primary source of the neurally mediated vasodilator activity that was required for initiation of an erection. NO became understood to be the non-adrenergic, non-cholinergic neurotransmitter in the penis (Iguarro et al 1990; Rajfer et al 1992), and was widely accepted as a pre-eminent mediator of corporeal relaxation as well as acting in the CNS to modulate the initiating mechanisms of erection (Melis et al 1994). The supporting evidence came from a wide range of experiments involving isolated smooth-muscle preparations, anesthetized rats and dogs with electrical stimulation of NO-dependent penile responses, and anatomical/histochemical studies of nitric oxide synthase (NOS) localization, mostly by NADPH-diaphorase staining (Brock et al 1994).

The development of other "concepts" has, at least in part, eroded our confidence in the "only NO theory", that is, the theory that NO is the only obligatory element of the system. An example of a conflicting finding was that apomorphine-induced erections in normal, conscious rats could not be persistently blocked after decreasing the production of NO by administering high doses of an NOS antagonist (Adams et al 1994). The evidence revealed that NOS activity (both neuronal and endothelial) could be reduced by >90% and yet full apomorphine-induced erectile function remained. In other types of studies, experiments have shown that within 24 hours, in castrated rats, erections are lost, whereas NO production is not yet decreased significantly. In the chronic phase of castration, a condition which markedly reduces NOS activity, testosterone replacement re-establishes erections within 24 hours, a time frame too brief for recovery of NOS activity (Heaton 1994). Successful reproductive capacity in NOS knockout rats has also presented a conceptual conundrum.

An explanation for the conflicting results is that the "only NO theory" is insufficient to explain all erectile mechanisms. Two decades of research have demonstrated the functional presence of other vasodilator factors such as vasoactive intestinal polypeptide (VIP), prostanoids and acetylcholine involved in both cGMP- and cAMP- mediated relaxation of the penile vasculature (Kim et al 1995; Tamura et al 1995). Erectile mechanisms can involve both of these cyclic nucleotide mechanisms, and adaptive processes can occur in the signaling pathways that counteract the decrease in the NO system.

These findings also suggest that NO, while playing a role in normal vasodilatation/erection, is not absolutely essential for erectile function, although other factors must clearly play more than supporting roles. This being the case it must be that other vasoactive systems have the capacity to play important roles in the production of neurally mediated erections under some conditions. Further, there is substantial interplay between local, neural and humoral systems involved in the regulation of vascular tone that will impact on overall function.

As a medical and scientific problem erectile dysfunction gained greatly in stature when Rajfer et al (1992) published their information linking NO with normal erectile function. In that same year NO was touted as "Molecule of the Year" by the journal *Science*. This kind of notoriety resulted, at least in part, from the plethora of findings that had accumulated in studies on vascular and neural as well as other systems. In the case of erectile dysfunction, this disclosure heralded a new maturity in the study of erectile function and dysfunction – suddenly the principles of normal vascular biology (NVB) became *de facto* the underpinnings of erectile physiology, i.e. the principles underlying the control of the circulation could be applied to penile function once anatomical differences were taken into account.

Concepts from normal vascular biology

In many situations in which a persistent abnormality of the circulation exists, the factor(s) involved in the maintenance of the "state" are often distinct from the initiating cause(s) (Lever 1986). A comprehensive understanding of the time course of change(s) in the neural, humoral and local vasoactive systems in these conditions is required in order to elucidate which mechanisms are involved in the initiation, the development and the established phases of the circulatory state. Investigations into the causal involvement of systems have, until recently, focused mostly on neural and humoral systems, not on local systems. Not surprisingly, the discovery of NO as the local, endothelium-derived relaxing factor has markedly altered the concepts of local system involvement (Ignarro et al 1990; Rajfer et al 1992). Further, the synthesis of compounds, such as arginine analogs, which inhibit the production of NO at the level of the enzyme NOS provided tools by which this local factor could be assessed.

Initial studies, using NOS antagonists, were aimed at revealing the circulatory control role(s) for NO in vivo (Gardiner et al 1990). Inhibition of the production of NO, via NOS inhibition, provokes a rapid and sustained increase in total peripheral resistance, impaired flow to regional circulations and a marked increase in the level of mean arterial pressure (MAP) (Gardiner et al 1990). The hierarchy of circulatory control systems that have the capacity to exert influences on the level of vascular tone can be described as combinations of the following: neuronal (for example, sympathetic nervous system – SNS), humoral (for example, angiotensin II, epinephrine) and local systems (for example NO, endothelin-1 and prostaglandins). Few studies have considered the quantitative contribution of "local" systems in vivo in the regulation of vascular tone and mean arterial pressure.

The proposed role of NO has been inferred largely from the hemodynamic consequences that occur in its absence and not by its contribution when it is active. Thus, the dramatic increases in regional vascular resistance and the rapid development of hypertension following decreased NO production have now been suggested by numerous investigators to represent the removal of the marked, chronic vasodilator function of this small molecule. Further, the increases in peripheral vasoconstriction have also been portrayed as a generalized hypersensitivity to vasoconstrictor systems (i.e. vasoconstrictors exert their effects "unopposed" following blockade of NO production). In some studies, experiments were designed to assess which of the neurohumoral-based mechanisms were playing the most significant role. In conflict with the "increased sensitivity" hypothesis, many of these studies did not find an enhanced contribution from a neural or humoral factor. For example, several studies have indicated a lack of involvement of the sympathetic nervous system in the NOS blockade-induced pressor response (Pucci et al 1992; Kumagai et al 1993; Banting et al 1996). Further, the contribution of the renin–angiotensin system (RAS) to the NOS blockade-induced hypertension has not been generally agreed upon. Pollock et al (1993) indicated a significant role of the RAS in the hypertension following decreased NO production, whereas several others (Pucci et al 1992; Arnal et al 1993; Banting et al 1996) have demonstrated a complete lack of involvement of the RAS. Still other studies have demonstrated an increased sensitivity to α_1-adrenoceptor activation (Deng et al 1993; Li and Schiffrin 1994), but not to angiotensin II receptor activation in blood vessels from rats treated chronically with an NOS antagonist (Arnal et al 1993).

Results of this type indicate that a substantially more complicated interaction exists between the countervailing vasoactive systems that

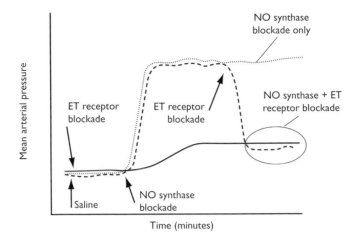

Figure 1
Reversal of NOS blockade hypertension by antagonizing the actions of endothelin.

dictate the level of vascular tone than has previously been proposed in the literature. Thus, the novel finding published in Banting et al (1996) which demonstrated that up to 90% of the hypertension following acute NOS blockade in conscious rats could be accounted for by a dramatic upregulation of endothelin-mediated vasoconstriction revealed yet another layer of complexity in the control system. This finding showed that administering an endothelin receptor (ET-R) antagonist to a conscious rat prior to NOS blockade prevented the development of the subsequent hypertension, and that the same ET-R antagonist could also reverse this form of hypertension after it had developed (Figure 1). In addition, the results further revealed that the role of endothelin in the normal circulation was minimal, in that administration of the ET-R antagonist in the resting state did not significantly alter systemic blood pressure.

Results obtained in chronic NOS blockade studies, again in conscious rats, have also shown that augmented endothelin-mediated vasoconstriction continues to play an important role in the pressor response. In a different way, however, the enhanced vasoconstrictor mechanism was demonstrated to be a consequence of two processes: (1) by direct actions of endothelin acting as a vasoconstrictor and (2) via indirect actions, involving a sensitization or "priming" action with respect to α_1-adrenoceptor-mediated constrictor effects. Specifically,

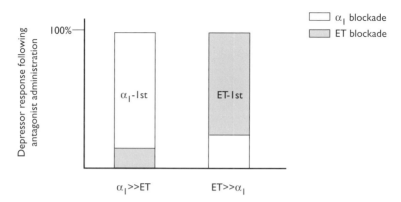

Figure 2
Contrasting responses with different order of administration of α_1 and ET-receptor blockers during chronic NOS blockade.

our findings (unpublished observations) have established that endothelin-mediated effects, via both direct and indirect actions, account for at least 60% of the hypertension induced by chronic NOS blockade. The indirect actions were exposed by comparing the depressor responses to ET and α_1-adrenoceptor antagonism. When the α_1-adrenoceptor antagonist was administered first (left-hand bar in Figure 2) there was a markedly increased depressor responsiveness. This hypersensitivity was determined to be largely mediated by enhanced endothelin activity, as blocking ET_A/ET_B receptors dramatically removed the signaling via α_1-adrenoceptors (right-hand bar in Figure 2). This capacity of endothelin to modulate the vascular sensitivity or "gain" to α_1-adrenoceptor activation may represent a mechanism by which vascular tone is differentially regulated in specific regions as a function of changes in local factors. Further, of particular importance would be the impact on circulations in which there is little capacity for compensatory changes or autoregulation.

Application of the concept in the control of erectile function

These experimental findings described above, involving both acute and chronic blood pressure responses in conscious rats, indicate that the chronic role of NO in the vasculature is more subtle than that of a chronic vasodilator. Further, the results, which are based on global systemic responses, suggest that a similar relationship between NO and vasoconstrictor systems is likely to be found in specialized circulations such as the penile vasculature, that is, that the principles of normal vascular biology are directly applicable to the penis. Methodology which can elucidate whether this NO–ET regulation concept is applicable uses the technique of Banting et al (1996) and involves isolating and perfusing the penile vasculature of the rat.

A fully functional penile erection is recognized as involving at least three sets of peripheral nerves (thoracolumbar sympathetic, sacral parasympathetic and pelvic somatic). At the level of penile tissue these operate as sympathetic and parasympathetic as well as non-adrenergic, non-cholinergic (NANC) nerve terminals (Zhang et al 1994). A component of the erectile control systems that has received much less attention is the balance that occurs at the local level between vasoactive substances derived from the vascular endothelium and smooth muscle or from the circulation.

Regardless of the mechanism that a particular system uses, if an alteration in function diminishes the capacity for smooth-muscle relaxation the consequence would be elevated penile vascular resistance. Increased resistance leads to insufficient arterial inflow and inadequate venous occlusion, ultimately resulting in erectile dysfunction (Krane et al 1989; Saenz de Tejada et al 1991; Anderson 1993; Lerner et al 1993). Thus, the level of vascular tone in vivo results from a critical balance of countervailing vasoactive systems at the neural, humoral and local levels. A widely discussed view in the current literature subscribes to the concept that an imbalance in countervailing systems, particularly NO, will result in vascular hypersensitivity to the other systems (Greenberg et al 1991; Ito et al 1991; Vo et al 1991; Lerman et al 1992; Shinozuka et al 1992; Jones et al 1993; Zhang et al 1994; Luscher and Noll 1995). Thus, as indicated earlier, the physiological response to a lack of NO would involve a "tipping of the balance" toward "unopposed" vasoconstrictor systems.

In experiments in which the specialized circulation of the penile vasculature was characterized for interactions between vasoconstrictor and vasodilators some features common to the systemic concepts were found. For example, in the artificially perfused penile bed, as expected, α_1-adrenoceptor signaling becomes hyperresponsive following decreases in NO production (dotted line in Figure 3). More important, however, is the fact that hypersensitivity is almost completely reversed by concomitant treatment with an ET_A/ET_B receptor antagonist (bold line in Figure 3). Thus, endothelin seems to "prime" or "sensitizes" the pudendal vasculature to the neural signaling.

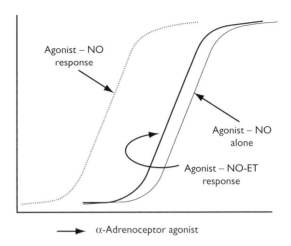

Figure 3
NO-ET regulation of vasoconstrictor responses.

Interestingly, the actions of the upregulated endothelin alone appear to be insufficient to induce vasoconstriction without the presence of α_1-adrenoceptor stimulation, i.e. the levels of endothelin required to produce this level of hyperreactivity are, in fact, sub-pressor (see trace in Figure 4).

In a number of different conditions it is likely that decreases in NO production could be a common feature of the pathophysiological process. It may be that, in certain pathophysiological conditions, insufficient NO production may provoke the upregulation of ET-1 activity. Even if this change is subtle, the potential priming action on neural signaling systems may be a major cause of erectile dysfunction, as it will shift the balance in favor of vasoconstrictor mechanisms. This shift in balance, even with normal constrictor stimuli, can lead to a high level of contractile tone in the penile vasculature, thereby preventing penile tumescence. In the penile circulation, which is dependent on active extrinsic neural stimuli for dynamic control (and less on autoregulation), a disturbance in the reciprocal relationship between NO and ET-1 may profoundly influence vascular tone, mediating erectile dysfunction.

The penile vasculature represents a specialized circulation that is subjected to extremes of hemodynamic conditions (i.e. tumescence and detumescence). In the penis, there is little to no intrinsic autoregulation or metabolic regulation, as in the vasculature of the kidney,

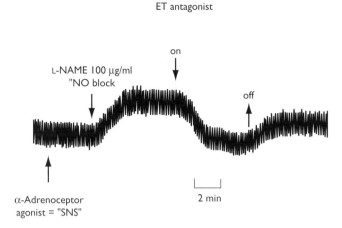

Figure 4
SNS hyperreactivity with low NO is reversed by ET blockade.

heart, brain, gut and skeletal muscle (Krane et al 1989). The dual action of neural systems in concert with local systems would appear to have most of the control of the smooth-muscle tone, and dictates resistance and therefore arterial inflow in this specialized circulation. A dramatic change in the local balance between NO and ET-1 could have a catastrophic impact on arterial inflow and thereby erections (Figure 5). A normalization of the balance between vasoconstrictor and vasodilator systems can be realized, however, by the inhibition of the specific system that underlies the abnormality. Thus, in the case of a dysfunction in the NO production system normalization of the balance of tone can be obtained by the administration of an endothelin receptor antagonist even though the levels of NO have not been returned to control levels (Figure 5).

   In conclusion, there is a local penile regulatory system that involves the countervailing influences of NO and ET. This system is very likely to be involved in the local regulation of penile vascular tone, which in turn will very probably impact on overall erectile function in vivo. This reciprocal control system is identical to that found in the systemic circulation. The dramatic functional difference between the two systems is that an abnormality in the penile vasculature could potentially induce a catastrophic impact on erectile function because of the limited presence of other systems capable of regulatory balance. The lack of compensatory penile autoregulatory systems is a harbinger of

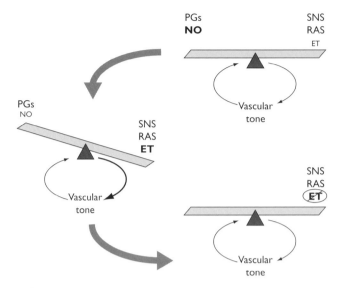

Figure 5
Impact of changes in local balance between NO and ET-1 on arterial inflow and hence on erections.

risk, that is, without intrinsic feedback systems the penile vasculature will always be a slave to the capacities of the extrinsic control systems to induce vasodilatation. In contrast, in the systemic circulation the NO–ET system is one of many control systems, so that the impact on the general circulation is markedly blunted as a consequence of numerous autoregulatory mechanisms. The full impact that abnormalities in the local penile vascular regulatory system will have on the complex etiologies of erectile function remains to be elucidated.

References

Adams MA, Mawani F, Okenka K, et al (1994). Prolonged high dose L-NAME does not abolish apomorphine-induced erections in rats. *Int J Impot Res* **6**(suppl. 1): A4 (abstract.).

Adams MA, Banting JD, Maurice DH, et al (1997). Vascular control mechanisms in penile erection: phylogeny and the inevitability of multiple and overlapping systems. *Int J Impot Res* **9**: 1–7.

Anderson KE (1993). Pharmacology of lower urinary tract smooth muscles and penile erectile tissues. *Pharmacol Rev* **45**: 253–308.

Arnal JF, Amrani AIE, Chatellier G, et al (1993). Cardiac weight in hypertension induced by nitric oxide synthase blockade. *Hypertension* **22**: 380–7.

Banting JD, Friberg P, Adams MA (1996). Acute hypertension after nitric oxide synthase inhibition is mediated primarily by increased endothelin mediated vasoconstriction. *J Hypertens* **14**: 975–81.

Brock GB, Zvara P, Sioufi R, et al (1994). Nitric oxide synthase is testosterone dependent *Int J Impot Res* **6**(S1): (D42).

Deng LY, Thibault G, Schiffrin EL (1993). Effect of hypertension induced by nitric oxide synthase inhibition on structure and function of resistance arteries in the rat. *Clin Exp Hypertens* **15**: 527–37.

Gardiner SM, Compton AM, Kemp PA, et al (1990). Regional and cardiac haemodynamic responses to glyceryl trinitrate, acetylcholine, bradykinin and endothelin-1 in conscious rats: effect of NGnitro-L-arginine methyl ester. *Br J Pharmacol* **101**: 632–9.

Greenberg SS, Cantor E, Diecke FP, et al (1991) Cyclic GMP modulates release of norepinephrine from adrenergic nerves innervating canine arteries. *Am J Hypertens* **4**: 173–6.

Heaton JP, Varrin SJ (1994). Effect of castration and exogenous testosterone supplementation in an animal model of penile erection. *J Urol* **151**: 797–800.

Ignarro LJ, Bush PA, Buga GM, et al (1990). Nitric oxide and cyclic GMP formation upon electrical field stimulation cause relaxation of corpus cavernosum smooth muscle. *Biochem Biophys Res Commun* **170**: 843–50.

Ito S, Johnson CS, Carretero OA (1991). Modulation of angiotensin II-induced vasoconstriction by endothelium-derived relaxing factor in the isolated microperfused rabbit afferent arteriole. *J Clin Invest* **87**: 1656–63.

Jones CJ, Defily DV, Patterson JL, et al (1993). Endothelium-dependent relaxation competes with a1- and a2-adrenergic constriction in the canine epicardial coronary microcirculation. *Circulation* **87**: 1264–74.

Kim YC, Kim JH, Davies MG, et al (1995). Modulation of vasoactive intestinal polypeptide (VIP)-mediated relaxation by nitric oxide and prostanoids in the rabbit corpus cavernosum. *J Urol* **153**: 807–10.

Krane RJ, Goldstein I, Saenz de Tejada I (1989). Impotence. *N Engl J Med* **321**: 1648–59.

Kumagai H, Averill DB, Khosla MC, et al (1993). Role of nitric oxide and angiotensin II in the regulation of sympathetic nerve activity in spontaneously hypertensive rats. *Hypertension* **21**: 476–84.

Lerman A, Sandok EK, Hildebrand FL, et al (1992). Inhibition of endothelium-derived relaxing factor enhances endothelin-mediated vasoconstriction. *Circulation* **85**: 1894–8.

Lerner SE, Melman A, Christ GJ (1993). A review of erectile dysfunction: new insights and more questions. *J Urol* **149**: 1246–55.

Lever AF (1986). Slow pressor mechanisms in hypertension: a role for hypertrophy of resistance vessels? *J Hypertens* **4**: 515–24.

Li JS, Schiffrin EL (1994). Resistance artery structure and neuroeffector mechanisms in hypertension induced by nitric oxide synthase. *Am J Hypertens* **7**: 996–1004.

Luscher TF, Noll G (1995). The endothelium as a regulator of vascular tone and growth. In: *The Endothelium in Cardiovascular Disease*, ed. TF Luscher, pp. 1–24. Springer, Heidelberg.

Melis MR, Mauri A, Argiolas A (1994). Apomorphine- and oxytocin-induced penile erection and yawning in intact and castrated male rats: effect of sexual steroids. *Neuroendocrinology* **59**: 349–54.

Pollock DM, Polakowski JS, Divish BJ, et al (1993). Angiotensin blockade reverses hypertension during long-term nitric oxide synthase inhibition. *Hypertension* **21**: 660–6.

Pucci ML, Lin L, Nasjletti A (1992). Pressor and renal effects of NG-nitro-L-arginine as effected by blockade of pressor mechanisms mediated by the sympathetic nervous system, angiotensin, prostanoids and vasopressin. *J Pharmacol Exp Ther* **261**: 240–5.

Rajfer J, Aronson WJ, Bush PA, et al (1992). Nitric oxide as a mediator of relaxation of the corpus cavernosum in response to nonadrenergic, noncholinergic neurotransmission. *N Engl J Med* **326**: 90–4.

Saenz de Tejada I, Moroukian P, Tessier J, et al (1991). Trabecular smooth muscle modulates the capitator function of the penis. Studies on a rabbit model. *Am J Physiol* **260**: H1590–5.

Shinozuka K, Kobayashi Y, Shimoura K, et al (1992). Role of nitric oxide from the endothelium on the neurogenic contractile responses of rabbit pulmonary artery. *Eur J Pharmacol* **222**: 113–20.

Tamura M, Kagawa S, Kimura K, et al (1995). Coexistence of nitric oxide synthase, tyrosine hydroxylase and vasoactive intestinal polypeptide in human penile tissue – a triple histochemical and immunohistochemical study. *J Urol* **153**: 530–4.

Vo PA, Reid JJ, Rand MJ (1991). Attenuation of vasoconstriction by endogenous nitric oxide in rat caudal artery. *Br J Pharmacol* **107**: 1121–8.

Zhang J, Van Meel JC, Pfaffendorf M, et al (1994). Endothelium-dependent, nitric oxide-mediated inhibition of angiotensin II-induced contractions in rabbit aorta. *Eur J Pharmacol* **262**: 247–53.

3

The male climacteric: fact or fiction?

J Lisa Tenover

In men there is no "andropause" that corresponds to the female menopause. The reproductive changes that occur in men as they age occur over a long period of time and are more subtle than the profound changes in gonadal function that occur in women at menopause. The term "male climacteric" has been used by a number of authors to designate adult Leydig cell failure (Heller and Myers 1944; McCullagh 1946). However, this term describes a syndrome that is characterized by serum testosterone levels well below the normal range (usually less than 150 ng/dl) and symptoms similar to those of a menopausal woman (including hot flashes, decreased libido, and irritability), which are thought to be due to androgen withdrawal. The syndrome can be associated with signs of feminization (gynecomastia, loss of secondary sexual hair), inability to concentrate, tiredness, and episodes of depression. This 'male climacteric' can be caused by Klinefelter's syndrome (XXY syndrome), pituitary ablation due to surgery or radiation, idiopathic Leydig cell failure, testicular atrophy secondary to mumps orchitis or disruptions of testicular blood supply during surgery, or the consequence of a number of systemic diseases such as the hepatopathies and arteriopathies. Since the term "male climacteric" has been used in this context, it does not appropriately apply to the changes that occur as a natural consequence of aging in men.

The more relevant clinical question is not whether older men experience a true climacteric, but, rather, whether many older men experience an age-associated decline in androgens and whether this has a negative impact on their sexual function. This issue will be addressed here.

Androgen changes with normal male aging

Although conflicting data pertaining to this point are found in the early medical literature, most studies within the past two decades have demonstrated an age-related decline in serum total testosterone levels in normal men (Vermeulen 1991). The decline in testosterone with age is due to a decrease in testosterone production; testosterone clearance actually slows with age. Young adult men exhibit a circadian rhythm in their serum levels of total testosterone, with peak levels occurring in the morning and falling slowly by about 35% during the day. This daily fluctuation in serum testosterone is attenuated in older men (Bremner et al 1983).

The physiologic causes for a decline in testosterone production with age are multifactorial. The predominant change appears to be at the level of the testes, where there is a decline in Leydig cell number and in the activity of the enzymes in the metabolic pathway governing testosterone production (Takahashi et al 1983; Neaves et al 1984). The ability of the testes to increase testosterone production in response to increased gonadotropin stimulation is also attenuated in older men (Harman and Tsitouras 1980).

There is evidence that age-related alterations in hypothalamo-pituitary function also contribute to the decline in testosterone production. An overview of available data supports the view that elderly men fail to demonstrate an appropriate increase in luteinizing hormone (LH) secretion in response to a hypoandrogenic state. Most older men with low testosterone levels have gonadotropin levels (especially LH levels) that are within the normal young male adult range, resulting in a relative hypogonadotropic hypogonadism. The precise mechanisms responsible for the blunted LH response to diminished steroid feedback inhibition are not defined, but several observations suggest involvement at the hypothalamic level (for a review see Tenover 1994). Table 1 outlines the reproductive hormonal changes seen with aging in men.

The decline in serum testosterone with age is not universal. Most studies evaluating testosterone levels with age have been carried out with a population of predominantly Caucasian men; few data are available as regards other ethnic populations. In addition, the rate of testosterone decline among individuals can vary greatly, is impacted by disease and medications, and does not inevitably result in hypogonadism.

Nearly all the testosterone circulating in blood is bound to proteins: sex hormone-binding globulin (SHBG) and albumin. The affinity of testosterone for SHBG is strong, while the affinity for albumin is not. Only a small portion of circulating testosterone

Table 1   Male reproductive hormone changes with normal aging

Decreased testosterone production; decreased testosterone clearance

Decreased levels of serum total and free testosterone

Increased sex hormone-binding globulin; decreased "bioavailable testosterone"

No change in serum levels of dihydrotestosterone

Increased serum estradiol levels

Small increase in serum gonadotropin (LH and follicle-stimulating hormone) levels

Decreased LH pulse amplitude

Increased hypothalamic sensitivity to sex steroid feedback

(usually 1–2%) is totally "free." Because SHBG binds testosterone tightly, some individuals have called the portion of testosterone that is not bound to SHBG the "bioavailable" testosterone (Manni et al 1985). Others have proposed that non-protein-bound (free) testosterone is the "active" fraction of testosterone (Vermeulen and Verdonck 1972). Exactly which testosterone measurement most accurately reflects the pool available to tissues has not been settled, however. As more data are collected, it seems likely that the portion of serum testosterone available to any given tissue may depend on the characteristics of that particular tissue and its blood supply (Sakiyama et al 1988).

Regardless of which fraction of testosterone is determined to be "biologically" available, most data support the view that serum levels of all three testosterone components (total, free, and non-SHBG-bound) decline with normal aging. Levels of SHBG increase with age, and the age-related increase in SHBG results in a steeper rate of decline in serum levels of non-SHBG-bound ("bioavailable") testosterone than that seen for total testosterone. In general, serum dihydrotestosterone levels do not decrease significantly with age.

The magnitude of the decline in testosterone with age and the prevalence of older men with "low" testosterone levels have not been well documented. There is a paucity of longitudinal population-based sampling studies that have evaluated androgen levels, and also there is no agreement on what level of serum testosterone establishes an older man as being "androgen-deficient". Table 2 lists some data on the "prevalence" of low testosterone levels in various populations.

Table 2   Examples of prevalence data for testosterone "deficiency" in older men

Study population	Age (years)	Number in study	Total testosterone (ng/dl)	Percentage of population
Rural Austria[a]	50–87	817	< 300	11.4
Belgium[b]	20–100	300	< 317	1 (20–40 years)
				7 (40–60 years)
				22 (60–80 years)
				36 (80–100 years)
USA[c]	60–83	379	< 350	36
			< 300	29
			< 250	8

[a], Lunglmayr (1997); [b], Vermeulen (from Tenover 1996); [c], Tenover (unpublished data).

Male sexual function changes with age

In 1948 Kinsey et al reported that the frequency of intercourse declined significantly with age. Since that time, many studies have reported a decline in sexual activity and strength of sexual desire with age. Coital activity is the most rapidly declining aspect of sexual function. The Duke Longitudinal Study reported that 95% of men aged 46–50 years had intercourse at least once a week, but only 28% of men aged 66–71 had intercourse that frequently (Pfeiffer et al 1968). Bretschneider and McCoy (1988) found that 63% of men aged 80–102 years reported themselves as being "sexually active," but for 83% of these men this was sexual activity without intercourse. Panser et al (1995) found that in 70–79-year-old men, compared with 40–49-year-old men, there was a higher prevalence of complete erectile dysfunction (ED) with sexual stimulation (27.4% vs 0.3%) and absent libido (25.9% vs 0.6%). The Massachusetts Male Aging Study, a community-based sample of 1290 men aged 40–70 years, found the reported prevalence of impotence to be 52% and that the variable most strongly associated with impotence was age (Feldman et al 1994). Mulligan et al (1988) in a survey of an older Veterans Administration outpatient population reported that erectile dysfunction (ED) and absence of libido occurred in 25% and 31%, respectively, in men 65–75 years of age and in 30% and 47%, respectively, in men 75 years and older.

More objective evidence for age-related changes in sexual function includes evidence that both frequency and duration of nocturnal penile tumescence (NPT) decrease progressively with age (from age 23 through 73 years) in healthy sexually non-dysfunctional men; these findings were independent of variations in sleep (Schiavi and Schreiner-Engel 1988). An age-related decline in cavernous arterial blood flow during prostaglandin E_1-induced erections has also been reported (Chung et al 1996).

For both ED and libido, as with many other medical problems, it is often difficult to differentiate which phenomena are due to non-pathologic aging and which are influenced by medical conditions and pharmacologic agents. In addition, normal aging effects on ED or libido could involve a number of systems, including hormonal, neural, and vascular, thus making the contribution of any one factor difficult to elucidate.

Certainly, as men age, chronic disease can impact on the prevalence of sexual dysfunction. In the Massachusetts Male Aging Study, after age the major risk factors for reported ED were diabetes mellitus, heart disease, and hypertension (Feldman et al 1994), while in the Veterans Administration study, diabetes mellitus and urinary incontinence were highly associated with ED (Mulligan et al 1988).

Many commonly used medications have been shown to impair sexual function, with the most common manifestation being ED. In young patients there is often a clear association of initiation of a new medication and onset of ED, while in older men there is often a subtle worsening of underlying ED problems with medication. The mechanisms by which medications produce ED or affect other aspects of sexual function are unclear. Categories of medication that have commonly been associated with sexual dysfunction include antihypertensives (especially central-acting agents, diuretics, and β-blockers), cardiac medications (especially nitrates and antiarrhythmics), and psychotropic agents such as antidepressants, major tranquilizers, and antipsychotics (Galbraith 1991).

Androgens and sexual function

Testosterone replacement studies in castrated animals and in truly hypogonadal young adult men have demonstrated that testosterone restores sexual function in these settings. Since aging is associated with a decline in both serum testosterone levels and parameters of sexual function, the major question is whether the two are related in any way and whether testosterone therapy would improve aspects of sexual function in this older age group. One approach to addressing this question is through clinical correlation data.

Davidson et al (1983), in a cross-sectional study of 220 men aged 41–93 years, found that increasing age was associated with a decline in the levels of sexual activity, libido, and potency. Serum total and free testosterone levels also decreased with age, and free testosterone levels independently and significantly correlated with all sexual functional measures except sexual enjoyment. Using data from the Baltimore Longitudinal Study, 183 men over the age of 60 years were evaluated by Tsitouras et al (1982), who reported that those men who were more sexually active tended to have higher serum testosterone levels than those who were less sexually active. Korenman et al (1990) explored the relationship between reproductive hormone levels and ED in 267 impotent men ≥ 50 years and compared their findings to those in young controls and age-matched older men without ED. When adjustment was made for age and body mass index, they found no difference in non-SHBG-bound testosterone levels between potent and impotent older men. In the Massachusetts Male Aging Study, there was no correlation found between any component of serum testosterone (total, free, or non-SHBG-bound) and the reported presence of ED (Feldman et al 1994). The Duke Longitudinal Study similarly demonstrated no correlation between levels of serum testosterone and levels of sexual activity in their healthy older men (Pfeiffer et al 1968). Schiavi et al (1990) studied 77 men, aged 45–74 years, who were healthy and in stable relationships, and reported that there was a positive correlation between serum levels of non-SHBG-bound testosterone and levels of sexual desire and sleep-related erections, but that there was no correlation with reported ED.

Overall, the data on the correlation of sexual function measures with levels of testosterone in older men present a mixed picture. While there is some support for a relationship between declining testosterone levels and sexual activity and/or sexual desire in this age group, there seems to be little to no support for a relationship between declining testosterone levels and ED.

Testosterone replacement therapy

Testosterone administration to young hypogonadal men increases libido, frequency of sexual activity, and erectile ability (Skakkeback et al 1981; Kwan et al 1983). Frequency of sexual thoughts and total number of erections per week have shown a dose–response relationship to testosterone replacement in these patients (Davidson et al 1979; O'Carroll et al 1985). Sleep-related erections, which are usually impaired in hypogonadal men, are restored by testosterone (O'Carroll et al 1985). In contrast, erections in response to visual erotic stimuli do not seem to be affected by testosterone replacement (Davidson et al 1979; Kwan et al 1983; O'Carroll et al 1985). Some (Skakkeback et al 1981; O'Carroll et al 1985), but not all (Davidson et al 1979; Salmimies et al 1982) studies have shown testosterone replacement positively affects well-being and mood in hypogonadal young men; the extent to which an improvement in mood may influence sexual interest, activity, or even erectile function is unclear.

Acute experimental induction of hypogonadism in previously eugonadal young men results in a marked decline in frequency of sexual desire, sexual fantasies, and coital activity (Bagatell et al 1994). Testosterone replacement at a dose that maintains serum testosterone at about half the baseline level was sufficient to sustain normal sexual function. On the other hand, variation of testosterone levels within the normal range in young adult men (Buena et al 1993) does not appear to have a major influence on sexual behavior.

There are no clinical trials that have evaluated the effect of testosterone therapy on aspects of sexual function in healthy older men with low or low–normal testosterone levels. There are, however, some studies which have evaluated the effects of raising serum testosterone levels in older adult men with various types of sexual dysfunction. O'Carroll and Bancroft (1984), in a double-blind, crossover study design, evaluated the effects of intramuscular injections of testosterone or placebo in eugonadal men up to 64 years of age who had either low libido or ED. Baseline testosterone levels were 490–662 ng/dl, and with testosterone therapy increased to 605–922 ng/dl. With this modest increase in serum testosterone level, the group with low libido demonstrated an improvement in sexual desire, while the group with ED showed no changes with testosterone therapy. Carani et al (1990) reported an improvement in sexual function with testosterone therapy for men with ED who had low levels of free testosterone prior to treatment, but no effect on those men who had initial free testosterone levels within the normal range. Raising the serum testosterone levels in 17 older men with ED and baseline serum testosterone levels < 275 ng/dl, Guay et al (1995) reported that 61% of the men had no improvement in ED or libido, 22% improved libido only, and 39% had a "complete response." The final testosterone levels achieved in this study lacked predictive value as to which men would improve their sexual function with androgen therapy.

Summary

To summarize what has been reviewed:

1. All components of serum testosterone decline with normal male aging, but the rate and extent of decline vary greatly among individuals.
2. Unless disease or medication intervenes, the majority of men will not reach serum testosterone levels that are in a truly 'hypogonadal' range.
3. Erectile dysfunction and decreased libido occur more frequently as men age.
4. In young adult men, there are few data to support an association between ED and serum testosterone except in men who are profoundly hypogonadal. Even fewer data support a relationship between the age-related decline of serum testosterone levels in older men and ED.
5. There are data to support a relationship between testosterone levels and sexual desire, but most studies in younger adult men suggest that subnormal testosterone levels are all that is needed for full libido in most men.
6. There are no studies evaluating the effect of testosterone replacement on sexual function in normal healthy older men, but some data from studies in which older men with sexual dysfunction were given testosterone demonstrated that, in certain cases, replacement therapy did improve sexual activity, and even occasionally ED.

At this point in time there are not enough data to support the hypothesis that the relative hypogonadism that occurs with normal aging in about 25–30% of older men contributes significantly to the majority of cases of sexual dysfunction in this age group. Individual cases may occur where testosterone therapy could be beneficial, however. Testosterone therapy is relatively inexpensive, and with proper screening at least a short-term therapeutic trial of replacment therapy may be warranted in selected older men with sexual dysfunction.

References

Bagatell CJ, Heiman JR, Rivier JE, et al (1994). Effects of endogenous testosterone and estradiol on sexual behavior in normal young men. *J Clin Endocrinol Metab* **78**:711–16.

Bremner WJ, Vitiello MV, Prinz PN (1983). Loss of circadian rhythmicity in blood testosterone levels with aging in normal men. *J Clin Endocrinol Metab* **56**:1278–81.

Bretschneider JG, McCoy NL (1988). Sexual interest and behavior in healthy 80 to 102 year olds. *Arch Sex Behav* **17**:109–29.

Buena F, Peterson MA, Swerdloff RS, et al (1993). Sexual function does not change when serum testosterone levels are pharmacologically varied within the normal male range. *Fertil Steril* **59**:1118–23.

Carani CM, Zini D, Baldini A, et al (1990). Effects of androgen treatment in impotent men with normal and low levels of free testosterone. *Arch Sex Behav* **19**:223–34.

Chung WS, Park YY, Kwon SW (1996). The impact of aging on penile hemodynamics in normal responders to pharmacological injection: a doppler sonographic study. *J Urol* **157**:2129–31.

Davidson JM, Camargo CA, Smith ER (1979). Effects of androgen on sexual behavior in hypogonadal men. *J Clin Endocrinol Metab* **48**:955–8.

Davidson JM, Chen JJ, Crapo L, et al (1983). Hormonal changes and sexual function in aging men. *J Clin Endocrinol Metab* **57**:71–7.

Feldman HA, Goldstein I, Hatzichristou DG, et al (1994). Impotence and its medical and psychosocial correlates: results of the Massachusetts male aging study. *J Urol* **151**:54–61.

Galbraith RA (1991). Sexual side effects of drugs. *Drug Therapy* March:38–41.

Guay AT, Bansal S, Heatley GJ (1995). Effect of raising endogenous testosterone levels in impotent men with secondary hypogonadism: double blind placebo-controlled trial with clomiphene citrate. *J Clin Endocrinol Metab* **80**:3546–52.

Harman SM, Tsitouras PD (1980). Reproductive hormones in aging men. I. Measurement of sex steroids, basal luteinizing hormone, and Leydig cell response to human chorionic gonadotropin. *J Clin Endocrinol Metab* **51**:35–40.

Heller CG, Myers GB (1944). The male climacteric, its symptomatology, diagnosis and treatment. *JAMA* **126**:472–8.

Kinsey AC, Pomeroy WB, Martin CE (1948). *Sexual Behavior in the Human Male*. WB Saunders, Philadelphia.

Korenman SG, Morley JE, Mooradian AD, et al (1990). Secondary hypogonadism in older men: its relation to impotence. *J Clin Endocrinol Metab* **71**:963–9.

Kwan M, Greenleaf WJ, Mann J, et al (1983). The nature of androgen action on male sexuality: a combined laboratory–self-report study on hypogonadal men. *J Clin Endocrinol Metab* **57**:557–62.

Lunglmayr G (1997). Trial of androgen supplementation in aging men. In: *Current Advances in Andrology*, eds GMH Waites, J Frick, GWH Baker, pp. 289–92. Monduzzi Editore, Bologna, Italy.

McCullagh EP (1946). Climacteric – male and female. *Cleveland Clin Q* **13**:166–73.

Manni A, Pardridge WM, Cefalu W, et al (1985). Bioavailability of albumin-bound testosterone. *J Clin Endocrinol Metab* **61**:705–10.

Mulligan T, Retchin SM, Chinchilli VM, et al (1988). The role of aging and chronic disease in sexual dysfunction. *J Am Geriatr Soc* **36**:520–4.

Neaves WB, Johnson L, Porter JC, et al (1984). Leydig cell numbers, daily sperm production, and serum gonadotropin levels in aging men. *J Clin Endocrinol Metab* **55**:756–63.

O'Carroll R, Bancroft J (1984). Testosterone therapy for low sexual interest and erectile dysfunction in men: a controlled study. *Br J Psychiatry* **145**:146–51.

O'Carroll R, Shapiro C, Bancroft J (1985). Androgens, behaviour and nocturnal erection in hypogonadal men: the effect of varying the replacement dose. *Clin Endocrinol* **23**:527–38.

Panser LA, Rhodes T, Girman CJ, et al (1995). Sexual function of men ages 40 to 79 years: the Olmsted county study of urinary symptoms and health status among men. *J Am Geriatr Soc* **43**:1107–11.

Pfeiffer E, Verwoerdt A, Wang HS (1968). Sexual behavior in aged men and women. *Arch Gen Psychiatry* **19**:753–8.

Sakiyama R, Pardridge WM, Musto NA (1988). Influx of testosterone-binding globulin (TeBG) and TeBG-bound sex steroid hormones into rat testis and prostate. *J Clin Endocrinol Metab* **67**:98–103.

Salmimies P, Kockott G, Pirke KW, et al (1982). Effects of testosterone replacement on sexual behavior in hypogonadal men. *Arch Sex Behav* **11**:345–53

Schiavi RC, Schreiner-Engel P (1988). Nocturnal penile tumescence in healthy aging men. *J Gerontol* **43**:M146–50.

Schiavi RC, Schreiner-Engel P, Mandeli J, et al (1990). Healthy aging and male sexual function. *Am J Psychiatry* **147**:766–71.

Skakkeback NE, Bancroft J, Davidson JM, et al (1981). Androgen replacement with oral testosterone undecanoate in hypogonadal men: a double-blind controlled study. *Clin Endocrinol* **14**:49–61.

Takahashi J, Higashi Y, Lanasa JA, et al (1983). Studies of the human testis. XVIII. Simultaneous measurement of nine intratesticular steroids: evidence for reduced mitochondrial function in testis of elderly men. *J Clin Endocrinol Metab* **56**:1178–87.

Tenover JS (1994). Androgen administration to aging men. In: *Endocrinology and Metabolism Clinics of North America*, Vol 23(4), ed. WJ Bremner, pp. 877–92. WB Saunders, Philadelphia, PA.

Tenover JL (1996). Effects of androgen supplementation in the aging male. In: *Androgens and the Aging Male*, eds B Oddens, A Vermeulen, pp. 191–204. Parthenon Publishing, Pearl River, NY.

Tsitouras PD, Martin CE, Harman SM (1982). Relationship of serum testosterone to sexual activity in healthy elderly men. *J Gerontol* **37**:288–93.

Vermeulen A (1991). Androgen administration to aging men. *Endocrinol Metab Clin North Am* **23**:877–92.

Vermeulen A, Verdonck L (1972). Some studies on the biological significance of free testosterone. *J Steroid Biochem* **3**:421–6.

4

A rational approach to investigation of the sexually dysfunctional man

Ahmed I El-Sakka and Tom F Lue

The therapeutic strategy of treating an impotent man is either to correct the cause of impotence or to bypass the cause and offer a non-specific, safe and effective treatment. The ultimate goal is to convert the sexually and mentally crippled patient and his frustrated partner to a satisfied, sexually practicing couple.

For a satisfactory and cost-effective outcome, we have used a patient's goal-directed approach (Figure 1) for the past 10 years. We recommend that every patient should have thorough medical and psychosexual history, physical examination and appropriate laboratory tests. Further diagnostic testing is tailored to the treatment chosen by the patient. Of course the physician should also take the following into consideration: patient's age, general health, concomitant medical diseases, and the goals and expectations of the patient and his partner. Nowadays, a variety of treatment options is available. The diagnostic approach for each treatment option is listed in Figure 2.

Medical and psychosexual history

Despite the explosion of new diagnostic tests, a detailed psychosexual and medical history remains the key to the diagnosis of erectile dysfunction. A detailed history also helps differentiate erectile failure from changes in sexual desire, and orgasmic or ejaculatory disturbances. Because of the sensitive nature of these issues, it is of paramount importance for the physician to establish a relationship of trust with his patient at an early stage.

dysfunction

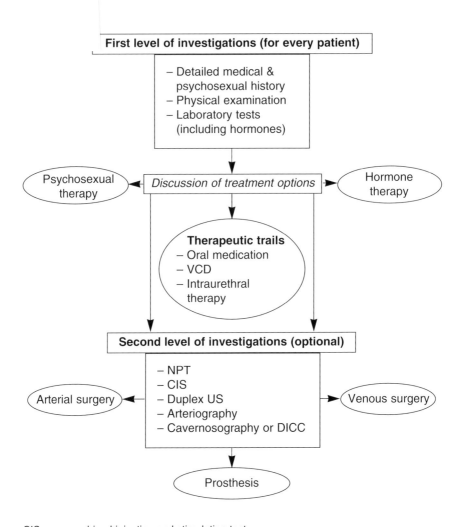

CIS = combined injection and stimulation test
NPT = nocturnal penile tumescence
VCD = vacuum constriction device
DICC = dynamic infusion cavernosometry and cavernosography
US   = ultrasound

Figure 1
Algorithm of diagnostic approach for impotent men.

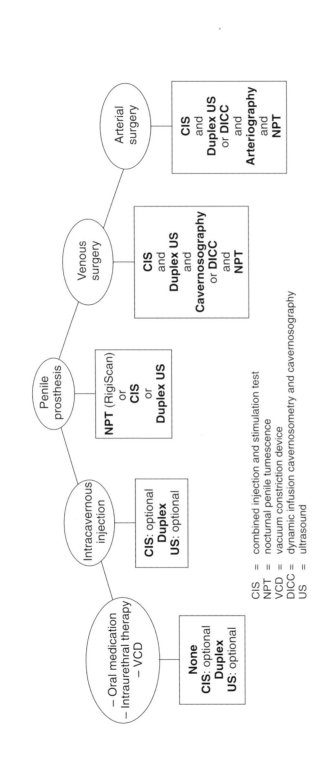

Figure 2
Diagnostic tests for chosen treatment options.

CIS = combined injection and stimulation test
NPT = nocturnal penile tumescence
VCD = vacuum constriction device
DICC = dynamic infusion cavernosometry and cavernosography
US = ultrasound

Table 1   Differentiation between psychogenic and organic erectile dysfunction

Characteristic	Organic	Psychogenic
Onset	Gradual	Acute
Circumstances	Global	Situational
Course	Constant	Varying
Non-coital erection	Poor	Rigid
Psychosexual problem	Secondary	Long history
Partner problem	Secondary	At onset
Anxiety and fear	Secondary	Primary

Modified from Hengeveld (1991).

A careful medical history with knowledge of concurrent illnesses and medications is essential. Because erectile dysfunction may have multiple causes, a detailed history and physical examination may help determine whether the dysfunction is a result of anatomic, psychogenic, endocrinologic, neurologic or vascular abnormalities.

The psychosexual history should include the quality of erection, the duration of impotence, the level of libido and a complete inventory of sexual partners. Although exceptions are not uncommon, an assessment of the onset of dysfunction, the presence or absence of morning erection and any psychological conflict may help determine whether the dysfunction is mostly psychogenic or organic (Table 1). Often the sexual history provides the most helpful information in directing further evaluation and treatment. For example, a patient who reports a recent history of impotence associated with a low libido may be suffering from an endocrinopathy that can easily be treated with hormone replacement.

A psychogenic disorder may occasionally be the primary cause of erectile dysfunction. Early recognition saves the patient from much unnecessary and costly diagnostic work-up. As erectile dysfunction is known to be associated with many common medical conditions and medications, careful questioning may yield clues: a history of peripheral vascular or coronary arterial disease, diabetes, renal failure, tobacco and alcohol use, or neurologic or chronic debilitating disease can direct further evaluation. Clinically, an older patient with a long history of diabetes and vascular disease is likely to have impotence secondary to vascular and neuropathic disease. On the other hand, a young patient with psychiatric illness is more likely to have psychogenic impotence or possibly impotence secondary to psychotropic medications. Neuroleptic treatment can restore desire, but may cause erectile, orgasmic and sexual satisfaction problems. A patient's past surgical history may similarly yield insights. Radical pelvic surgery (prostatectomy, abdominoperineal resection), radiation and pelvic trauma are well known to be associated with impotence (Armenakas et al 1993; Walsh et al 1994).

Physical examination

A thorough physical examination with particular attention to sexual and genital development may occasionally reveal an obvious cause (for example, micropenis, chordee or Peyronie's plaque). The finding of small soft atrophic testes or gynecomastia should prompt an endocrine evaluation for hypogonadism or hyperprolactinemia. Patients with certain genetic syndromes, such as Kallmann's or Klinefelter's, may present with obvious physical signs of hypogonadism or a distinctive body habitus. A careful neurologic examination should also be performed. Testing for genital and perineal sensation and the bulbocavernosus reflex is also useful in assessing possible neurogenic impotence. Care should be taken to look for signs of either thyroid under-activity or over-activity, as well as for stigmata of liver failure, renal failure or anemia. Hypertension, cardiac murmurs and arrhythmia should also be assessed. However, Davis-Joseph et al (1995) reported that history and physical examination had a 95% sensitivity but only a 50% specificity in diagnosing organic erectile dysfunction, and concluded that a multifaceted comprehensive approach is required for a definitive diagnosis of erectile dysfunction. In many cases, a careful history and physical examination will direct the physician to the most expedient and cost-effective approach and eliminate the need for unnecessary diagnostic tests.

Laboratory investigation

The laboratory investigation is directed at identifying treatable conditions or previously undetected medical illnesses that may be contributory, such as metabolic disturbances or endocrine abnormalities. A basic laboratory evaluation includes complete blood count, urinalysis, renal and liver function, lipid profile and morning testosterone.

Discussion of the available options

Informing the patient and partner of the available diagnostic and therapeutic options is an important aspect of the office consultation. The treatment options currently available, and their costs, advantages and disadvantages are listed in Table 2.

In the late 1970s and early 1980s, the penile prosthesis and psychosexual therapy were the only two effective treatments for erectile dysfunction. The introduction of the less invasive but highly effective intracavernous injection and vacuum constriction device, and more recently intraurethral therapy and new oral medication, have dramatically changed management. The success of these non-specific treatments has some investigators questioning the wisdom of the traditional medical approach of making an accurate diagnosis and following it up with a specific treatment. Although finding and correcting the exact cause seems to be the most logical

Table 2   Treatment options for erectile dysfunction: costs, advantages and disadvantages

Treatment	Cost (US$)	Advantages	Disadvantages/ side-effects
Psychosexual therapy	500–2 000	Non-invasive, resolves conflict	Moderately successful High recurrence rate
Oral drugs	15–45/month	Non-invasive	Poor efficacy; frequent systemic side-effects
Vacuum constriction device	350–450	Low cost, non-invasive	Unnatural erection; petechiae, pain
Intraurethral therapy	200/month	Minimally invasive	Low success rate; urethral bleeding, penile pain
Intracavernous injection	40–200/month	Natural erection, highly successful	More invasive; priapism, fibrosis, pain
Prosthesis	6 000–15 000	Highly successful	Requires surgery, anesthesia; infection, fibrosis
Vascular surgery	8 000–15 000	Restores natural erection	Moderate success rate; requires surgery, anesthesia

approach, the current socioeconomic climate argues strongly against it. Therefore, we have proposed a patient's goal-directed approach (Lue 1990), which determines the extent of further work-up according to the patient's age, general health and treatment goal.

Additional investigations when needed

Nocturnal penile tumescence testing

The nocturnal penile tumescence (NPT) test was one of the earliest devised to study erectile dysfunction. Nocturnal penile tumescence or sleep-related erection is a recurring cycle of penile erections associated with rapid eye movement (REM) sleep in virtually all potent men. In 1970, Karacan suggested that NPT could be used to evaluate erectile dysfunction, as its mechanism is presumed to rely on neurovascular responses similar to those of erotically induced erections. The primary goal of NPT testing is to distinguish psychogenic from organic causes of impotence.

Although NPT testing is non-invasive, its usefulness has been questioned. Anxiety and depression can at times influence the content of the dream state, negatively affecting spontaneous nocturnal erections. In addition, sleep disturbances such as apnea and motor agitation can also induce erroneous recordings. Dysfunctions at the level of the cortex and spine may still permit nocturnal tumescence while causing an erectile deficit in the awake state. Moreover, normal NPT may also occur in patients with a mild vascular problem (such as the "pelvic steal syndrome") who often lose an erection during pelvic thrusts. Clinically, all these factors question the effectiveness of the NPT test in the study of the cause of impotence (Colombo et al 1994). Moreover, NPT evaluation has proved to be quite costly, as it is often done in a specially equipped sleep center.

In 1985 the RigiScan was introduced. This combines the sophisticated monitoring of rigidity, tumescence, and number and duration of events with the convenience and economic advantage of an ambulatory monitoring system (Bradley et al 1985). Cilurzo et al (1992) suggested the following as normal parameters for an NPT evaluation: four to five erectile episodes per night; mean duration > 30 min; an increase in circumference of > 3 cm at the base and > 2 cm at the tip; and > 70% maximal rigidity at both base and tip. In a study of 16 healthy men aged 24–44 years, Kaneko et al (1991) found that the mean duration of tumescence (i.e. circumference expansion > 10 mm) was 23.0 ± 6.9 min at the tip and 38.3 ± 12.0 min at the base. The maximum rigidity lasting > 10 min was $82.9\pm10.1\%$ at the tip and 85.4 ± 8.4 at the base.

Because the RigiScan measures radial rigidity (compressibility), the validity of this measurement has been questioned. Allen et al (1993) reported that, when RigiScan base and tip radial rigidity exceeded 60% of maximum, correlation with axial rigidity and observer ratings was poor. In this range, the RigiScan failed to discriminate axial rigidities between 450 and 900 g of buckling force. As an axial rigidity of more than 550 g is necessary for vaginal penetration, the RigiScan may not be able to detect mild abnormalities in erectile function.

Many investigators have advocated the use of NPT studies, particularly in selecting outpatients with psychogenic impotence (Shabsigh et al 1990; Allen et al 1994). A normal finding in a patient in whom a psychologic cause is suspected may help reduce the cost of the evaluation by preventing unnecessary endocrine and vascular evaluation. However, because of the problems associated with various NPT tests, findings often need to be confirmed independently by other studies. For these reasons, we have abandoned NPT testing as a routine part of the impotence evaluation. However, in some selected cases (patients with complex and confusing histories and those involved in litigation in which compensation or guilt hinges on erectile status–Hirshkowitz and Ware 1994), we would agree that NPT is a useful tool in confirming the clinical diagnosis. In these cases, for financial reasons, we will begin with a RigiScan test, because a normal result practically rules out significant vascular insufficiency. When abnormal NPT is noted on RigiScan and the clinical diagnosis is uncertain, a formal sleep laboratory study with polysomnography may be indicated to rule out sleep apnea and nocturnal myoclonus as the cause of impaired erection.

Psychometry and psychologic interview

Several psychometric instruments are available for the evaluation of erectile dysfunction: (1) standardized personality questionnaires; (2) the depression inventory; and (3) questionnaires for sexual dysfunction and relationship factors. Currently, a skilful diagnostic interview remains the mainstay of psychologic evaluation. Traditional psychoanalytic theory has not been replaced by a newer concept popularized by Kaplan (1983) who theorizes that the determinants of psychogenic impotence operate on different levels of causation, ranging from superficial and mild problems to those deeply rooted in early life. Hartmann (1991) suggests that the interview should be focused on the following: (1) current sexual problem and its history; (2) deeper causes of sexual dysfunction; (3) dyadic relationship causes; and (4) psychiatric symptoms.

In obtaining the current sexual history, the interviewer should strive to determine whether the dysfunction is primary or secondary, constant, phasic or situational, and partner-specific. The interviewer should also obtain information on the extent of non-coital erections (masturbatory, nocturnal or morning), and history related to traumatic experience, cultural or educational indoctrination, and neurotic processes in which the sexual symptoms serve as a defense against unconscious fear. In assessing a partner-related problem, the couple should be interviewed both together and apart if possible.

Although psychologic consultation is not indicated for most patients with non-psychogenic causes of erectile dysfunction, it is very useful in directing treatment in patients with deep-seated psychologic problems. For example, a patient with severe depression, a strained relationship or unrealistic expectations will probably not enjoy a satisfactory outcome, even with a perfectly functioning penile prosthesis.

Neurologic testing

In a broader sense, neurologic testing should assess peripheral, spinal and supraspinal centers, and both somatic and autonomic pathways. However, the effect of neurologic deficit on penile erection is a complicated phenomenon and, with a few exceptions, neurologic testing will rarely change management. Moreover, there is no reliable test to assess neurotransmitter release, which leaves a major gap in the current assessment of overall neurologic function associated with penile erection. In our opinion, the aim of neuro-urologic testing is to: (1) uncover reversible neurologic disease, such as dorsal nerve neuropathy secondary to long-distance bicycling; (2) assess the extent of neurologic deficit from a known neurologic disease, such as diabetes mellitus or pelvic injury; and (3) determine whether a referral to a neurologist is necessary (for example, for work-up for a possible spinal cord tumor).

Somatic nervous system

Biothesiometry
This test is designed to measure the sensory perception threshold to various amplitudes of vibratory stimulation produce by a hand-held

electromagnetic device (biothesiometer) placed on the pulp of the index fingers, both sides of the penile shaft and the glans penis. However, Bemelmans et al (1995) argue that biothesiometric investigation of penile glans sensitivity is unsuited for the evaluation of penile innervation and cannot replace neurophysiologic tests.

Sacral evoked response–bulbocavernous reflex latency
This test is performed by placing two stimulating ring electrodes around the penis, one near the corona and the other 3 cm proximal. Concentric needle electrodes are placed in the right and left bulbocavernous muscles to record the response. Square-wave impulses are delivered via a direct current stimulator. The latency period for each stimulus response is measured from the beginning of the stimulus to the beginning of the response. An abnormal bulbocavernous reflex (BCR) latency time, defined as a value greater than three standard deviations above the mean (30–40 ms), carries a high probability of neuropathology (Padma-Nathan 1994).

Dorsal nerve conduction velocity
In patients with adequate penile length, it is possible to use two BCR latency measurements, one from the glans and one from the base of the penis, to determine the conduction velocity of the dorsal nerve. Gerstenberg and Bradley (1983) have determined an average conduction velocity of 23.5 m/s with a range of 21.4–29.1 m/s in normal subjects.

Genitocerebral evoked potential studies
This test involves electrical stimulation of the dorsal nerve of the penis as described for the BCR latency test. Instead of recording electromyographic (EMG) responses, this study records the evoked potential waveforms overlying the sacral spinal cord and cerebral cortex (Goldstein and Krane 1992). This study can provide an objective assessment of the presence, location and nature of afferent penile sensory dysfunction.

Autonomic nervous system

Heart rate variability and sympathetic skin response
Although autonomic neuropathy is an important cause of erectile dysfunction, direct testing is not available. The tests of heart rate control and blood pressure control are indirect methods of assessment. Because heart rate and blood pressure responses can be affected by many external factors, these tests must be done under standardized conditions (Abicht 1991).

Smooth-muscle EMG and single potential analysis of cavernous electrical activity
Direct recording of cavernous electrical activity with a needle electrode during flaccidity and with visual sexual stimulation was first reported by Wagner et al (1989). The normal resting flaccid electrical activity from the corpora cavernosa was a rhythmic slow wave with an intermittent burst of activity. Patients with suspected autonomic neuropathy demonstrated a discoordination pattern with continuing electrical activity during visual sexual stimulation or after intracavernous injection of a smooth-muscle relaxant.

Djamilian et al (1993) reported that, in normal subjects, single potential analysis of cavernous electrical activity (SPACE) shows a regular pattern of activity with long phases of electrical silence at the usual amplification interrupted by synchronous, low-frequency, high-amplitude potentials. In patents with disruption of the peripheral autonomic supply, asynchronous potentials with higher frequencies and an irregular shape are typical. In those with complete spinal cord lesions, abnormal as well as normal electrical activity is found. More studies are needed to define the clinical utility.

Hormonal assessment

It is well known that endocrinopathy leading to impotence may be a manifestation of a more serious, possibly life-threatening disease, such as a prolactin-secreting tumor (Carter et al 1978; Mattman and Montague 1986). For these reasons, some routinely perform testosterone and prolactin measurements as an initial evaluation. Because testosterone-binding globulin (TeBG) is known to be decreased in hypothyroidism, obesity and acromegaly, and increased in hyperthyroidism and estrogen therapy, it is necessary to measure the free biologically active hormone in these conditions, when total testosterone can be misleading. For practical reasons, we usually obtain a single morning testosterone (normal 300–1000 ng/dl). If the result is abnormal, we repeat the test and obtain prolactin, luteinizing hormone (LH) (normal, 1–15 mIU/ml) and follicle-stimulating hormone (FSH) (normal, 1–15 mIU/ml) to differentiate primary from secondary hypogonadism. Only men with clearly documented hypogonadism are candidates for testosterone replacement therapy. We prefer to refer patients with secondary hypogonasim to an endrocrinologist for further work-up of possible pituitary or hypothalamic dysfunction.

Abnormally elevated prolactin levels (> 22 ng/ml) can lower testosterone secretion through inhibition of LH-releasing hormone (LHRH) secretion by the hypothalamus, and thus result in impotence.

Although the incidence of a prolactin-secreting tumor is extremely low in most series of impotent patients, a large number of these patients (> 90%) will have impotence and decreased libido as the presenting complaint (Carter et al 1978; Maatman and Montague 1986). Hyperprolactinemia may also be caused by certain drugs, or medical conditions such as renal insufficiency and hypothyroidism, or it may be idiopathic (Weideman and Northcutt 1981).

Some men with gynecomastia or suspected androgen resistance (high serum testosterone and LH with undermasculinization) should undergo determination of serum estradiol and androgen receptors on the genital skin. Patients with a rapid loss of secondary sex characteristics may have both testicular and adrenal failure, and should also be tested for adrenal function (McClure and Marshall 1994). Other endocrine disorders, such as hyper- and hypothyroidism and adrenocortical dysfunction or tumor, may affect sexual function and should be investigated if suspected.

Vascular evaluation

Penile brachial pressure index

The penile brachial index (PBI) represents the penile systolic blood pressure divided by the brachial systolic blood pressure. A penile brachial index of 0.7 or less has been used to indicate arteriogenic impotence (Metz and Bengtsson 1981). However, this test has many limitations. For example, measurement in the flaccid state will not reveal the full functional capacity of the cavernous arteries in the erect state. Secondly, the continuous-wave Doppler probe does not discriminately select the arterial flow of the paired cavernous arteries, as the probe detects all pulsatile flow within its path, and usually detects the higher blood flow of the dorsal penile artery, which is located superficially. Therefore, a normal PBI cannot be relied upon to exclude arteriogenic impotence. Aitchison et al (1990) reported that the PBI is inaccurate and poorly reproducible and suggests no justification for its continued use.

Penile plethysmography (penile pulse volume recording)

This test is performed by connecting a 2.5- or 3-cm cuff to an air plethysmograph. The cuff is inflated to a pressure above brachial systolic pressure, which is then decreased by 10 mmHg increments, and tracings are obtained at each level. The pressure demonstrating the best waveform is recorded. The normal waveform is similar to a normal arterial waveform obtained from a finger: a rapid upstroke, a sharp peak, a lower downstroke and occasionally a dicrotic notch. In patients with vasculogenic erectile dysfunction the waveform shows a slow upstroke, a low rounded peak, slow downstroke and no dicrotic notch.

Combined intracavernous injection and stimulation test

Differentiation among psychogenic, neurogenic and vascular causes is often difficult, even after obtaining a detailed history, a physical examination and endocrine evaluation. Additional information regarding the vascular status of the penis is often helpful. Intracorporeal injection (ICI) of papaverine, first introduced by Virag and associates (1984), was found to be a useful diagnostic tool, both inexpensive and minimally invasive, in patients with suspected vasculogenic impotence (Virag et al 1984; Abber et al 1986). The pharmacologic screening test allows the clinician to bypass neurogenic and hormonal influences and to evaluate the vascular status of the penis directly and objectively.

We currently use alprostadil (prostaglandin E_1), a potent vasodilating agent that is metabolized locally in the penis. The technique involves injecting 10 mg through a 28-gauge half-inch needle into the corpus cavernosum. The erectile response is periodically evaluated for both rigidity and duration. Normally, a full erection is achieved within 15 min (i.e. an erection of > 90° that is firm to palpation) and lasts longer than 15 min (Lue and Tanagho 1987).

A normal finding rules out the possibility of venous leakage (although about 20% of patients with arterial insufficiency may achieve a rigid erection owing to an intact veno-occlusive mechanism) (Pescatori et al 1994). An abnormal pharmacologic test result suggests penile vascular disease (arterial, venous, cavernous) and warrants further evaluation, although it may not always be indicative (Lue and Tanagho 1987; Steers 1993). The patient's fear of injection often produces a heightened sympathetic response, which may produce a false-positive result. To obtain better results, patients are also instructed to perform self-stimulation if a rigid erection does not occur within 15 min. This technique is known as the combined injection and stimulation (CIS) test. In our experience, many patients (about 75%) who initially have a subnormal response to intracavernous injection will have significant improvement in their erections after self-stimulation (Donatucci and Lue 1992).

Doppler waveform analysis

Duplex ultrasonography (gray scale and color coded)
In 1985, high-resolution sonography and pulsed Doppler blood flow analysis (duplex ultrasonography) with intracavernous injection of

papaverine was introduced as a means of evaluating penile arterial insufficiency (Lue et al 1985). Duplex sonography provided clear advantages over previous techniques: first, in contrast to pudendal arteriography, duplex sonography is non-invasive and can be performed in the office setting; secondly, the high-resolution duplex ultrasound probe allows the ultrasonographer to image the individual cavernous arteries selectively and to perform Doppler blood flow analysis simultaneously within these vessels. Arteriography is most useful as a detailed roadmap of the penile arterial system, including the recipient and donor arteries in patients who are candidates for penile revascularization. The color-coded Doppler device provides an additional advantage of easier assessment of direction of blood flow and communication among the cavernous, dorsal and spongiosal arteries, which are crucial in penile vascular and reconstructive surgery.

The study is performed by first obtaining a baseline study of the flaccid penis. High-resolution ultrasonography is used to image the corpora cavernosa, the corpus spongiosum and the tunica albuginea. The cavernous arteries are usually identified near the septum at the base in the midshaft. The arterial diameter of the flaccid penis and the presence of any calcifications within the vessel wall are noted.

A pharmacologic erection is then induced by the intracavernous injection of a vasodilating agent such as papaverine (15–30 mg) or alprostadil (10 mg). Sonographic assessment of the penis is then repeated 3–5 min after the injection. Each main cavernous and dorsal artery is individually assessed. Cavernous arterial diameter and pulsation are recorded. The presence of a communication between the paired cavernous arteries or between the dorsal and cavernous arteries should also be noted. An asymmetrical appearance and response of the cavernous arteries or the lack of arterial pulsation may indicate a significant lesion (Benson and Vickers 1989). We encourage all patients to perform manual self-stimulation in a private setting. Scanning is then repeated and, if necessary, repeated again after the second injection and self-stimulation.

Cavernous arterial occlusion pressure
This variation of penile blood pressure determination was introduced by Padma-Nathan in 1989. It involves infusing saline solution into the corpora cavernosa at a rate sufficient to raise the intracavernous pressure above the systolic blood pressure. A Doppler transducer is then applied to the side of the penile base. The saline infusion is stopped, and the intracavernous pressure is allowed to fall. The pressure at which the cavernous arterial flow becomes detectable is defined as

the cavernous artery systolic occlusion pressure (CASOP). A gradient between the cavernous and brachial artery pressures of less than 35 mmHg and equal pressure between the right and left cavernous arteries have been defined as normal. Results have been shown to correlate well with those of arteriography (Padma-Nathan et al 1988) and peak systolic velocity obtained by high-resolution duplex Doppler ultrasonography (Rhee et al 1995). However, dynamic infusion cavernosometry is nevertheless a more invasive procedure, and thus more prone to psychologic inhibition. Moreover, in many patients with severe venous leakage, the cavernous artery occlusion pressure becomes unmeasurable, because the intracavernous pressure often cannot be raised above the systolic blood pressure.

Cavernosometry and cavernosography

The current standard diagnostic study for veno-occlusive dysfunction is pharmacologic cavernosometry and cavernosography. Cavernosography performed during visual sexual stimulation was introduced by Wagner (1981) and Shirai and Ishii (1981) to visualize veno-occlusive dysfunction. This technique was modified by Virag (1981) and Wespes et al (1984), who introduced dynamic cavernosometry during artificial erection produced by saline infusion.

Cavernosometry involves simultaneous saline infusion and intracorporeal pressure monitoring. A more physiologic refinement is the addition of intracavernous injection of vasodilating agents such as papaverine + phentolamine, alprostadil or a combination of the three drugs. The saline infusion rate necessary to maintain erection is thus directly related to the degree of venous leakage (Wepes et al 1986). Veno-occlusive dysfunction is indicated by either the inability to increase intracorporeal pressure to the level of the mean systolic blood pressure with saline infusion or a rapid drop of intracorporeal pressure after cessation of infusion (Puyau and Lewis 1983; Rudnick et al 1991). Puech-Leao and colleagues (1990) introduced a gravity saline infusion set. They found that gravity infusion cavernosometry correlates well with pump infusion cavernosometry and may provide a simpler and more economical alternative.

Cavernosography involves the infusion of radiocontrast solution into the corpora cavernosa during an artificial erection to visualize the site of venous leakage. Both cavernosometry and cavernosography should always be performed after activation of the veno-occlusive mechanism by intracavernous injection of vasodilators (Lue et al 1986); various leakage sites to the glans, corpus spongiosum, superficial and deep dorsal veins, and cavernous and crural veins can then

be detected. Technical factors may influence the findings on cavernosometry and cavernosography. The study is done in a non-sexual
setting with little privacy, leading to patient anxiety and an adverse
effect on the erectile response. The phenomenon of incomplete trabecular smooth-muscle relaxation will falsely suggest veno-occlusive
dysfunction in some normal subjects (Montague and Lakin 1992).
Therefore repeated injections of vasodilators may be necessary to
achieve a complete smooth-muscle relaxation (Hatzichristou et al
1995). The normal maintenance rate in patients with complete
smooth-muscle relaxation is reported to be less than 5 ml/min, with a
pressure decrease from 150 mmHg of less than 45 mmHg in 30 s.

Arteriography

Penile arteriography was introduced by the pioneering work of
Michal and Pospichal (1978). Currently, selective pudendal arteriography performed with the aid of intracavernous injection is considered by many to be the gold standard for evaluating penile arterial
anatomy (Stuyven et al 1979; Rajfer et al 1990; Rosen et al 1990).
    Although angiography is probably the most accurate single test for
evaluating the anatomy of the cavernous arteries, significant limitations to its application have been pointed out. Like all invasive radiographic tests, the study is performed under artificial conditions, which
may produce a significant sympathetic response and inhibit the erectile response. Inadequate vasodilatation of the cavernous arteries,
vasospasm induced by cannulation and injection of contrast solution
may result in an abnormal radiographic appearance.
    Arteriography is most useful in providing anatomic rather than
functional information. Owing to the relatively high cost and invasive
nature of the study, only a small percentage of impotent patients are
appropriate candidates (generally, only those who are candidates for
arterial revascularization). Perhaps the strongest indication is in the
young man with impotence secondary to a traumatic arterial disruption or in the rare patient with pelvic steal syndrome. In these very
selected cases, a detailed roadmap of the arterial anatomy is essential
for planning surgical reconstruction.

Cavernous assessment

Cavernous smooth muscle

Wespes et al have advocated corporeal biopsies with light microscopy
and computerized morphometric analysis as an adjunctive technique

in the diagnosis of vascular impotence. They have observed an age-related decrease in smooth-muscle content within the corpora cavernosa (Wespes et al 1992). When computerized morphometry was used to compare young patients with hemodynamically adequate erection in elderly patients with erectile dysfunction, the corpora cavernosa were composed of: 40–52% smooth muscle in the young; 19–36% in the elderly with corporal veno-occlusive dysfunction; and 10–25% in those with arterial impotence (collagen was correspondingly increased) (Wespes et al 1991). Malovrouvas et al (1994) reported that the biopsy gun specimens were as representative as the open biopsy specimens. The most severe lesions were observed in the erectile tissue, in particular in the smooth muscle of the trabeculae and the helicine arteries, which had been reduced and replaced by connective tissue.

Nitric oxide synthase

Brock et al (1986) determined the presence of nitric oxide synthase (NOS) (as shown by nicotinamide adenine dinucleotide phosphate [NADPH] diaphorase staining) in nerve fibers, smooth muscle and sinusoidal endothelium. Positive staining for NOS correlated significantly with a clinical history of cavernous nerve integrity.

At present cavernous biopsy remains a controversial issue. The proponents believe that it is essential for examining the cavernous tissue before arterial or venous surgery is contemplated. However, we feel that the less invasive tests, such as CIS and duplex ultrasonography, are adequate in predicting the integrity of the cavernous smooth muscle (Persson et al 1989) and more studies are needed before the routine use of cavernous biopsy can be recommended.

Summary

We have used a patient's goal-directed approach to impotence for the past 10 years. We feel that every patient should have a thorough medical and psychosexual history, physical examination and appropriate laboratory tests. Further diagnostic testing is tailored to the treatment option chosen by the patient. The physician should also consider the patient's age, general health, concomitant medical diseases, and the goals and expectations of the patient and his partner in recommending tests or treatment for the patient. Various established and developing tests were also discussed.

References

Abber JC, Lue TF, Orvis BR, et al (1986). Diagnostic tests for impotence: a comparison of papaverine injection with the penile-brachial index and nocturnal penile tumescence monitoring. *J Urol* **135**:923–5.

Abichet JH (1991). Testing the autonomic system. In: *Erectile Dysfunction*, eds U Jonas, WF Thon, CG Stief, pp. 187–93. Springer-Verlag, Berlin.

Aitchison M, Aitchison J, Carter R (1990). Is the penile brachial index a reproducible and useful measurement? *Br J Urol* **66**:202–4.

Allen RP, Smolev JK, Engel RM, et al (1993). Comparison of RigiScan and formal nocturnal penile tumescence testing in the evaluation of erectile rigidity. *J Urol* **149**:1265–8.

Allen RP, Engel RM, Smolev JK, et al (1994). Comparison of duplex ultrasonography and nocturnal penile tumescence in evaluation of impotence. *J Urol* **151**:1525–9.

Armenakas NA, McAninch JW, Lue TF, et al (1993). Posttraumatic impotence: magnetic resonance imaging and duplex ultrasound in diagnosis and management. *J Urol* **149**:1272–5.

Bemelmans BL, Hendrick LB, Koldewijn EL, et al (1995). Comparison of biothesiometry and neuro-urophysiological investigations for the clinical evaluation of patients with rectile dysfunction. *J Urol* **153**:1483–6.

Benson CB, Vickers MA (1989). Sexual impotence caused by vascular disease: diagnosis with duplex sonography. *AJR Am J Roentgenol* **153**:1149–53.

Bradley WE, Timm GW, Gallagher JM, et al (1985). New method for continuous measurement of nocturnal penile tumescence and rigidity. *Urology* **26**:4–9.

Brock G, Nunes L, Padma-Nathan H, et al (1986). Nitric oxide synthase: a new diagnostic tool for neurogenic impotence. *Urology* **42**:412–17.

Carter JN, Tyson JE, Tolis G, et al (1978). Prolactin-screeing tumors and hypogonadism in 22 men. *N Engl J Med* **299**:847–52.

Cilurzo P, Canale D, Turchi P, et al (1992). Rigiscan system in the diagnosis of male sexual impotence. *Arch Ital Urol Nefrol Androl* **64**(Suppl 2):81–5.

Colombo F, Fenice O, Austoni E (1994). NPT: nocturnal penile tumescence test. *Arch Ital Urol Nefrol Androl* **66**:159–64.

Davis-Joseph B, Tiefer L, Melman A (1995). Accuracy of the initial history and physical examination to establish the etiology of erectile dysfunction. *Urology* **45**:498–502.

Djamilian M, Stief CG, Hartmann U, et al (1993). Predictive value of real-time RigiScan monitoring for the etiology of organogenic impotence. *J Urol* **149**:1269–71.

Donatucci CDF, Lue TF (1992). The combined intracavernous injection and stimulation test: diagnostic acuracy. *J Urol* **148**:61–2.

Gerstenberg TC, Bradley W (1983). Nerve conduction velocity measurements of dorsal nerve of the penis in normal and impotent males. *Urology* **21**:90–2.

Goldstein I, Krane RJ (1992). Diagnosis and therapy of erectile dysfunction.In: *Campbell's Urology*, eds PC Walsh, AB Retik, TA Stamey, ED Vaughan Jr. WB Saunders, Philadelphia.

Hatzichristou DG, Saenz de Tejada I, Kupferman S, et al (1995). In vivo assessment of trabecular smooth muscle tone, its application in pharmaco-cavernosometry and analysis of intracavernous pressure determinants. *J Urol* **153**:1126–35.

Hengeveld MW (1991). Erectile disorder: a psychosexological review. In: *Erectile Dysfunction*, eds U Jonas, WF Thon, CG Stief, Springer-Verlag, Berlin.

Hirshkowitz M, Ware JC (1994). Studies of nocturnal penile tumescence and rigidity. In: *Sexual Dysfunction: A neuro-medical approach*, eds C Singer, WJ Weiner, Futura Publishing Co, Armonk, NY.

Kaneko S, Yachiku S, Miyata M, et al (1991). Continuous monitoring of penile rigidity and tumescence in Japanese without erectile dysfunction. *Nippon Hinyokika Gakkai Zasshi (Japanese Journal of Urology)* **83**:955–60.

Kaplan HS (1983). *The Evaluation of Sexual Disorders*. Brunner/Mazel, New York.

Karacan I (1970). Clinical value of nocturnal penile erection in the prognosis of impotence. *Med Aspects Hum Sex* **4**:27.

Lue TF (1990). Impotence: A patient's goal-directed approach to treatment. *World J Urol* **8**:67.

Lue TF, Tanagho EA (1987). Physiology of erection and pharmacological management of impotence. *J Urol* **137**:829–36.

Lue TF, Hricak H, Marich KW, et al (1985). Vasculogenic impotence evaluated by high-resolution ultraonography and pulsed Doppler spectrum analysis. *Radiology* **155**:777–81.

Lue TF, Hricak H, Schmidt RA, et al (1986). Functional evaluation of penile veins by cavernosography in papaverine-induced erection. *J Urol* **135**:479–82.

Maatman TJ, Montague DK (1986). Routine endocrine screening in impotence. *Urology* **27**:499–502.

McClure RD, Marshall L (1994). Endocrinologic sexual dysfunction. In: *Sexual Dysfunction: A neuro-medical approach*, eds C Singer, WJ Weiner, pp. 245–73. Futura Publishing Co, Armonk, NY.

Malovrouvas D, Petraki C, Constantinidis E, et al (1994). The contribution of cavernous body biopsy in the diagnosis and treatment of male impotence. *Histol Histopathol* **9**:427–31.

Metz P, Bengtsson J (1981). Penile blood pressure. *Scand J Urol Nephrol* **15**:161–4.

Michal V, Pospichal J (1978). Phalloarteriography in the diagnosis of erectile impotence. *World J Urol* **2**:239–48.

Montague DK, Lakin MM (1992). False diagnoses of venous leak impotence. *J Urol* **148**:148–9.

Padma-Nathan H (1989). Evaluation of the corporal veno-occlusive mechanism: dynamic infusion cavernosometry. *Semin Intervent Rad* **6**:205.

Padma-Nathan H (1994). Neurophysiological studies of sexual dysfunction. In: *Sexual Dysfunction: A neuro-medical approach*, eds C Singer, WJ Weiner, pp. 101–15. Futura Publishing Co, Armonk, NY.

Padma-Nathan H, Klavans S, Goldstein I, et al (1988). The screening efficacy of PBI versus duplex ultrasound versus cavernosal artery systolic occlusion pressure. In: *Proceedings of the Third Biennial World Meeting on Impotence*, Boston, 6 October, p. 32.

Persson C, Diederichs W, Lue TF, et al (1989). Correlation of altered penile ultrastructure with clinical arterial evaluation. *J Urol* **142**:1462–8.

Pescatori ES, Hatzichristou DG, Namburi S, et al (1994). A positive intracavernous injection test implies normal veno-occlusive but not necessarily normal arterial function: a hemodynamic study. *J Urol* **151**:1209–16.

Puech-Leao P, Chao S, Glina S, et al (1990). Gravity cavernosometry – a simple diagnostic test for cavernosal incompetence. *Br J Urol* **65**:391–4.

Puyau FA, Lewis RW (1983). Corpus cavernosography. Pressure flow and radiography. *Invest Radiol* **18**:517–22.

Rajfer J, Rosciszewski A, Mehringer M (1988). Prevalence of corporeal venous leakage in impotent men. *J Urol* **140**:69–71.

Rajfer J, Canan V, Dorey EJ, et al (1990). Correlation between penile angiography and duplex scanning of cavernous arteries in impotent men. *J Urol* **143**:1128–30.

Rhee B, Osborn A, Witt M (1995). The correlation of cavernous systolic occlusion pressure with peak velocity flow using color duplex Doppler ultrasound. *J Urol* **153**:358–60.

Rosen MP, Greenfield AJ, Walker TG, et al (1990). Arteriogenic impotence: findings in 195 impotent men examined with selective internal pudendal angiography. Young Investigator's Award. *Radiology* **174**:1043–8.

Rudnick J, Bodecker R, Weidner W (1991). Significance of the intracavernosal pharmacological injection test, pharmacocavernosography, artificial erection and cavernosometry in the diagnosis of venous leakage. *Urol Int* **46**:338–43.

Shabsigh R, Fishman IJ, Shotland Y, et al (1990). Comparison of penile duplex ultrasonography with nocturnal penile tumescence monitoring for the evaluation of erectile impotence. *J Urol* **143**:924–7.

Shabsigh R, Fishman IJ, Toombs RD, et al (1991). Venous leaks: anatomical and physiological observations. *J Urol* **146**:1260–5.

Shirai M, Ishii N (1981). Hemodynamics of erection in man. *Arch Androl* **6**:27–32.

Steers WD (1993). Impotence evaluation [editorial]. *J Urol* **149**:1284.

Struyven J, Gregoir Ws Giannakopoulos S, et al (1979). Selective pudendal arteriography. *Eur Urol* **5**:233–42.

Virag R (1981). Syndrome d'érection instable par insuffisance veineuse. Diagnostic et correction chirurgicale. A propos de 10 cas avec un recul moyen de 12 mois. *J Mal Vasc* **6**:121–4.

Virag R, Frydman D, Legman M, et al (1984). Intracavernous injection of papaverine as a diagnostic and therapeutic method in erectile failure. *Angiology* **35**:79–87.

Wagner G (1981). Methods of differential diagnosis of psychogenic and organic erectile failure. In: *Impotence*, eds G Wagner, R Green, pp. 89–130. Plenum, New York.

Wagner G, Gerstenberg T, Levin RJ (1989). Electrical activity of corpus cavernosum during flaccidity and erection of the human penis: a new diagnostic method? *J Urol* **142**:723–5.

Walsh PC, Partin AW, Epstein JI (1994). Cancer control and quality of life following anatomical radical retropubic prostatectomy: results at 10 years. *J Urol* **152**:1831–6.

Weideman CL, Northcutt RC (1981). Endocrine aspects of impotence. *Urol Clin North Am* **8**:143–51.

Wespes E, Delcour C, Struyen J, et al (1984). Cavernometry–cavernography: its role in organic impotence. *Eur Urol* **10**:229–32.

Wespes E, Delcour C, Struyven J, et al (1986). Pharmacocavernometry–cavernography in impotence. *Br J Urol* **58**:429–33.

Wespes E, Goes PM, Schiffmann S, et al (1991). Computerized analysis of smooth muscle fibers in potent and impotent patients. *J Urol* **146**:1015–17.

Wespes E, Moreira de Goes P, Schulman C (1992). Vascular impotence: focal or diffuse penile disease. *J Urol* **148**:1435–6.

5

The role of audiovisual sexual stimulation in the evaluation of the impotent man

Francesco Montorsi, Giorgio Guazzoni, Andrea Cestari, Patrizio Rigatti

Penile erection is a complex psychoneurovascular phenomenon initiated by a central or peripheral stimulus leading to cavernous arterial and sinusoidal dilatation followed by the activation of the veno-occlusive mechanism of the corpora cavernosa. Relaxation of the smooth muscle fibers of the arterial and sinusoidal walls is essential to cause penile engorgement with blood and subsequent penile rigidity. Thus, while assessing the erectogenic response of a patient complaining of erectile dysfunction (ED), it is of critical importance to obtain complete cavernous smooth muscle relaxation in order to avoid false-positive diagnoses of vasculogenic impotence. An intracavernous injection of vasoactive agents is the most widely used method to assess the erectogenic response of a patient with ED. However, there is general consensus that although a rigid erection lasting 30 minutes after an intracavernous vasoactive injection indicates the correct function of the cavernous veno-occlusive mechanism, this does not necessarily exclude an abnormality of the cavernous arterial inflow (Pescatori et al 1994). On the contrary, a lack of erectile response after an intracavernous vasoactive injection not only implies significant vascular alterations of the corpora cavernosa; it is now known that a significant sympathetic discharge induced by patient-related anxiety to the injection test may inhibit or reduce corporeal smooth muscle relaxation and subsequently impair the erectile response (Nehra et al 1996). In this case, the potential risk of a false-positive diagnosis of vasculogenic ED due to sympathetic override would certainly be high. In order to reduce the patient's anxiety during the test and subsequently limit sympathetic discharge and facilitate the occurrence of penile erection the use of audiovisual sexual stimulation (AVSS) has been considered.

AVSS and vasoactive drugs

Although the use of AVSS has become popular in association with intracavernous vasoactive injections, the first reports regarding the use of AVSS to evaluate impotent patient came from investigators who used this procedure by itself as a first screening for patients with ED. Nocturnal penile tumescence (NPT) testing and AVSS were initially used to evaluate impotent diabetics and non-diabetics (Zuckerman et al 1985; Wincze et al 1988). Diabetic and healthy men were likewise studied with penile diameter and penile pulse monitoring while viewing erotic movies (Bancroft and Bell 1985; Bancroft et al 1985). They suggested that the degree of erection in response to erotic films may help distinguish between organic and psychogenic impotence. In their normal control group, an increase in penile diameter was seen in all 22 subjects. However, no mention of rigidity was made. Earls et al (1988) studied 19 normal subjects with AVSS. All men developed tumescence; however, seven indicated that the rigidity was not maximal. Slob et al (1990) reported on the use of AVSS in conjunction with NPT and an erection meter: they concluded that this procedure could be useful as an initial screening test. Overall data reported in literature regarding the actual clinical value of AVSS used by itself in the evaluation of patients with ED are controversial. Opsomer et al (1990) obtained an 80% erection rate among "normal" subjects, and a 20% full erectile response from "impotent" subjects. This differed widely from the experience of Cahill et al (1988), who reported the lack of any meaningful erection in 25 patients using AVSS. Fouda et al (1989) found a 6.6% positive response rate to AVSS without intracavernous injection. Mellinger and Vaughan (1990) suggested that changes in arterial diameter, blood flow velocity and acceleration values differed according to whether the erection was drug induced or AVSS induced.

AVSS and tactile sexual stimulation

Incrocci and Slob (1994) and Incrocci et al (1996) first compared the erectogenic effects of AVSS alone or combined with tactile stimulation and intracavernous vasoactive injections. In a group of 406 consecutive impotent patients they demonstrated that a partial or full erection was obtained in 34% of cases with visual erotic stimulation, 52% with associated visual erotic and vibrotactile stimulation and 82% with visual erotic stimulation plus intracavernous vasoactive injection. They suggested that a positive response to visual erotic stimulation or to combined visual erotic and vibrotactile stimulation should be positively reinforced by the doctor. According to these investigators, this finding shows that nothing is seriously wrong and that the genital apparatus is basically capable of responding sexually. They also suggested that, when no response occurs, one should be quick to reassure the patient and explain that such a response has no diagnostic significance (Slob et al 1990). Failure to respond may result from lack of interest, dislike of the film, anxiety or fear of loosing control (Buvat et al 1990; Incrocci and Slob 1994).

As mentioned earlier, AVSS has gained ground in the diagnostic algorithm of a patient with ED when used in association with intracavernous vasoactive injections. Katlowitz et al (1993a) demonstrated the possibility of improving the erectile response induced by an intracavernous injection with the addition of AVSS in 56.5% of 25 consecutive impotent patients. In 13% of these cases, the addition of AVSS induced an adequate erection when intracavernous injection alone had failed. The same group of investigators (Katlowitz et al 1993b) studied a series of 33 impotent patients with suspected vasculogenic impotence using pulsed Doppler ultrasound performed after the injection of multiple doses of Trimix (a mixture of papaverine, phentolamine and prostaglandin E_1). AVSS was applied after maximal response to Trimix. Seventeen patients (51%) responded to multidose with grade IV and V erection. When AVSS was initiated, five more patients responded and seven were upgraded to grade V, with an overall response of 40%. The authors suggested that AVSS can augment the in-office response to pharmacologic testing over that obtained by "maximal" pharmacologic dosing, thereby increasing the sensitivity and specificity of the test.

Of clear practical importance was the demonstration that a combination of tactile stimulation and AVSS caused greater erectogenic effects than AVSS alone (Donatucci and Lue 1992; Rowland et al 1994). It is known that tactile stimulation of the genitalia elicits a reflexogenic erection (De Groat and Steers 1988): impulses reach the spinal erection center (S2–4 and T10–L2), with some of the signals following the ascending tract to result in sensory perception and others activating the autonomic nuclei that release neurotransmitters to initiate the erectile process (Goldstein 1988). Reflexive stimuli are much stronger than psychogenic elicitations: masturbation often induces erection and ejaculation, but visual or psychic stimuli usually do not result in ejaculation (Donatucci and Lue 1992; Rowland et al 1994).

Authors' experience

On the basis of our clinical experience with impotent patients, we had the feeling that an intracavernous injection followed by a combination of tactile stimulation and AVSS produced maximal erectile response; this combination was therefore always used both during a simple injection test and during penile color Doppler sonography. At our center, we initially investigated the diagnostic value of erotically enhanced penile color Doppler sonography as a minimally invasive tool to evaluate penile hemodynamics (Montorsi et al 1995). Color Doppler sonography was used to study the cavernosal arteries of 135 consecutive impotent patients following an intracavernous injection of a vasoactive mixture (injection phase) with subsequent tactile stimulation and AVSS (stimulation phase). We found that in 36% of patients the erectile response was upgraded after the adjunct of tactile stimulation and AVSS. Color Doppler assessment performed after the stimulation phase identified 16% of patients as arteriogenic despite normal erections, with 7% falsely diagnosed as venogenic after the injection phase. These data led us to conclude that when color Doppler sonography and the injection-stimulation test were performed together as a single diagnostic procedure, the overall diagnostic accuracy was significantly enhanced.

In the meantime, several investigators advocated the use of multiple consecutive vasoactive injections, that is, re-dosing, in order to enhance corporeal smooth muscle relaxation during vascular testing and reduce the risk of false-positive diagnoses of vasculogenic ED (Barrett et al 1997; Ho et al 1997). We thus became interested in investigating the effect of the injection plus tactile and AVSS versus re-dosing during penile color Doppler sonography. In order to do so we designed a study in which we assessed 50 consecutive impotent patients using penile color Doppler sonography before and after an intracorporeal injection (phase 1), subsequent tactile stimulation and AVSS (phase 2), a second injection (phase 3) and repeat tactile stimulation (TS) and AVSS (phase 4). In our study, following the first injection penile erection was upgraded in 41 patients (82%) through the use of TS and AVSS. Further upgrading as a result of the second injection with stimulation was noted in 11 patients (22%). Among the patients who completed the four phases of the test the maximal peak systolic velocity was noted after the first and second injection in 20 (59%) and 14 (41%) cases, respectively. Compared with post-injection values the resistive index was always increased by TS and AVSS. The maximal resistive index occurred after initial and repeat TS plus AVSS in 15 (48%) and 16 (52%) patients, respectively. Following the first injection plus TS and AVSS, impotence was diagnosed as non-vasculogenic in 14 patients (28%), arteriogenic in nine (18%), venogenic in 17 (34%) or mixed arterio-venogenic in 10 (20%). Following the second injection plus stimulation the same results were noted in 18 (36%), 9 (18%), 13 (26%) and 10 (20%) patients, respectively. Thus, there were four false-positive cases (8%) of venogenic impotence. These results confirmed that, in order to study cavernous artery inflow and veno-occlusive function, color Doppler sonography should be performed following an injection plus TS and AVSS. We suggested that, when the erectile response does not match the best-quality erection obtained during sexual activity at home, a second injection should be given with stimulation (Montorsi et al 1996).

To explain further the erectogenic effects of the combination injection plus AVSS versus reducing (that is, in order to understand which of the two procedures exerted the greatest impact on cavernous smooth muscle relaxation), we also studied 20 consecutive patients with erectile dysfunction using real-time evaluation of penile tumescence and rigidity in different settings. RigiScan monitoring was performed in two sessions that took place within a time interval of one week in randomized order. Patients were positioned on an examination couch in a quiet and semi-obscured room; the RigiScan device was applied and activated, and the patient was left alone for 10 minutes (adaptation period). An intracavernous injection of alprostadil 10 µg was then given and the patient was left alone for 10 minutes subject to real-time recording of penile activity. After 10 minutes the patient was told to stimulate his penis manually while watching an erotic video (without ejaculating). The test was stopped after 10 minutes for a total 30-minute test duration. The second session consisted of the initial 10 minutes of adaptation under RigiScan real-time recording, followed by an intracavernous injection of alprostadil 10 µg, which was subsequently repeated after 10 minutes. This was then followed by a 10-minute period of observation for a total length of the session of 30 minutes. During this session, genital stimulation was never attempted. All patients were subjected to both in a randomized order. Morphometric analysis of the RigiScan traces was performed by an examiner who was unaware of the type of session from which the graphs were obtained. A statistical analysis of results was conducted using the Student's *t*-test for paired data or the McNemar test, as appropriate. Before making a comparison between the sessions, the possibility of a period effect was tested by means of a two-sample *t*-test, aimed at comparing the differences between the periods in the two groups of patients. The possibility of a treatment–period interaction was tested by a two-sample *t*-test comparing the patient's average response with the two treatments in the two groups. Five patients (20%) achieved full rigid erection after the first injection of alprostadil.

Owing to the fact that the complete activation of the cavernous smooth muscle mechanism had already been achieved, they did not undergo either genital stimulation or re-dosing, and were thus excluded from the study. Fifteen patients (80%) did not achieve a rigid erection after the first injection of alprostadil; these patients completed both sessions and underwent a morphometric analysis of the RigiScan traces, thus being considered for the final evaluation. Both genital stimulation and re-dosing caused a significant increase in the erectile response when compared with the effect of the first injection of alprostadil (injection plus stimulation: $p < 0.01$; re-dosing $p < 0.05$). Before comparing the two treatments for each parameter we verified that neither the period effect nor the treatment–period interaction was statistically significant. The values of tip tumescence, base rigidity and tip rigidity seen after the first injection of alprostadil did not differ significantly in the two sessions (tumescence tip: $p = 0.05$; rigidity base: $p = 0.16$; rigidity tip: $p = 0.55$), and only base tumescence was slightly higher in the re-dosing session ($p = 0.04$). However, genital stimulation caused an increase in erectile response which was significantly greater than that observed after re-dosing.

At the end of each session patients were asked to compare the quality of the erection obtained during the test with the erection usually achieved during sexual activity at home. After the injection plus stimulation session, 13 patients (87%) achieved an erection that was either comparable with or greater than their usual maximum erection; the same occurred in seven patients (47%) after the re-dosing session. This difference was statistically significant ($p < 0.01$). The final conclusion obtained by this study was that a combination of an intracavernous vasoactive injection plus TS and AVSS should be always used during color Doppler sonography in order to maximize corporeal smooth muscle relaxation and accurately to investigate both the cavernous arterial inflow and the veno-occlusive mechanism. We believe that this study reconfirmed the advisability of re-dosing the patient in the event of an erection during the injection-stimulation test not matching the best-quality erection usually obtained during sexual activity at home. In our experience, during the last consecutive 300 color Doppler sonographies performed using this technique, re-dosing was only necessary in 29 cases (9%) in which complete smooth muscle relaxation was not achieved after the injection plus stimulation phase. We are aware that watching an erotic video may not be well accepted by all patients, and we believe that is essential to take into consideration the patient's personal preference (such as heterosexual vs homosexual). These factors should always be discussed during the preliminary patient interview. However, one of the patients in our color Doppler sonography series refused to undergo the genital stimulation phase of the test and only 10

(3%) considered the video as not stimulating or depressing their erectile response. Finally another potential advantage of reducing the number of consecutive vasoactive injections was that, by limiting the total
dose of drug injected intracavernously, the rate of prolonged erections
requiring treatment to detumescence could potentially be reduced
(Montorsi et al 1998).

It is known that the most precise method to investigate the cavernous
veno-occlusive mechanism is pharmaco-cavernosometry; this is made
possible by the presence of a linear relationship between the intracavernous pressure and flow to maintain the erection, which is indicative
of complete cavernous smooth muscle relaxation (Nehra et al 1996).
Recently Pescatori et al (1997) were the first to suggest the use of AVSS
as a method to increase the erectogenic response to the intracavernous
vasoactive injection during pharmaco-cavernosometry. From their preliminary data they showed that AVSS can be administered to a patient
undergoing pharmaco-cavernosometry by means of virtual glasses
with headphones connected to a standard videotape recorder playing
an erotic movie. With this method the need for re-dosing was significantly reduced, thus confirming our color Doppler sonography data.

Conclusions

We conclude that at present AVSS plays a significant role in the evaluation of a patient with ED. It should be emphasized that AVSS should
always be associated with TS of the genitalia in order to maximize the
relaxation of corporeal smooth muscle and subsequently to obtain the
greatest erectile response. We believe that TS plus AVSS should
always be used in conjunction with vasoactive agents given intracavernously. This should be done both in the case of a simple office injection test and during penile color Doppler sonography. Although the
use of AVSS during pharmaco-cavernosometry might also be of value,
this nevertheless needs to be confirmed by future studies.

References

Bancroft J, Bell C (1985). Simultaneous recording of penile diameter and
    penile arterial pulse during laboratory-based erotic stimulation of normal
    subjects. *J Psychosom Res* **29**:303–6.

Bancroft J, Bell C, Ewing DJ et al (1985). Assessment of erectile function in diabetic and non-diabetic impotence by simultaneous recording of penile diameter and penile arterial pulse. *J Psychosom Res* **29**:315–24.

Barrett DM, Nehra A, King BF (1997). Hemodynamic interpretation following redosing during Doppler ultrasonography: is there a change in diagnosis? *J Urol* **157**:179(abstract 695).

Buvat J et al (1990). Recent developments in the clinical assessment and diagnosis of erectile dysfunction. *Annu Rev Sex Res* **1**:265–308.

Cahill BE, Ross EV, Pielet RW et al (1988). Measurement of impotence by laser Doppler flowmetry and conventional methodology. *J Urol* **140**:749–50.

De Groat WC, Steers WD (1988). Neuroanatomy and neurophysiology of penile erection. In: *Contemporary Management of Impotence and Infertility*, eds EA Tanagho, TF Lue, RD McClure, pp. 3–27. Williams & Wilkins, Baltimore.

Donatucci CF, Lue TF (1992). The combined intracavernous injection and stimulation test: diagnostic accuracy. *J Urol* **148**:61–2.

Earls CM, Morales A, Marshall WL (1988). Penile sufficiency: an operational definition. *J Urol* **139**:536–9.

Fouda A, Hassouna M, Beddoe E et al (1989). Priapism: an avoidable complication of pharmacologically induced erection. *J Urol* **142**:995–7.

Goldstein I (1988). Evaluation of penile nerves. In: *Contemporary Management of Impotence and Infertility*, eds EA Tanagho, TF Lue, RD McClure, pp. 70–83. Williams & Wilkins, Baltimore.

Ho LV, Lewis RW, Sathyanarayana K (1997). Two-injection color duplex Doppler studies. *J Urol* **157**:178(abstract 690).

Incrocci L, Slob AK (1994). Visual sexual stimulation and penile vibration in screening men with erectile dysfunction. *Int J Impot Res* **6**:227–9.

Incrocci L, Hop WCJ, Slob AK (1996). Visual erotic and vibrotactile stimulation and intracavernous injection in screening men with erectile dysfunction: a 3-year experience with 406 cases. *Int J Impot Res* **8**:227–32.

Katlowitz NM, Albano GJ, Morales P, et al (1993a). Potentiation of drug-induced erection with audiovisual sexual stimulation. *Urology* **41**:431–4.

Katlowitz NM, Albano GJ, Patrias G, et al (1993b). Effect of multidose intracorpreal injection and audiovisual sexual stimulation in vasculogenic impotence. *Urology* **42**:695–7.

Mellinger BC, Vaughan ED (1990). Penile blood flow changes in the flaccid and erect state in potent young men measured by duplex scanning. *J Urol* **144**:894–7.

Montorsi F, Guazzoni G, Bocciardi A, et al (1995). Improved minimally-invasive assessment of penile hemodynamics: the combination of color Doppler sonography and injection-stimulation test. *Int J Impot Res* **7**:33–40.

Montorsi F, Guazzoni G, Barbieri L, et al (1996). The effect of intracorporeal injection plus genital and audio-visual sexual stimulation versus second injection on penile color Doppler sonography parameters. *J Urol* **155**:536–40.

Montorsi F, Guazzoni G, Barbieri L et al (1998). Genital plus audio-visual sexual stimulation following intracavernous vasoactive injection is significantly more erectogenic than redosing: results of a prospective study. *J Urol* **159**:113–15.

Nehra A, Goldstein I, Pabby A, et al (1996). Mechanisms of venous leakage: a prospective clinicopathological correlation of corporeal function and structure. *J Urol* **156**:1320–9.

Opsomer RJ, Wese FX, Van Cangh PJ (1990). Visual sexual stimulation plethysmography: complementary test to nocturnal penile plethysmography. *Urology* **35**:504–8.

Pescatori ES, Hatzichristou DG, Namburi S, et al (1994). A positive intra-caverous injection implies normal veno-occlusive but not necessarily normal arterial function: a hemodynamic study. *J Urol* **151**:1209–11.

Pescatori ES, Silingardi V, Galeazzi GM, et al (1997). AVSS through virtual glasses: a pilot study. *2nd Meeting of European Society for Impotence Research, Madrid October 1–4, 1997.* Abstract Book, p. 20.

Rowland DL, Den Ouden AH, Slob Ak (1994). The use of vibrotactile stimulation for determining sexual potency in the laboratory in men with erectile problems: methodological considerations. *Int J Impot Res* **6**:153–61.

Slob AK, Blom JMH, Bosch JW (1990). Erection problems in medical practice: differential diagnosis with relatively simple method. *J Urol* **143**:46–9.

Wincze JP, Bansal S, Malhotra C, et al (1988). A comparison of nocturnal penile tumescence penile response to erotic stimulation during waking states in comprehensively diagnosed groups of males experiencing erectile difficulties. *Arch Sex Behav* **17**:333–48.

Zuckerman M, Neeb M, Ficher M et al (1985). Nocturnal penile tumescence and penile responses in the waking state in diabetic and nondiabetic sexual dysfunctionals. *Arch Sex Behav* **14**:109–29.

6

Current concepts in the treatment of erectile dysfunction

The when and how of vascular testing of the patient with erectile dysfunction

Eric J H Meuleman

Introduction

Erectile dysfunction (ED) is broadly classified into two categories: organic and psychologic. In reality, most of the patients demonstrate a combination of both components (Meuleman and Diemont 1995). Organic ED may be classified into neurogenic ED, arteriogenic ED and veno-occlusive dysfunction. The latter two are the causes of the clinical entity known as vascular ED. Because combinations of etiologies are common, the term vascular ED does not rule out the presence of contributing psychologic or neurologic factors, but merely means that vascular factors are the predominant cause of ED. The two principal causes of arteriogenic ED, that is, obstruction within the penile inflow tract, are atherosclerotic vascular disease (Queral et al 1979; Padma-Nathan et al 1986), and traumatic arterial occlusion, following blunt perineal trauma (St Louis et al 1983; Goldstein et al 1984). The most widespread cause for atherosclerotic vascular disease in patients with ED is exposure to cigarette smoking. The causal concept for neurologic ED is a disturbance in the mechanisms responsible for the integration of mental and physical impulses in the central nervous system, resulting in an uncoordinated motor outflow along autonomic and somatic neural pathways to the cavernous body (Krane and Siroky 1981; de Groat and Steers 1988): erotic fantasy and sexual stimuli of various origins (tactile, audiovisual, gustatory and olfactory) arouse psychologic mechanisms, which in their turn generate neurologic impulses in the autonomic motor tracts (pelvic nerves) necessary for cavernous smooth muscle relaxation. In this concept direct mechanical stimulation of penile sensory nerves and the reflex activation of pelvic floor muscles are of supportive value (Herbert 1973; Lavoisier et al 1986, 1988; Wespes et al 1990). The most common causes of neurogenic ED are spinal cord tiple sclerosis and pelvic surgery. Veno-occlusion is a ᠎ocess depending on volume and pressure changes mediat᠎tions in the tone of the cavernous smooth muscle cells. of this hydraulic process may have several causes, such as ᠎᠎ᴊ neurogenic changes (Lincoln et al 1987); (2) altered intercellular communication (Christ et al 1997); (3a) heightened contractility of corporeal smooth muscle secondary to increased reactivity to α_1-adrenoceptor activation with age and disease (Christ et al 1991); (3b) impaired relaxation of corporeal smooth muscle (Saenz de Tejada et al 1989); and (4) parenchymal changes at the level of the extracellular matrix or the corporeal smooth muscle cells (Van der Ven et al 1995).

Before embarking on any diagnostic test, it should be noted that current treatments are beneficial for almost all types of ED. This fact may make one wonder if it is necessary to perform any vascular test at all. The principles of a goal-directed approach are therefore briefly described, followed by a discussion of the currently available vascular tests in detail. In Figure 1 the algorithm of a goal-directed approach towards the diagnosis and treatment of ED is depicted.

Goal-directed approach

In a goal-directed approach the clinical diagnostic algorithm is primarily directed towards treatment. On the basis of the history, a physical examination and an explanation of diagnostic and treatment options, the patient and his partner decide on further diagnostic procedures or on primary treatment. Preferably, this is effected in dialogue with the partner. Motivation and expectations with respect to diagnosis and treatment are addressed extensively. In cases where the history reveals explicit clues for psychogenicity, the patient may be referred to a sexologist or a professional psychotherapist. Auto intra cavernous injection (ICI) therapy, vacuum therapy or an oral α_2-sympathicolytic drug may be proposed as first-line treatment options. For ICI therapy, an experimental period may be arranged, before the patient decides to embark on this method on a more permanent basis. An ICI test may be utilized in preparation for ICI treatment. At this stage, in our clinic, the treatment is to a large extent supervised by specialized nurses. If primary treatment does not produce the desired result one can switch to another treatment or decide on further diagnostic evaluation. In some cases, the patient will decide that treatment does not fit with his expectations and abandon further treatment.

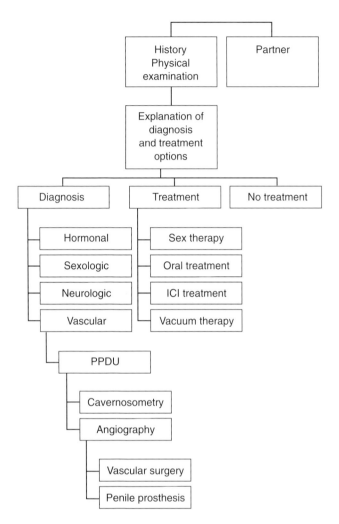

Figure 1
Algorithm for goal-directed approach diagnosis and treatment of erectile dysfunction. PDDU, penile pharmaco-duplex ultrasonography.

Vascular tests

Several tests are available for the evaluation of the penile inflow tract and the veno-occlusive mechanism, such as the ICI test and the enhanced ICI test, such as penile pharmaco-duplex ultrasonography (PPDU), cavernosometry and selective penile angiography. Each test has its pros and cons, related to validity, costs, invasiveness and availability. All tests have in common the feature that the cavernous body is pharmacologically stimulated by an intracavernous injection of a vasoactive agent. The choice of the vascular test depends on the purpose of testing: assessing either (1) erectile capacity or (2) arterial response, or subsequently (3) locating a specific vascular lesion for surgical management or (4) defining the vascular status in groups of patients with a specific disease. Because the purpose of testing differs in various circumstances there is no commonly agreed diagnostic work-up procedure that applies for all purposes.

ICI test

A major breakthrough in the diagnosis of male sexual dysfunction was accomplished with the discovery of pharmacologically inducible erection by ICI of vasoactive agents (Virag 1982). Theoretically, vasoactive substances substitute for the neurotransmitter to activate arterial and sinusoidal mechanisms. A practical purpose for an ICI test is the assessment of erectile capacity. The question in that case is: are arterial response and veno-occlusion, together resulting in erectile response, sufficient for ICI therapy, to date the most effective and frequently used non-surgical treatment modality? As an adequate test for this purpose we recommend an ICI test using either prostaglandin E_1 (PGE_1) or the combination of papaverine/phentolamine in a single dose or a dose titration in the office or at home. Other ICI drugs, such as calcitonin gene-related peptide (Truss et al 1994), nitric oxide donors (Porst 1993) and vasoactive intestinal peptide (VIP), or combinations of drugs and alternative routes for administration, such as the intraurethral application of high dosages of PGE_1, are currently under investigation (Padma-Nathan et al 1997).

Although, theoretically, ICI testing seems to be straightforward, in practice its interpretation is complicated. Formerly, a positive erectile response, defined as a rigid erection, has been presumed to signify a normal vascular status; if only a partial, short-lived or absent erectile response resulted, vascular ED was presumed (Lue and Tanagho 1987). To date, we know that a normal erectile response defined as a rigid erection implies normal veno-occlusive function, but not necessarily normal arterial function. There are several reasons for the fact that normal arterial function can*not* be discriminated by a "simple" ICI test. First, a positive erectile response merely reflects an intracavernous pressure equal to or greater than 50–80 mmHg, depending on penile geometry, whereas the maximum erectile response is as high as the systemic blood pressure. Secondly, a negative erectile response, defined as tumescence without enough rigidity or no response at all, may be due to excessive adrenergic constrictor tone as a result of anxiety. Finally, the result of the ICI test performed at home may be better than if it is done in the office (Buvat et al 1986).

A single ICI test, using 50 mg papaverine, may lead to a false-negative erectile response (Meuleman et al 1990) in 25% of non-selected impotent men, whereas prolonged erection may occur in 5.3% (Porst 1990). In a multi-center study comparing papaverine, papaverine–phentolamine and PGE_1, PGE_1 emerged as the most accurate diagnostic drug, with an overall erection rate of 74% and a prolonged erection rate of only 0.1%. Recently, in a review of the literature, Jünemann found the following rates of prolonged erections during diagnostic work-up: papaverine 9.5%, papaverine–phentolamine 5.3% and PGE_1 2.4%. Non-responders bear a high probability of a vascular etiology with a predominance of veno-occlusive insufficiency (Jünemann and Alken 1989).

If the purpose of an ICI test is to evaluate whether the patient is a candidate for ICI treatment, we advise a low-dose test, combined with masturbation, visual erotic stimulation and eventually the application of a penoscrotal tourniquet. Additionally, a post-investigation questionnaire may be used to rate erection following the test, when the patient has left the office (Vruggink et al 1995). A negative test is followed by repeated tests up to a maximum dose of 30 mg/1 mg papaverine–phentolamine or 20 μg PGE_1 in an ICI trial at home. Under these circumstances, the ICI will provide an ultimate assessment of the patients' maximal responsiveness to treatment by auto-ICI, and may make more invasive diagnostic tests redundant. The most feared complication of ICI tests is prolonged erection. The group most prone to prolonged erection is younger patients with non-vascular ED and a better baseline erectile function. Therefore the dose used for initial testing should be adapted to the historical characteristics of the patients and lowered with suspected neurogenic or psychological ED.

Enhanced vascular tests

If the purpose of testing is assessing arterial response and locating a vascular lesion for specific surgical treatment, such as penile revascularization or venorestrictive surgery, or defining the vascular status in groups of patients with a specific disease, the most commonly used first-line test is PPDU, eventually followed by cavernosometry and selective pudendal angiography. To determine candidacy for vascular surgery, the ideal patient would exhibit a single mechanism, namely failure of cavernosal perfusion, and a segmental correctable arterial lesion amenable to bypass, endarterectomy, or stenting or localized veno-occlusive dysfunction (De Palma 1997).

PPDU

The development and application of sonographic equipment have experienced tremendous growth since Gaskell introduced a Doppler device for evaluating penile blood pressure in 1971. Early Doppler systems were non-directional, i.e. no distinction could be made between blood moving away from the probe and blood moving toward the probe. Nor could a distinction be made between the cavernous and dorsal arteries. The systems could only detect the presence of flow, and were used in measurements of penile arterial pressure (Abelson 1975; Kempczinski 1979). In 1980, the pulsed-Doppler device was introduced for evaluating erectile dysfunction (Velcek et al 1980). This device can detect the direction of blood flow and uses various depths of sampling. Coupling of the device to a spectral analyzer made it possible to obtain a printed Doppler velocity waveform of the vessel under study. In the latest development, PPDU, blood flow velocity waveform analysis and ultrasonographic imaging are combined to assess anatomical and functional parameters of pharmacologically stimulated penile circulation simultaneously (Meuleman et al 1992a).

Technique

A duplex scanner with color flow imaging capabilities is used. B-mode color images and Doppler spectra are obtained with a 7.5 MHz linear-array transducer. B-mode ultrasonography provides visualization of cavernous arteries and bodies. Electronic cursors are used to measure diameters of cavernous arteries in longitudinal projection in the proximal penile shaft up to an axial resolution of 0.1 mm. By using color images as a guide to the localization and direction of blood flow, the Doppler sample volume cursor is placed in the cavernous artery as proximal as possible in the infrapubic region, and the Doppler angle correction cursor is adjusted to match the correct axis of flow. The resulting angle-corrected Doppler spectrum is displayed on the monitor, and acceleration time, peak flow velocity and diastolic flow

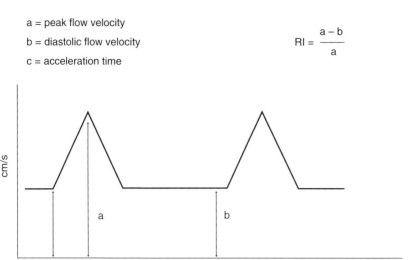

a = peak flow velocity

b = diastolic flow velocity

c = acceleration time

$$RI = \frac{a - b}{a}$$

Figure 2
Doppler spectrum analysis.

velocity are measured directly from the recorded velocity tracing. That information is used to calculate resistance index (RI):

$$RI = \frac{\text{peak flow velocity} - \text{diastolic flow velocity}}{\text{peak flow velocity}}$$

(Figure 2). Knowledge of these parameters provides an estimate of penile blood flow and is a useful indicator of arterial inflow capacity and venous outflow. Furthermore, pathological conditions, such as vascular calcifications or fibrosis associated with Peyronie's disease, can be located. Additionally, PPDU may be helpful in staging penile carcinoma.

In PPDU, the sampling location and interval after pharmacological stimulation are critical (Meuleman et al 1992b; Kim et al 1994). In healthy controls there is a mean reduction of flow velocity between the crural and distal subcoronal cavernous artery of about 20%, whereas in patients with peripheral arterial occlusive disease velocity may be reduced by 50% (Montorsi et al 1993). With respect to location the consensus in the literature is that velocity tracings should be obtained in the most proximal part of the cavernous arteries, i.e. in the crural part. With respect to timing, the consensus is that arterial response is to be determined in the phase of erection with highest flow rates, i.e. in the first minutes following intracavernous pharmacological stimulation (Bongaerts et al 1992). Following the original study by Lue et al (1985) of less than a peak flow velocity < 25 cm/s and a dilatation of the cavernous artery of less than

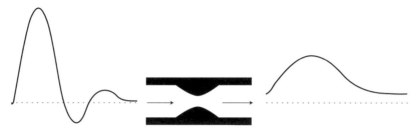

Figure 3
The hemodynamic effect of an arterial stenosis. Note the dampened velocity waveform with low peak flow velocity and long acceleration time.

75% have been considered to indicate arterial disease. To date, cavernous arterial dilatation is apparently an unreliable parameter, and measurement of the single Doppler parameter peak flow velocity is an inadequate discriminant of arterial disease. Current parameters are: peak flow velocity and acceleration time; an acceleration time of > 72 ms is considered to be an indicator of arterial disease. Mellinger has added the category of penile blood flow acceleration (peak flow velocity/acceleration time) to the list of duplex data (Mellinger et al 1990).

In the literature, controversies exist on reference values. The differences may be attributed to the different standards that were used for the selection of patients and healthy controls. Moreover, the large ranges of values may indicate that there is a large surplus capacity in arterial supply. This means that the arterial supply must be severely compromised before it becomes a predominant cause of ED. It should be noted that arterial response has been shown *not* to depend on the type of any currently used vasoactive agent or on external factors such as anxiety and stress, as long as supraphysiological dosages are used. We recently demonstrated that peak flow velocity and acceleration time do not change in a dose range of 1–10 μg PGE_1, whereas erectile response improves in the higher dose ranges (Benet et al 1997). These data justify the use of a standard of 10 μg PGE_1 in the diagnostic evaluation of patients with ED. As a rule of thumb, a dampened velocity waveform, with long systolic acceleration time (> 72 ms) and a low peak flow velocity (< 25–30 cm/s), indicate arterial disease (Figure 3).

Veno-occlusion and erectile response are two closely related phenomena. In fact, veno-occlusive function is presumed sufficient when an adequate erectile response occurs. Because cavernous venous outflow is not quantifiable by PPDU, veno-occlusive function is indirectly estimated by assessing cavernous venous resistance in the phase of maximal erectile response. Parameters are diastolic flow velocity (Kropman et al 1992), and its derivative resistance index (RI). In our opinion, RI is the superior parameter, because the most important variable associated with the process of sampling, the probe–vessel angle, is filtered out in the formula RI = (peak flow velocity – diastolic flow velocity)/(peak flow velocity). Following pharmacological stimulation the value of RI adjusts to a level depending on intracavernous pressure. As soon as intracavernous pressure equals or exceeds systemic diastolic blood pressure, diastolic blood flow velocity will equal zero and the value for RI equals 1.00. As long as intracavernous pressure remains below systemic diastolic pressure, diastolic flow will persist and the value for RI will remain below 1.00. It has been estimated that an intracavernous pressure of 50–80 mmHg is necessary for full erection, depending on the volume of the cavernous body (Saenz de Tejada et al 1991). As a consequence, a post-injection value of 1.00 indicates full erection, whereas a post-injection value < 1.00 indicates incomplete erection, depending on penile geometry. In conclusion, veno-occlusive dysfunction is characterized by RI < 1.00 in the phase of maximal erectile response (Figure 4).

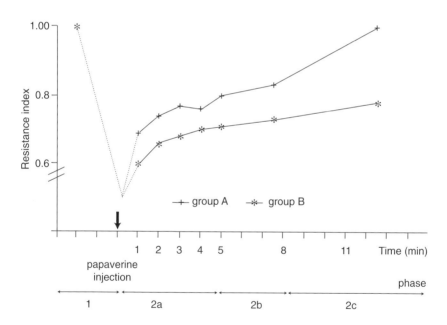

Figure 4
Resistance index before and after (arrow) ICI of 12.5 mg papaverine in men without (group A) and with (group B) veno-occlusive dysfunction. Note the sharp decrease of RI immediately following the ICI and the return of RI towards 1.00 in the group without veno-occlusive dysfunction.

One aspect in the evaluation of the veno-occlusive mechanism is particularly troublesome: in contrast to arterial response, erectile response is influenced by the type and dosage of the vasoactive agent and by the psychological impact of the test setting on the patient. This may lead to a false diagnosis of veno-occlusive dysfunction. This may be decreased by starting with a high dose of vasoactive agent(s) or by repeated dosing. Both strategies, however, carry the risk of prolonged erection. Furthermore, the incorporation of visual sexual stimulation, genital self-stimulation or vibrotactile stimulation may decrease psychological inhibition and enhance erectile response (Rowland and Slob 1992; Vruggink et al 1995). Our experience is that these additions interfere with PPDU. We found the patient's self-report on erectile response and/or his experience of satisfactory sexual intercourse following the examination to be the most valid test for veno-occlusive sufficiency.

Cavernosometry

Cavernosometry is the primary modality available for quantifying and mapping veno-occlusive dysfunction in men with erectile failure, although its ability to differentiate between the types of veno-occlusive dysfunction is limited. Because it is an invasive test, at our institution it is reserved for selected patients suspected of having veno-occlusive dysfunction, in whom surgical repair directed at limiting venous outflow is under consideration. Usually, these are younger patients with a low resistance to venous outflow due to anatomical abnormalities such as ectopic veins or abnormal communications between the corpora and the spongiosum, mostly following a blunt perineal trauma.

In cavernosometry, venous outflow resistance is assessed by determining the intracavernous flow rate required to sustain erection (intracavernous pressure > 80 mmHg) in a state of controlled complete cavernous smooth muscle relaxation (Krane et al 1989). Since its introduction by Newman in 1964, several modifications of technique have evolved. In the earliest publications, a rollerpump was used to regulate the infusion flow rates. In 1988, Puech Leao introduced an alternative technique that required less complicated technology and is less expensive: gravity cavernosometry. Instead of using a rollerpump, a simple infusion set is used to generate a steady infusion pressure (Puech Leao et al 1990; Meuleman et al 1991) (Figure 5). Although the concepts of veno-occlusive function and cavernosometry seem to be straightforward, methodology and interpretation of results have long been subject to debate. In particular, the need for controlled complete smooth muscle relaxation has frustrated physicians performing cavernosometry. Anxiety and embarrassment in a non-sexual situation with little privacy appeared to be

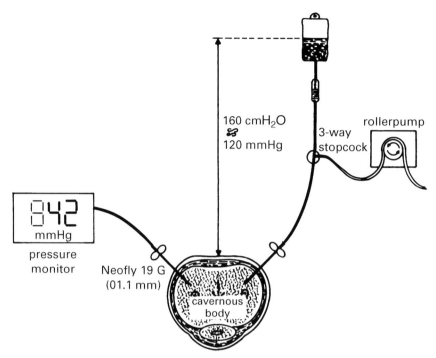

Figure 5

The concept of pump and gravity cavernosometry. Cavernous inflow of heparized saline is generated by a rollerpump or an infusion set at a level of 160 cmH$_2$O above the cavernous body pressure. Pressure is monitored synchronously.

almost incompatible with a state of drug-induced complete cavernous relaxation. Inevitably, cavernosometry has overestimated the degree of structural veno-occlusive dysfunction (Montague and Lakin 1992; Vickers et al 1992). This and the inability to identify individual subtypes of veno-occlusive dysfunction account for the disappointingly low long-term success rate of venous restrictive surgery (30–50%) (Petrou and Lewis 1992). Recently, Hatzichristou et al have developed a promising new methodology that enables cavernosometry under conditions of known corporeal smooth muscle relaxation, making it more reliable for clinical practice (Hatzichristou et al 1995). When, following a first ICI challenge, incomplete corporeal smooth muscle relaxation ensues, a second and eventually a third dose can be administered. In this way about 25% of patients can be rescued from a false-positive diagnosis of veno-occlusive dysfunction (Udelson et al 1994).

Treatment of prolonged erection

The most common complication during the diagnostic work-up and especially during pharmacocavernosometry with redosing is a prolonged erection. Not all pharmacologically induced prolonged erections necessitate a specific treatment, since penis detumescence generally occurs within a few hours. Lue demonstrated that, in pharmacologically induced prolonged erection, blood gas values manifest inadequate blood supply to the erectile tissue after 6 hours (Lue et al 1986).

To prevent this, the patients are not allowed to leave the office before the erection has subsided. In case erection recurs after drainage of the cavernous body, aspiration of cavernous contents is repeated to decrease cavernous body pressure and an adrenergic agonist is injected intracavernously to induce cavernous smooth muscle contraction, effective venous drainage and restriction of arterial inflow. We use 10 μg adrenaline. The correct dose is prepared by adding 1 mg adrenaline to 100 ml physiological saline, to make a solution of 10 μg adrenaline/1 ml. A standard 2-ml syringe is utilized to deliver 1 ml (10 μg) intracavernously. After a compressive bandage has been applied, the penis is fixed to the inner dorsal site of the thigh. After 30 minutes the bandage is removed. In case an erection has recurred the procedure is repeated. The blood pressure and pulse should be monitored during and following adrenergic agonist administration.

Pharmaco-penile angiography

Selective pudendal angiography has long been considered to be the gold standard for the evaluation of penile arterial integrity. Genestie and Romieux (1978) first performed selective penile angiography on impotent patients. To date, with the advent of non-invasive tests, penile angiography is performed in selected cases of patients suspected of having isolated arterial disease, in whom surgical repair is considered. The study is utilized to define the anatomical pattern of arterial occlusive disease and allows the planning of an appropriate vascular surgical approach. Four major technical improvements have greatly modified penile angiography: intracavernous injection of vasoactive agents, inducing maximal vasodilatation; new low-osmolality contrast media, preventing pain; digital subtraction angiography; and new catheters that enable this procedure to be performed with one single femoral artery puncture (Delcour et al 1989). The introduction of low-osmolality contrast media that are less painful has led us to perform penile angiography under local anesthesia.

Technique of penile angiography

A urethral catheter is inserted in all cases to provide for bladder drainage in face of the diuretic effect of the high osmolar angiographic contrast load. A lead shield is placed on the scrotum to protect the genitalia from exposure to x-rays. Angiography is performed with 5 French catheters. The aortic bifurcation and proximal common iliac arteries are always studied, as are the external iliac arteries, in order to visualize the hypogastric arteries and not to miss an accessory pudendal artery. Both internal pudendal arteries are selectively catheterized, by a right femoral approach, except in cases in which selective catheterization is not feasible because of severe and diffuse atherosclerotic lesions. Once the pudendal artery is selectively catheterized we produce vasodilatation by intracavernous injection of a mixture of up to 50 mg papaverine, 2.5 mg phentolamine and 10 µg PGE$_1$. The exact dosage depends on preangiographic testing. The rationale for a polypharmaceutical approach is based on the concept that maximal inflow may be more efficiently effected by the use of a combination of drugs that differ in their mechanisms of action. Non-ionic contrast agents carrying 35–37% iodine are used. Magnification studies are performed routinely, and various projections are obtained for adequate visualization of all the penile branches. Patients are usually fully evaluated in 2 hours and are required to remain on bed rest following the procedure for an additional 6 hours. The absence of opacification of penile vascularization always results from a technical failure in the angiographic technique: suboptimal vasodilatation, no injection of collateral pathways, etc. If the internal pudendal angiogram fails to opacify the penile arteries, all collateral networks must be opacified to exclude a variant origin of the penile arteries or collateralization for an occluded part of the penile pudendal arteries.

Summary

Several tests for diagnosing vascular ED may be chosen. In a goal-directed approach, one should bear in mind that treatment may be effective without diagnostic testing and that it is necessary to be well aware of the purpose of testing: global assessment of erectile capacity in preparation for auto-injection therapy, or detailed assessment of arterial and erectile response in preparation for surgical treatment. ICI testing may be sufficient for the majority of patients. Other, more invasive tests are reserved for preparing surgical treatment or for scientific studies.

References

Abelson D (1975). Diagnostic value of penile pulse and blood pressure. *J Urol* **113**:636–9.

Benet A, Melman A, Seftel A, et al (1997) Standardization of PGE1 dose in pharmaco-penile Duplex ultrasound: a Multicenter Study. *J Urol* **157**:A712.

Bongaerts AH, de Korte PJ, Delaere KP, et al (1992). Erectile dysfunction: timing of spectral wave-form analysis in the assessment of the function of the cavernosal arteries. *Eur J Radiol* **15**:140–5.

Buvat J, Buvat-Herbaut M, Dehaene JL, et al (1986). Is intracavernous injection of papaverine a reliable screening test for vascular impotence? *J Urol* **135**:476–8.

Christ GJ, Stone B, Melman A (1991). Age-dependent alterations in the efficacy of phenylephrine-induced contractions in human corpus cavernosum of impotent men. *Can J Physiol Pharmacol* **69**:909–13.

Christ GJ, Richards S, Winkler A (1997). Integrative erectile biology: the role of signal transduction and cell-to-cell communication in coordinating corporal smooth muscle tone and penile erection. *Int J Impot Res* **9**:69–84.

De Palma RG (1997). Vascular surgery for impotence: a review. *Int J Impot Res* **9**:61–7.

Delcour C, Katoto RM, Richoz B, et al (1989). Penile arteriography: technical improvements. *Int J Impot Res* **1**:43.

Gaskell P (1971). The importance of penile blood pressure in cases of impotence. *Can Med Assoc J* **105**:1047–51.

Ginestie JF, Romieux A (1978). *Radiologic Exploration of Impotence*. Martinus Nijhoff Medical Division, The Hague.

Goldstein I, Mortara R, Krane RJ (1984). Impotence following blunt trauma. *J Urol* **13**:200A.

de Groat WC, Steers WD (1988). Neuroanatomy and neurophysiology of penile erection. In: *Contemporary Management of Impotence and Infertility*, eds EA Tanagho, TF Lue, RD McClure, p. 3. Williams & Wilkins, Baltimore.

Hatzichristou DG, Saenz de Tejada I, Kupferman S, et al (1995). In vivo assessment of trabecular smooth muscle tone, its application in pharmacocavernosometry and analysis of intracavernous pressure determinants. *J Urol* **153**:1126–35.

Herbert J (1973). The role of the dorsal nerves of the penis in the sexual behaviour of the male rhesus monkey. *Physiol Behav* **10**:293–300.

Jünemann KP, Alken P (1989). Pharmacotherapy of ED: A review. *Int J Impot Res* **1**:71.

Kempczinski RF (1979). Role of the vascular diagnostic laboratory in the evaluation of male impotence. *Am J Surg* **138**:278–82.

Kim SH, Paick JS, Lee SE, et al (1994). Doppler sonography of deep cavernosal artery of the penis: variation of peak systolic velocity according to sampling location. *J Ultrasound Med* **13**:591–4.

Krane RJ, Siroky MB (1981) Neurophysiology of erection. *Urol Clin North Am* **8**:91–102.

Krane RJ, Goldstein I, Saenz de Tejada I (1989). Impotence. *N Engl J Med* **321**:1648–59.

Kropman RF, Schipper J, van Oostayen JA, et al (1992). The value of increased end diastolic velocity during penile duplex sonography in relation to pathological venous leakage in erectile dysfunction. *J Urol* **148**:314–17.

Lavoisier P, Courtois F, Barres D, et al (1986). Correlation between intracavernous pressure and contraction of the ischio-cavernosus muscle in man. *J Urol* **136**:936–9.

Lavoisier P, Proulx J, Courtois F, et al (1988). Relationship between perineal muscle contractions, penile tumescence, and penile rigidity during nocturnal erections. *J Urol* **139**:176–9.

Lincoln J, Crowe R, Blacklay PF, et al (1987). Changes in the vipergic, cholinergic, and adrenergic innervation of human penile tissue in diabetic and non-diabetic impotent males. *J Urol* **137**:1053–9.

Lue TF, Tanagho EA (1987). Physiology of erection and pharmacological management of impotence. *J Urol* **137**:829–36.

Lue TF, Hricak H, Marich KW, et al (1985). Vasculogenic impotence evaluated by high-resolution ultrasonography and pulsed Doppler analysis. *Radiology* **55**:777–81.

Lue TF, Hellstrom WJ, McAninch JW, et al (1986). Priapism: a refined approach to diagnosis and treatment. *J Urol* **136**:104–8.

Mellinger BC, Fried JJ, Vaughn ED (1990) Papaverine-induced penile blood flow acceleration in impotent men measured by duplex scanning. *J Urol* **144**:897–9.

Meuleman EJ, Diemont WL (1995). Investigation of erectile dysfunction. *Urol Clin North Am* **22**:803–19.

Meuleman EJ, Bemelmans BL, van Asten WN, et al (1990). The value of combined papaverine testing and duplexscanning in men with erectile dysfunction. *Int J Impot Res* **2**:87.

Meuleman EJ, Wijkstra H, Doesburg WH, et al (1991). Comparison of the diagnostic value of gravity- and pump cavernosometry in the evaluation of the cavernous venoocclusive mechanism. *J Urol* **146**:1266–70.

Meuleman EJ, Bemelmans BL, van Asten WN, et al (1992a). Assessment of penile blood flow by duplex ultrasonography in 44 men with normal erectile potency in different phases of erection. *J Urol* **147**:51–6.

Meuleman EJ, Bemelmans BL, Doesburg WH, et al (1992b). Penile pharmacological duplex ultrasonography: a dose–effect study comparing papaverine, papaverine/phentolamine and prostaglandin E1. *J Urol* **148**:63–6.

Montague DK, Lakin MM (1992). False diagnoses of venous leak impotence. *J Urol* **148**:148–9.

Montorsi F, Bergamaschi F, Guazzoni G, et al (1993). Velocity and flow volume gradients along the cavernosal artery: a duplex and color Doppler sonography study. *Eur Urol* **23**:357–60.

Newman H, Nortrup JD, Delvin J (1964). Mechanism of human penile erection *Invest Urol* **1**:350.

Padma-Nathan H, Azadzoi K, Blanco R (1986). Development of an animal model of atherosclerotic impotence. *Surg Forum* **37**:640.

Padma-Nathan H, Hellstrom WJ, Kaiser FE et al (1997). Treatment of men with erectile dysfunction with transurethral Alprostadil. *N Engl J Med* **336**:1–7.

Petrou S, Lewis RW (1992). Management of corporeal veno-occlusive dysfunction. *Urol Int* **49**:48–55.

Porst H (1990). Diagnostic use and side-effects of vaso-active drugs: A report on over 2100 patients with erectile failure. *Int J Impot Res* **1**(suppl 2):222 (Abstract).

Porst H (1993). Prostaglandin E1 and the nitric oxide donor linsidomine for erectile failure: a diagnostic comparative study of 40 patients. *J Urol* **149**:1280–3.

Puech-Leao P, Chao S, Glina S, et al (1990). Gravity cavernosometry – a simple diagnostic test for cavernosal incompetence. *Br J Urol* **65**:391–4.

Queral LA, Whitehouse WM Jr, Flinn WR (1979). Pelvic hemodynamics after aorto-iliac reconstruction. *Surgery* **86**:799–809.

Rowland DL, Slob AK (1992). Vibrotactile stimulation enhances sexual response in sexually functional men: a study using concomitant measures of erection. *Arch Sex Behav* **21**:387–400.

Saenz de Tejada I, Goldstein I, Azadzoi K, et al (1989). Impaired neurogenic and endothelium-dependent relaxation of human penile smooth muscle from diabetic men with impotence. *N Engl J Med* **320**:1025–30.

Saenz de Tejada I, Moroukian P, Tessier J (1991). Trabecular smooth muscle modulates the capacitor function of the penis. Studies on a rabbit model. *Am J Physiol* **260**:1590–5.

St Louis EL, Jewett MA, Gray RR (1983). Basketball-related impotence. *N Engl J Med* **308**:595–6.

Truss MC, Becker AJ, Thon WF, et al (1994). Intracavernous calcitonin gene-related peptide plus prostaglandin E1: possible alternative to penile implants in selected patients. *Eur Urol* **26**:40–5.

Udelson D, Hatzichristou D, Saenz de Tejada I, et al (1994). A new methodology of pharmacocavernosometry which enables hemodynamic analysis under conditions of known corporal smooth muscle relaxation. *Int J Impot Res* **6** (suppl 1):A17.

van der Ven PFM, Wei AY, Jap PHK, et al (1995). Increased expression of a 68-kDA protein in the corpus cavernosum of some men with erectile dysfunction. *J Androl* **16**:242–7.

Velcek D, Sniderman KW, Darracot Vaughan E, et al (1980). Penile flow index utilizing a Doppler pulse wave analysis to identify penile vascular insufficiency. *J Urol* **123**:669–73.

Vickers MA Jr, Benson CB, Dluhy RG, et al (1992). The current cavernosometric criteria for corporovenous dysfunction are too strict. *J Urol* **147**:614–17.

Virag R (1982). Intracavernous injection of papaverine for erectile failure. *Lancet* **ii**:938.

Vruggink PA, Diemont WL, Debruyne FM, et al (1995). Enhanced pharmacological testing in patients with erectile dysfunction. *J Androl* **16**:163–8.

Wespes E, Nogueira MC, Herbaut AG, et al (1990). Role of the bulbocavernosis muscle in the mechanism of human erection. *Eur Urol* **18**:45–8.

7

The pharmacological basis of sexual therapeutics

Karl-Erik Andersson, William D Steers

Introduction

The introduction of intracavernous injection of papaverine as a treatment of erectile dysfunction (Virag 1982) stimulated research interest not only in the mechanisms of penile erection, but also in vasodilator drugs that can be used for injection therapy. However, intracavernous administration of vasoactive drugs has inevitable drawbacks, reflected by the relatively large number of drop-outs from therapy, and the need for non-intracavernous treatment alternatives has been stressed repeatedly. Recent progress concerning both the central (Steers 1990; de Groat and Booth 1993; Andersson and Wagner 1995; Argiolas and Melis 1995; Giuliano et al 1995) and peripheral (Andersson 1993; Andersson and Wagner 1995; Giuliano et al 1997) control mechanisms of penile erection has made it possible to define several new targets for pharmacological treatment of the disorder.

Drugs and treatments used for treatment of erectile dysfunction can be classified in different ways. Heaton et al (1997) recently suggested a classification based on the mode of action, dividing drugs into central initiators, peripheral initiators, central conditioners, peripheral conditioners, and others. Such a classification is attractive, but assumes that the modes of action of the different drugs used are known, which at present is not always the case. In this review, the pharmacological bases of some of the drugs currently used for intracavernous and non-intracavernous initiation of erection are briefly discussed.

Drugs for intracavernous administration

Among the many drugs and/or drug combinations tested (for reviews, see for example Jünemann and Alken 1989; Jünemann 1992; Gregoire 1992; Linet and Ogrinc 1996; Porst 1996), only three, used alone or in combination, have become widely clinically accepted and administered on a long-term basis, namely papaverine, phentolamine, and prostaglandin (PG) E_1 (alprostadil). The experimental and clinical experiences with several other agents used for treatment and discussed below are limited.

Papaverine

Papaverine is often classified as a phosphodiesterase inhibitor, but the drug has a very complex mode of action (Ferrari 1974) and may be regarded as a "multilevel acting drug" (Andersson 1994). Which of its several possible mechanisms of action is the dominating one at the high concentrations that can be expected when the drug is injected intracavernously is difficult to establish. In vitro, it has been shown that papaverine relaxes the penile arteries, the cavernous sinusoids, and the penile veins (Kirkeby et al 1990). In dogs, Jünemann et al (1986) demonstrated that papaverine had a dual hemodynamic effect, decreasing the resistance to arterial inflow and increasing the resistance to venous outflow. The latter effect, which has also been demonstrated in men (Delcour et al 1987), may be related to activation by papaverine of the veno-occlusive mechanism.

Injected intracavernously, papaverine will reach maximal concentrations in the systemic circulation within 10–30 minutes (Hakenberg et al 1990; Tanaka 1990). Hakenberg et al (1990) injected 15 mg papaverine (plus 0.5 mg phentolamine) intravenously and intracavernously. The maximum serum concentration of papaverine obtained was approximately five times higher when the drug was given intravenously than when it was given into the penis. Papaverine has a relatively short plasma half-life (1–2 h) and is extensively metabolized in the liver. Since elimination was much slower from the corpus cavernosum than from the systemic circulation (Tanaka 1990), intracavernous administration seems to reduce the risk of obtaining systemic side-effects.

Intracavernosal injection of papaverine can produce local and systemic side-effects. Even lethal complications have been described (Hasmat et al 1991). A common local effect is intracavernous fibrosis. Jünemann and Alken (1989), surveying the literature, reported that the occurrence of intracavernous fibrosis in patients receiving papaverine or papaverine–phentolamine was approximately 5%. Most of these lesions were reversible. The cause of the lesions has not been clarified, but it has been suggested that the pH of the papaverine solution (which is between 3 and 4 for a 2% solution of papaverine in water) is of importance (Seidmon and Samaha 1989). However, Stackl (1992) suggested that neither the pH nor the osmolarity of the solution was responsible for the fibrotic reactions, but rather a property inherent to papaverine. Others propose that the scarring is due to the "superrigidity" that is induced. Another side-effect is priapism and prolonged erections, which may occur in 5–10% of cases (Jünemann and Alken 1989). At particular risk for developing papaverine-induced priapism were younger patients with better-quality baseline erection, patients with neurological disorders, and patients without evidence of vascular disease (Lomas and Jarow 1992).

Papaverine is known to be hepatotoxic; this characteristic may manifest itself either as an increase in liver transaminases or, in rare cases, as a drug-induced hepatitis.

According to Jünemann (1992), the present experiences with papaverine show that papaverine–phentolamine is superior to papaverine alone in the therapy of erectile dysfunction, and he suggested that papaverine monosubstance should be excluded from the pharmacotherapy owing to its low efficacy (papaverine produces erection in 36% of patients, compared with 65% for papaverine–phentolamine) and its high risk of side-effects, including cavernous fibrosis.

α-Adrenoceptor antagonists

Sympathetic nervous activity via release of norepinephrine and stimulation of α-adrenoceptors is of central importance for keeping the penis in the flaccid state (Andersson and Wagner 1995). Receptor-binding studies have revealed that the number of α-adrenoceptors is 10 times higher than the number of β-adrenoceptors (Levin and Wein 1980). The presence of both α_1- and α_2-adrenoceptors has been demonstrated in human corpus cavernosum tissue, but available information supports the view of a functional predominance of α_1-adrenoceptors. This may be the case also in the penile vasculature, although a contribution of α_2-adrenoceptors to the contraction induced by norepinephrine and electrical stimulation of nerves cannot be excluded (Andersson and Wagner 1995).

Receptor cloning and pharmacological studies in human tissues have revealed the existence of at least three subtypes of α_1-adrenoceptor, and consensus has been reached on classification and nomenclature

(Hieble et al 1995). Currently, three native subtypes have been recognized, which have been designated as α_{1A}, α_{1B}, and α_{1D}. The cloned counterparts are termed α_{1a}, α_{1b}, and α_{1d}. When reviewing historical data, it is important to be aware of this re-classification, as many different classifications have been used previously. There is increasing evidence that an additional α_1-adrenoceptor subtype with a low affinity for prazosin (α_{1L}), which is not yet fully characterized, may occur in, for example, vascular smooth muscle (Muramatsu et al 1995).

As mentioned above, α_1-adrenoceptors seem to predominate functionally in penile tissues. An important question, then, is whether or not one of the α_1-adrenoceptor subtypes is more important than the others. In a preliminary communication, Price et al (1993) reported that in human corporeal tissue three subtypes of α_1-adrenoceptor mRNA (α_{1a}, α_{1b}, and α_{1d} – current terminology) could be identified, the α_{1a}- and α_{1d}-adrenoceptors predominating. This was confirmed by other investigators (Traish et al 1996). However, it is known that the levels of mRNA expression do not always parallel the expression of a functional receptor protein. Traish et al (1995) characterized the functional α_1-adrenoceptor proteins in human corpus cavernosum tissue, using receptor binding and isometric tension experiments. Their results demonstrated the presence of α_{1A}-, α_{1B}-, and α_{1D}-adrenoceptors, and suggested that the norepinephrine-induced contraction in this tissue is mediated by two or possibly three receptor subtypes. The possibility that the α_{1L}-adrenoceptor subtype may be of importance in penile erectile tissues has apparently not been explored. Whether or not antagonists, selectively acting at any of the α_1-adrenoceptor subtypes, would offer any advantages over the currently used drugs (phentolamine, thymoxamine) in the treatment of erectile dysfunction remains to be established.

Phentolamine

Beside being a competitive α-adrenoceptor antagonist with similar affinity for α_1- and α_2-adrenoceptors, which is its main mechanism of action, phentolamine can also block receptors for 5-hydroxytryptamine (5-HT, serotonin) and cause release of histamine from mast cells. Phentolamine may also have a direct, non-specific, relaxant effect on blood vessels (Taylor et al 1965). Since phentolamine non-selectively blocks α-adrenoceptors, it can be expected that, by blocking prejunctional α_2-adrenoceptors, it would increase the norepinephrine release from adrenergic nerves, thus counteracting its own post-junctional α_1-adrenoceptor blocking actions. Whether such an action contributes to the limited efficacy of intracavernously administered phentolamine in producing erection is not known.

In dogs, phentolamine, like papaverine, decreased the resistance to arterial inflow to the penis. However, papaverine, but not phentolamine, increased the resistance to venous outflow (Jünemann et al 1986). The lack of effect on venous outflow of intracavernous phentolamine has also been demonstrated in men (Wespes et al 1989).

There is a general lack of information about the pharmacokinetics of phentolamine. The drug has a reduced efficacy when given orally, probably due to extensive first-pass metabolism. A discrepancy between the plasma half-life (30 min) and effect duration (2.5–4.0 h) has been demonstrated (Imhof et al 1975); whether this can be attributed to active metabolites is not known. When the drug is given intracavernously, the serum concentration of phentolamine will reach a maximum within 20–30 minutes, and then rapidly decline to undetectable values (Hakenberg et al 1990).

The most common side-effects of phentolamine after intravenous administration are orthostatic hypotension and tachycardia. Cardiac arrhythmias and myocardial infarction have been reported, but these are very rare events. Theoretically, such effects may be encountered also after intracorporeal administration, but so far this does not seem to be the case.

Since a single intracavernous phentolamine injection does not result in a satisfactory erectile response in most cases, the drug is widely used in combination with papaverine (Zorgniotti and Lafleur 1985; Jünemann and Alken 1989), or with vasoactive intestinal polypeptide (VIP): (Gerstenberg et al 1992).

Thymoxamine

Thymoxamine has a competitive and relatively selective blocking action on α_1-adrenoceptors. In addition, it may have antihistaminic actions. Little is known about its pharmacokinetics, but after systemic administration it has an effect duration of 3–4 h. In vitro, thymoxamine caused relaxation of norepinephrine-contracted human corpus cavernosum preparations (Imagawa et al 1989), but was less potent than prazosin and phentolamine.

Thymoxamine was shown to produce erection when injected intracavernously (Brindley 1986), and in a double-blind crossover study Buvat et al (1989) showed it to be more active than saline, but less active than papaverine. Buvat et al (1989) reported on the experiences of intracavernous injections of thymoxamine in 170 patients with impotence, and pointed out that the drug did not produce, but facilitated, erection by inducing prolonged tumescence. They also stressed that the main advantage of the drug was its safety. Only 2 out of the

170 patients injected had prolonged erections. Buvat et al (1991), comparing papaverine and thymoxamine, also found that thymoxamine had less tendency to produce corporeal fibrosis than papaverine (1.3% vs 32.0%). The positive safety aspects were underlined by Arvis et al (1996), who reported no serious side-effects among 104 men followed for 11 months and performing 7507 self-administrations.

In a comparative study between thymoxamine and PGE_1, Buvat et al (1996) showed that PGE_1 was significantly more effective than thymoxamine (71% vs 50% responders), especially in patients with arteriogenic dysfunction (96% vs 46%). However, thymoxamine was significantly better tolerated than PGE_1, causing fewer prolonged erections and fewer painful reactions.

As a facilitating drug, thymoxamine may be a reasonable alternative for treatment of erectile dysfunction.

Prostaglandin E_1

Human penile tissues have the ability to synthesize various prostanoids, and it has been suggested that arachidonate cascade products may be involved in the control of penile erection (Miller and Morgan 1994). $PGF_{2\alpha}$, PGI_2 (prostacyclin), high concentrations of PGE_2, and, most potently among the prostanoids tested, the thromboxane (Tx) A_2 analogues U46619 and U44069 caused contraction of isolated preparations of corpus cavernosum and the cavernous artery (Hedlund and Andersson 1985). The contraction-mediating prostanoid receptor in the human corpus cavernosum is most probably a TxA_2-sensitive receptor, even if the presence of more than one contraction-mediating prostanoid receptor cannot be excluded (Hedlund et al 1989a, 1989b). However, it is not known if prostanoids contribute to tone in penile erectile tissues.

Hedlund and Andersson (1985) found PGE_1 to relax human trabecular tissue and segments of the cavernous artery contracted by norepinephrine and $PGF_{2\alpha}$ effectively. Such an effect is probably mediated via stimulation of adenylate cyclase in the smooth muscle and associated with an increase in cyclic adenosine monophosphate (cAMP) (Miller and Morgan 1994). Contributing to a direct smooth muscle effect of PGE_1, the prostanoid has been shown to inhibit release of norepinephrine from penile adrenergic nerves (Molderings et al 1992). Such an effect may contribute to PGE_1's relaxant effect on penile erectile tissues when it is injected intracorporeally. Recent data suggest that PGs and transforming growth factor-β_1 (TGF-β_1) may have a role in modulation of collagen synthesis and in the production of fibrosis of the corpus cavernosum (Moreland et al 1995).

PGE$_1$ is known to have a variety of pharmacological effects. For instance, it produces systemic vasodilatation, prevents platelet aggregation, and stimulates intestinal activity. Administered systemically, the drug has been used clinically to a limited extent. Little is known about its pharmacokinetics, but it has a short duration of action and is extensively metabolized. As much as 70% may be metabolized in one pass through the lungs (Gloub et al 1975), which may partly explain why it seldom causes circulatory side-effects when injected intracavernously.

Ishii et al (1986) demonstrated that intracavernously administered PGE$_1$ is effective for treatment of impotence of various causes, a finding confirmed in a large number of studies (Linet and Ogrinc 1996; Porst 1996). Compared with papaverine, PGE$_1$ was shown to produce a slower onset of action, a longer duration of action and fewer side-effects (Chen et al 1992).

PGE$_1$ seems to be at least as effective as papaverine or the papaverine–phentolamine combination, with a success rate of more than 70% (for a review, see Jünemann and Alken 1989; Linet and Ogrinc 1996; Porst 1996). The principal side-effect of locally injected PGE$_1$ is pain at the injection site (10–20%), whereas prolonged erections seem to be a rare complication (Jünemann and Alken 1989; Porst 1996). Priapism and prolonged duration of action are also more dose-related with PGE$_1$ than with papaverine or phentolamine. Contributing to the low incidence of prolonged erection and priapism may be the fact that PGE$_1$ can be metabolized in the penis by a prostaglandin dehydrogenase (Roy et al 1989). This should also decrease the risk of systemic side-effects.

Penile scarring may occur during PGE$_1$ therapy. This complication was found to be unrelated to the dose, number and frequency of injections, and the presence of baseline penile scarring, and was considered sporadic and unpredictable (Chen et al 1995).

Available information (see Porst 1996) suggests that PGE$_1$ currently represents the most efficacious and the safest drug currently used for intracavernous injection treatment of erectile dysfunction.

Other drugs

Vasoactive intestinal polypeptide

A role for VIP as neurotransmitter and/or neuromodulator in the penis has been postulated by several investigators, but its importance for penile erection has not been established (Andersson and Wagner 1995; Andersson and Stief 1997). However, the inability of VIP to produce erection when injected intracavernously in potent (Wagner and Gerstenberg 1988) or impotent men (Adaikan et al 1986; Kiely et al 1989; Roy et al 1990) indicates that it cannot be the main non-adrenergic, non-cholinergic mediator for relaxation of penile erectile tissues.

VIP has been shown to produce a wide range of effects. It is a potent vasodilator, inhibits contractile activity in many types of smooth muscle, and stimulates cardiac contractility and many exocrine secretions. It stimulates adenylate cyclase and the formation of cAMP (Fahrenkrug 1989).

Wagner and Gerstenberg (1988) found that even in high doses (60 µg), VIP was unable to induce erection on intracavernous injection in potent men. On the other hand, when used in conjunction with visual or vibratory stimulation, intracavernous VIP facilitated normal erection. Kiely et al (1989) injected VIP, papaverine, and combinations of these drugs with phentolamine intracorporeally in 12 men with impotence of varying etiology. They confirmed that VIP alone is poor at inducing human penile erections. However, in combination with papaverine and phentolamine Gerstenberg et al (1992) administered VIP together with phentolamine intracavernously to 52 patients with erectile failure. Forty per cent of the patients had previously received treatment with papaverine alone or with papaverine together with phentolamine. After sexual stimulation, all patients obtained erection sufficient for penetration. Those patients previously treated with papaverine or papaverine–phentolamine stated that the action of the VIP combination was more like the normal coital cycle. No patient developed priapism, corporeal fibrosis, or any other serious complication (Gerstenberg et al 1992). McMahon (1996) performed a pilot study in 20 men with erectile dysfunction of various etiologies using a VIP–phentolamine combination. Sixteen of the patients responded favorably, and side-effects were few.

VIP given intravenously can produce hypotension, tachycardia, and flushing (Palmer et al 1986; Krejs 1988). However, the plasma half-life of the peptide is short, which may contribute to the fact that systemic side-effects are rare when it is administered intracavernously.

It seems that VIP administered intracavernously together with phentolamine may be an alternative to the more established treatments with papaverine–phentolamine or PGE_1, but more experience is needed to give a fair evaluation of the advantages and disadvantages of this combination.

Calcitonin gene-related peptide

Stief et al (1990) demonstrated calcitonin gene-related peptide (CGRP) in nerves of the human corpus cavernosum, and suggested its use in erectile dysfunction. In human blood vessels from various regions, CGRP is known to be a potent vasodilator. Its effect may be dependent on or independent of the vascular endothelium (Crossman et al 1987; Persson et al 1991). The peptide relaxed the bovine penile artery by a direct action on the smooth muscle cells (Alaranta et al 1991), which suggests that it may have important effects on the penile vasculature.

In patients, intracavernous injection of CGRP induced dose-related increases in penile arterial inflow, cavernous smooth muscle relaxation, cavernous outflow occlusion, and erectile responses. The combination of CGRP and PGE_1 may be more effective than PGE_1 alone (Stief et al 1991b; Truss et al 1994a).

It cannot be excluded that CGRP, alone as a facilitating drug, or in combination with other drugs as an initiator of erection, can be useful for therapeutic purposes, but to assess its potential, more experiences are needed.

Linsidomine chlorhydrate

An important role for nitric oxide (NO) in the relaxation of corpus cavernosum smooth muscle and vasculature is widely accepted. In vitro, several investigators have shown that both acetylcholine and neuronally mediated relaxation in animal and human corpora cavernosa involves release of NO, or of an NO-like substance (Andersson and Wagner 1995). Both the endothelium and/or the nerves innervating the corpus cavernosum may be the source of the NO involved in erection, and thus more than one isoform of nitric oxide synthase (NOS) can be involved. There seems to be no doubt about the presence of NOS in the cavernous nerves and their terminal endings within the corpora cavernosa, and in the branches of the dorsal penile nerves and nerve plexus in the adventitia of the deep cavernous artery.

Mice lacking nervous NOS (nNOS) have erections, show normal mating behavior, and respond with erection to electrical stimulation of the cavernous nerves (Huang et al 1993; Burnett et al 1996). Surprisingly, isolated corporeal tissue from both wild-type and nNOS-deleted animals showed similar responses to electrical stimulation (Burnett et al 1996). It was suggested that electrically generated NOS is essential for erection, not only in nNOS-deleted, but also in normal mice. Several investigators have shown that isolated human cavernous tissue responds with relaxation to electrical stimulation of nerves after destruction of the endothelium, while responses to acetylcholine, bradykinin, and substance P are abolished (Kimoto et al 1990; Azadzoi et al 1992). In anesthetized dogs, destruction of the sinusoidal endothelium abolished the erectile response to acetylcholine, but only partially inhibited the response to electrostimulation (Trigo-Rocha et al 1993). The NOS demonstrated in rabbit corpus cavernosum was shown to be a cytosolic, constitutive isoform of NOS (Bush et al 1992), whereas the endothelium-derived NOS is known to be primarily membrane bound (Derouet et al 1994). If this is the case also in humans, it would suggest that the most important source of NO in penile tissue is neuronal.

It is reasonable to assume that drugs acting via NO may be useful for treatment of erectile dysfunction. Linsidomine, the active metabolite of the antianginal drug molsidomine, is believed to act by non-enzymatic liberation of NO (Feelisch 1992; Rosenkranz et al 1996), which by stimulating soluble guanylate cyclase increases the content of cyclic guanosine monophosphate (cGMP) in the smooth muscle cells and produces relaxation. Linsidomine also inhibits platelet aggregation (Reden 1990), and in some countries it is registered for treatment of coronary vasospasm and coronary angiography. The drug was reported to have a plasma half-life of approximately 1–2 h (Wildgrube et al 1986; Rosenkranz et al 1996).

Linsidomine was found effectively to relax preparations of rabbit and human corpora cavernosa contracted by norepinephrine or endothelin-1 in a concentration-dependent way (Holmquist et al 1992). In preliminary studies, Stief et al (1991a, 1992) and Truss et al (1994b) studied the effect of linsidomine injected intracorporeally in impotent patients, and found that the drug induced an erectile response by increasing the arterial inflow and relaxing cavernous smooth muscle. There were no systemic or local side-effects, and no patient had a prolonged erection. These promising results have not been confirmed by other investigators (Ports 1993; Wegner et al 1994). Placebo-controlled, randomized clinical trials must be performed to ascertain whether linsidomine is a useful therapeutic alternative to existing drugs available for intracorporeal injection.

Another NO donor, sodium nitroprusside (SNP), has been given intracorporeally for treatment of erectile dysfunction, but has been shown not to be effective (Martinez-Pineiro et al 1995; Tarhan et al 1996) and to cause profound hypotension. These rather discouraging results with donors of NO do not rule out that drugs acting through the L-arginine/NO/guanylate cyclase/cGMP pathway can be effective for treatment of erectile dysfunction (see below).

Drugs for non-intracavernous administration

There is a generally a high placebo response (40–50%) to non-intracavernously administered drugs. Therefore, placebo-controlled trials and valid instruments to measure response are mandatory to assess effects adequately.

Organic nitrates

Nitroglycerin and other organic nitrates are believed to cause smooth muscle relaxation by stimulating soluble guanylate cyclase via enzymatic liberation of NO (Feelisch 1992). Both nitroglycerin and isosorbide nitrate were found to relax isolated strips of human corpus cavernosum (Heaton 1989).

Transdermal administration of nitroglycerin is well established in the treatment of angina pectoris. The observation that topical application of nitroglycerin to the penis may lead to erection adequate for sexual intercourse (Talley and Crawley 1985) has stimulated several investigations on the efficacy of this potential mode of treatment of erectile dysfunction.

Owen et al (1989) performed a placebo-controlled, double-blind study on the effect of nitroglycerin ointment applied on the penises of 26 impotent patients with diagnosis of organic, psychogenic, or mixed-type impotence. Nitroglycerin increased, relative to placebo, penile circumference significantly in 18 out 26 patients, and in 7 out of 20 patients it increased blood flow in the cavernous arteries. Hypotension and headache were observed in one patient. In a double-blind, randomized, placebo-controlled trial, Claes and Baert (1989) treated 26 impotent men with nitroglycerin patches. They observed a positive response to nitroglycerin, with return to satisfactory sexual function, in 12 patients (46%), and some erectile improvement in 9 (35%). Only one patient of the 26 reported restoration of potency with placebo patches. Twelve of the patients reported mild to moderate headaches during nitroglycerin treatment.

The effects of nitroglycerin paste applied to the penis were also investigated in 10 impotent patients by Meyhoff et al (1992). They found that, when tested in the laboratory, all patients achieved an erectile response. When the paste was self-administered, potency was restored in four, semirigidity insufficient for intercourse was seen in two, tumescence in three, and no effect in one. Seven patients complained of headaches. A sufficient erectile response to the same nitroglycerin was found in 5 out of 17 patients with spinal cord injury (Sønksen and Biering-Sørensen 1992).

Comparing transdermal nitroglycerin and intracavernous injection of papaverine in 28 patients with spinal cord lesions and erectile dysfunction, Renganathan et al (1997) found that 61% responded to

nitroglycerin and 93% to papaverine. Nine patients had complications with papaverine, while the only side-effect of transdermal nitroglycerin was a mild headache (21%).

Even if the efficacy of transdermal nitroglycerin is limited, and
headaches seem to be a common side-effect, it may be an effective
treatment in selected patients.

Phosphodiesterase inhibitors

The L-arginine/NO/guanylate cyclase/cGMP pathway seems to be
the most important for penile erection in some species (see above),
and recent results with sildenafil, a selective inhibitor of the cGMP-
specific phosphodiesterase (PDE-5) found in the human corpus cavernosum (Stief et al 1995; Boolell et al 1996), further support the view
that this may also be the case in humans (Boolell et al 1996).
Sildenafil, which is rapidly absorbed after oral administration
(bioavailability 41%), has a plasma half-life of 3–5 h.

In a double-blind, placebo-controlled study on 416 patients with
erectile dysfunctions of various categories, Lue et al (1997) found that
sildenafil 5–100 mg improved erectile function dose dependently in
up to 77.8% of patients with organic impotence. Side-effects
(headache, vasodilatation, dyspepsia, and diarrhea) were mild and
well tolerated. In another placebo-controlled study on 27 patients
with erectile dysfunction caused by traumatic spinal cord injury,
Derry et al (1997) found a positive response to oral sildenafil (50 mg)
in 65%. Steers et al (1997) reported that sildenafil can produce erection sufficient for intercourse in about 50% of men with severe erectile dysfunction. The positive effects of sildenafil on erection seem to
be maintained for at least 1 year (Buvat et al 1997).

Sildenafil appears to be one of the most promising orally active
agents for the treatment of erectile dysfunction. The high response
rate and good tolerance make it an attractive first alternative for
patients who would have been considered candidates for injection
therapy. The efficacy of sildenafil compared with that of injection
therapy with, for instance, papaverine–phentolamine or PGE_1, will
help to decide its place in the therapeutic armamentarium.

Prostaglandin E_1

Vasoactive agents can be administered topically to the urethral
mucosa and can apparently be absorbed into the corpus spongiosum

and transferred to the corpora cavernosa. PGE_1 (alprostadil) and a PGE_1–prazosin combination were demonstrated to produce erections in a majority of patients with chronic, organic, erectile dysfunction (Padma-Nathan et al 1995). In a prospective, multicenter, double-blind, placebo-controlled study on 68 patients with long-standing erectile dysfunction of primarily organic origin (Hellstrom et al 1996), transurethrally administered alprostadil produced 75.5% full enlargement of the penis, and 63.6% of the patients reported intercourse. However, the frequency of intercourse or ability to perform in men who had no erection prior to drug therapy was not addressed. The most common side-effect was penile pain, experienced by 9.1–18.3% of the patients receiving alprostadil. There were no episodes of priapism. In another double-blind, placebo-controlled study on 1511 men with chronic erectile dysfunction from various causes, 64.9% had intercourse successfully when taking transurethral alprostadil compared with 18.6% on placebo (Padma-Nathan et al 1997). Again the most common side-effect was mild penile pain (10.8%).

Despite early encouraging results, some suggest that the true efficacy is nearer to 30–40% and the quality of erection deteriorates over time. Penile pain remains a problem in many patients. For men finding intracavernous injections problematic, the ease of intraurethral administration is an option. However, optimism should be tempered in those with severe dysfunction and those who have failed intracavernous therapy.

K⁺ channel openers

K^+ channel openers exert their main vasodilatatory effect by increasing the opening probability of an ATP-dependent K^+ channel in the smooth muscle membrane. This will lead to an efflux of K^+ and hyperpolarization of the cell, which, in turn, will prevent the opening of voltage-dependent calcium channels involved in activation. Additional mechanisms may be involved in the relaxation (Andersson 1992; Longman and Hamilton 1992).

Several K^+ channel openers (pinacidil, lemakalim, and nicorandil) have been shown to be effective in causing relaxation of isolated cavernous tissue from both animals and humans, and to produce erection when injected intracavernously in monkeys (Andersson 1993). However, only minoxidil, an arteriolar vasodilator used as an antihypertensive agent in patients with severe hypertension, seems to have been tried in men. Minoxidil is a pro-drug, not active in vitro but metabolized in the liver to the active molecule, minoxidil N-O sulfate

(McCall et al 1983). It has been shown that minoxidil sulfate has the properties of a K^+ channel opener.

Minoxidil is well absorbed, both from the gastrointestinal tract and transdermally, but its biotransformation to the active metabolite has not been evaluated in men. The drug has a half-life in plasma of 3–4 h, but the duration of its vascular effects is 24 h or even longer.

In a double-blind trial, minoxidil was given to 33 patients with neurogenic and/or arterial impotence, and compared with placebo (lubricating gel) and nitroglycerin (2.5 g 10% ointment). Minoxidil was applied on the glans penis as 1 ml of a 2% solution. Minoxidil was superior to both placebo and nitroglycerin in increasing penile rigidity, and it was suggested that the drug might be considered for long-term treatment of organic impotence (Cavallini 1991).

The main side-effects of the drug, when used in the treatment of hypertension, are fluid and salt retention, cardiovascular effects secondary to baroreflex activation, and hypertrichosis. Side-effects have so far not been reported when the drug is used for treatment of erectile dysfunction, but the experiences are limited.

The principle of K^+ channel opening is interesting, and the preliminary experiences with minoxidil seem promising, but further controlled clinical trials are needed to confirm and assess the efficacy and side-effects of the drug in patients with erectile dysfunction.

α-Adrenoceptor antagonists

Phentolamine

In a placebo-controlled study (16 patients), oral phentolamine (50 mg) was tried with some success in patients with non-specific erectile insufficiency (Gwinup 1988). These results were confirmed by Zorgniotti (1992) in a preliminary report. He also found (in 31 patients) that buccal administration of phentolamine (20 mg) was clearly more effective than placebo. Zorgniotti (1992) considered non-intracavernous, "on demand" administration of phentolamine a promising approach for treatment of impotence. Becker et al (1997) performed a double-blind placebo-controlled trial with oral phentolamine 20, 40, and 60 mg in patients with erectile dysfunction and a high likelihood of organogenic etiology, and found the drug to be of benefit. There were no serious complications, but some circulatory side-effects were seen after 60 mg.

Whether or not phentolamine is a competitive alternative to other oral treatments of erectile dysfunction has to be demonstrated in comparative clinical trials.

Yohimbine

In animals, α_2-adrenoceptor blockers such as yohimbine, idazoxan, and imiloxan may increase sexual arousal (Clark et al 1984; Smith et al 1987a, 1987b), and in men, yohimbine has for a long time been considered an aphrodisiac. Yohimbine is a relatively selective antagonist of α_2-adrenoceptors, and even if other actions have been demonstrated (Goldberg and Robertson 1983), these can be demonstrated only in concentrations that most probably cannot be obtained in men. The site of action of yohimbine is most probably not peripheral, since the predominant subtype of α-adrenoceptors in penile erectile tissue is of α_1-type (Andersson 1993), and since intracavernosal injection of another, more potent, α_2-adrenoceptor antagonist, idazoxan, did not produce penile erection in men (Brindley 1986). In normal healthy volunteers, Danjou et al (1988) found that intravenous infusion of yohimbine had no erectogenic effects. This does not exclude the idea that orally administered yohimbine may be effective (see below). In a randomized, double-blind, placebo-controlled study, Montorsi et al (1994) found that combination treatment with yohimbine and trazodone was more effective than placebo for the treatment of psychogenic impotence. Jacobsen (1992) found in a pilot study that eight out of nine patients with impotence associated with antidepressive treatment with the serotonin re-uptake blocker, fluoxetine, responded favorably to oral yohimbine. A potentiation of yohimbine effects by the opioid receptor antagonist naltrexone has been demonstrated (Charney and Heninger 1986).

The effects of yohimbine have been investigated in controlled trials on patients with organic (Morales et al 1987), psychogenic (Reid et al 1987), and mixed (Riley et al 1989; Susset et al 1989) etiology for their impotence. In organically impotent patients, a marginal effect of the drug was demonstrated: 43% responded (complete or partial response) to yohimbine and 28% to placebo (difference non-significant: Morales et al 1987). In studies of the same design in patients with psychogenic impotence, similar figures were obtained, although this time the difference between active treatment and placebo was significant (Morales et al 1987; Reid et al 1987). Positive responses in patients with impotence of mixed etiologies were reported in approximately one-third of the cases (Riley et al 1989; Susset et al 1989).

A crossover, double-blind study on 62 patients with impotence, where the efficacy of yohimbine ointment administered locally on the penis was compared with that of placebo, suggested positive results in a subgroup of patients (Turchi et al 1992), but in the total material no significant effects were found.

High-dose yohimbine (36 mg per day) was found to have no positive effect in a prospective, randomized, controlled, double-blind, crossover study of 29 patients with mixed-type erectile dysfunction (Kunelius et al 1997). Another double-blind, placebo-controlled study of 86 patients without clearly detectable organic or psychological causes (Vogt et al 1997) revealed that yohimbine was significantly more effective than placebo (71% vs 45%) in terms of response rate.

The plasma half-life of yohimbine was found to be 0.6 h (Owen et al 1987), whereas the plasma norepinephrine-increasing effects of the drug lasted for 12 h (Galitzky et al 1990). This discrepancy may be explained by the presence of an active metabolite (Owen et al 1987). The side-effects reported included increases in heart rate and blood pressure, but in addition orthostatic hypotension, anxiety, agitation, and manic reactions have also been described (Charney et al 1982, 1983; Price et al 1984).

It cannot be excluded that orally administered yohimbine can have a beneficial effect in some patients with erectile dysfunction. The conflicting results available may be attributed to differences in drug design, patient selection, and definitions of positive response. However, generally, available results of treatment are not impressive.

Opioid receptor antagonists

In men, it is well known that chronic injection of opioids can lead to impotence (Parr 1976; Crowley and Simpson 1978). It has also been suggested that endogenous opioids can be involved in sexual dysfunction, and that opioid antagonists would be effective as a treatment (Fabbri et al 1989).

Intravenous naloxone, which is a pure antagonist at opioid receptors, was found to have no effect on arousal in normal subjects (Goldstein and Hansteen 1977). Naltrexone has effects similar to those of naloxone, but can be given orally, and has a higher potency and a longer duration of action (24–72 h) than naloxone. It is well absorbed from the gastrointestinal tract, but is subject to an extensive first-pass metabolism, metabolized in the liver, and recycled by enterohepatic circulation. The major metabolite of naltrexone 6β-naltrexone also possesses opioid receptor antagonist activity and probably contributes to the effects of naltrexone. The plasma half-life of naltrexone is about 4 h and that of 6β-naltrexone 13 h.

In an open pilot study, Goldstein (1986) found that naltrexone (25–50 mg/day) restored erectile function in six out of seven men with "idiopathic" erectile dysfunction. Fabbri et al (1989) compared, in a single-blind randomized study, naltrexone to placebo in 30 men with idiopathic erectile impotence. It was found that sexual performance was improved in 11 out of the 15 naltrexone-treated patients, whereas placebo had no significant effects. Libido was not affected and there were no side-effects. In general, the adverse effects of naltrexone are transient and mild, but hepatocellular injury may be produced with high doses.

In a randomized, placebo-controlled, double-blind pilot study of 20 patients with idiopathic, non-vascular, non-neurogenic, erectile dys-function, van Ahlen et al (1995) found no significant effect on libido or frequency of sexual intercourse, but early morning erections increased significantly.

It cannot be excluded that increased inhibition by opioid peptides may be a factor contributing to non-organic erectile failure, and that naltrexone therapy in these cases may be a useful therapeutic agent. However, well-controlled studies confirming this are lacking.

Dopamine receptor agonists

It is well established that dopaminergic mechanisms may be involved in the regulation of male sexual behavior in animals (Bitran and Hull 1987; Foreman and Hall 1987). Apomorphine, a dopamine receptor agonist that stimulates both dopamine D_1 and D_2 receptors, has been shown to induce penile erection in rats (Lal et al 1984) and impotent (Lal et al 1987, 1989) men. L-Dopa may also stimulate erection in patients with Parkinson's disease (see, for example, Vogel and Schoffter 1983). It has been suggested that dopamine D_2 receptor stimulation may induce penile erection in rats, while activation of D_1 receptors has the opposite effect (Zarrindast et al 1992). In rhesus monkeys, quinelorane, a dopamine D_2 receptor agonist, produced penile erection (Pomerantz 1991), favoring the view that D_2 receptor stimulation is important for this response. This may be the case also in men (Lal et al 1989). However, clinical trials with quinelorane were discontinued prematurely before its efficacy could be assessed.

Injected apomorphine

Lal et al (1984) showed in a placebo-controlled, double-blind study on healthy volunteers that apomorphine, injected subcutaneously

(0.25–0.75 mg), was able to induce erection. This was confirmed by Danjou et al (1988), showing that apomorphine induced erection and potentiated the erection induced by visual erotic stimulation. There was no increase in libido, which was in agreement with previous observations (Julien and Over 1984). In 28 patients with impotence, Lal et al (1989) found that 17 responded with erection after subcutaneous apomorphine (0.25–1.0 g); no erection developed after placebo. Segraves et al (1991) also administered apomorphine subcutaneously (0.25–1.0 g) to 12 men with psychogenic impotence in a double-blind and placebo-controlled study. They found a dose-related increase in maximal penile circumference. An erection exceeding 1 cm was obtained in 11 of the 12 patients.

It cannot be excluded that a subgroup of impotent patients may have an impairment of central dopaminergic functions, and that the principle of dopamine receptor stimulation may be used not only diagnostically, but also therapeutically. The therapeutic potential of apomorphine, however, seems to be limited mainly because of frequently occurring side-effects. High doses (up to 5–6 mg in adult patients) may cause respiratory depression and, in the low-dose range (0.25–0.75 mg), where effects on penile erection can be demonstrated, emesis, yawning, drowsiness, transient nausea, lacrimation, flushing, and dizziness (Lal et al 1984; Segraves et al 1991) may occur. In addition, apomorphine is not effective orally and has a short duration of action. Even if Lal et al (1987) observed that non-responders, experienced side-effects, agents representing the principle of dopamine stimulation other than apomorphine may be useful.

Oral apomorphine

Heaton and coworkers (1995) reported that apomorphine, absorbed through the oral mucosa, will act as an erectogenic agent. In 12 impotent patients with no documentable organic disease, but with proven erectile potential, 3 or 4 mg apomorphine in a sublingual controlled-release form produced significantly durable erections in 67% without adverse effects. These results suggest that sublingual apomorphine has a potential to be an effective agent for some patients with erectile dysfunction.

Trazodone

Trazodone is an "atypical" antidepressive agent, which has been shown to selectively inhibit central 5-HT uptake. It increases the turnover of brain dopamine, but does not prevent the peripheral re-uptake of norepinephrine (Gergotas et al 1982). In addition, tra-zodone has been demonstrated to block receptors for 5-HT and dopamine, whereas its major metabolite, *m*-chlorophenylpiperazine (*m*-CCP), has agonist activity at 5-HT_{2C} receptors (Monsma et al 1993). This metabolite induces erection in rats and selectively increases the spontaneous firing rate of the cavernous nerves (Steers and de Groat 1989). The mode of action of trazodone in depression is not fully understood; it has a marked sedative action. Trazodone has a serum half-life of about 6 h and is extensively metabolized.

Blanco and Azadzoi (1987) showed that trazodone and its major metabolite had an α-adrenoceptor-blocking effect in isolated human cavernous tissue. Later investigations confirmed that trazodone, in concentrations obtained in blood after intake of clinically relevant doses, had an inhibitory effect on isolated corpus cavernosum prepa-rations contracted by norepinephrine or electrical stimulation (Saenz de Tejada et al 1991). However, the active metabolite, *m*-CCP, seemed to have no significant peripheral effects.

Orally administered trazodone has been associated with priapism in potent men (Azadzoi et al 1990), and with increased nocturnal erectile activity in healthy volunteers (Saenz de Tejada et al 1991). When injected intracavernously into patients with impotence, trazodone caused tumescence, but not full erection (Azadzoi et al 1990). Intracavernous trazodone acted as an α-adrenoceptor antagonist, but was not as effective as papaverine or a combination of papaverine and phentolamine (Azadzoi et al 1990). Positive clinical experience with the drug has been reported (Lance et al 1995). However, in a double-blind, placebo-controlled trial on 69 patients with erectile dysfunction of different etiologies, no effect of trazodone (150 mg/day) could be demonstrated (Meinhardt et al 1997).

The potential of trazodone in the treatment of penile erectile dys-function has not been fully explored. The drug may be an alternative in some anxious or depressed men.

Conclusions and future aspects

Even if intracavernous treatment of erectile dysfunction has made great progress since the introduction of papaverine and phenoxybenzamine, there is still room for improvement. Local, non-injection administration may be developed to an effective on-demand therapy for inducing erec-tion. Oral treatment with apomorphine, and particularly with sildenafil, is promising, and these drugs may be important in the strategy of future treatment of erectile dysfunction. One could look forward to a rational approach to erectile disorders based on the proposed etiology of dysfunction. Following failure of one or more oral agents, intraurethral or intracavernous drug treatment could be tried.

Acknowledgement

This study was supported by the Swedish Medical Research Council (grant no. 6837).

References

Adaikan PG, Kottegoda SR, Ratnam AA (1986). Is vasoactive intestinal polypeptide the principal transmitter involved in human penile erection? *J Urol* **135**:638–40.

van Ahlen H, Piechota HJ, Kias HJ, et al (1995). Opiate antagonist in erectile dysfunction: a possible new treatment option? Results of a pilot study with naltrexone. *Eur Urol* **268**:246–50.

Alaranta S, Uusitalo H, Hautamäki AM, et al (1991). Calcitonin gene-related peptide: immunohistochemical localization in, and effects on, the bovine penile artery. *Int J Impot Res* **3**:49–59.

Andersson K-E (1992). Clinical pharmacology of potassium channel openers. *Pharmacol Toxicol* **70**:244–54.

Andersson K-E (1993). The pharmacology of lower urinary tract smooth muscles and penile erectile tissues. *Pharmacol Rev* **45**:253–308.

Andersson K-E (1994). Pharmacology of erection: agents which initiate and terminate erection. *Sexuality and Disability* **12**:53–79.

Andersson K-E, Stief CG (1997). Neurotransmission, contraction and relaxation of penile erectile tissues. *World J Urol* **15**:14–20.

Andersson K-E, Wagner G (1995). Physiology of penile erection. *Physiol Rev* **75**:191–236.

Argiolas A, Melis MR (1995). Neuromodulation of penile erection: an overview of the role of neurotransmitters and neuropeptides. *Prog Neurobiol* **47**:235–55.

Arvis G, Rivet G, Schwent B (1996). Utilisation prolongée de chlorhydrate de moxisylyte (Icavex®) en auto-injections intra-caverneuses dans le traitement de l'impuissance. *J Urol (Paris)* **102**:151–6.

Azadzoi KM, Payton T, Krane RJ, et al (1990). Effects of intracavernosal trazodone hydrochloride: animal and human studies. *J Urol* **144**:1277–82.

Azadzoi KM, Kim N, Brown LM, et al (1992). Endothelium-derived nitric oxide and cyclooxygenase products modulate corpus cavernosum smooth muscle tone. *J Urol* **147**:220–5.

Becker AJ, Stief CG, Schulthesis D, et al (1997). Double blind study on oral phentolamine as treatment for erectile dysfunction. *J Urol* **157**:202 (abstract 785).

Benassi-Benelli A, Ferrari F, Pellegrini-Quarantotti B (1979). Penile erection induced by apomorphine and N-n-propylnorapomorphine in rats. *Arch Int Psychodyn Ther* **242**:241–7.

Bitran D, Hull EM (1987). Pharmacological analysis of male rat sexual behavior. *Neurosci Biobehav Rev* **11**:365–89.

Blanco R, Azadzoi KM (1987). Characterization of trazodone-associated priapism. *J Urol* **136**:203A.

Boolell M, Allen M, Ballard S, et al (1996). Sildenafil: an orally active type 5 cyclic CMP-specific phosphodiesterase inhibitor for the treatment of penile erectile dysfunction. *Int J Impot Res* **8**:47–52.

Brindley GS (1986). Pilot experiments on the actions of drugs injected into the human corpus cavernosum penis. *Br J Pharmacol* **87**:495–500.

Burnett AL, Nelson RJ, Calvin DC, et al (1996). Nitric oxide-dependent penile erection in mice lacking neuronal nitric oxide synthase. *Mol Med* **2**:288–96.

Bush PA, Aronson WJ, Buga GM, et al (1992). Nitric oxide is a potent relaxant of human and rabbit corpus cavernosum *J Urol* **147**:1650–5.

Buvat J and the Multicenter Study Group (1997). Sildenafil (Viagra), an oral treatment for erectile dysfunction; a 1-year open-label, extension study. *J Urol* **157**:204 (abstract 793).

Buvat J, Lemaire A, Buvat-Herbaut M, et al (1989). Safety of intracavernous injections using an alpha-blocking agent. *J Urol* **141**:1364–7.

Buvat J, Buvat-Herbaut M, Lemaire A, et al (1991). Reduced rate of fibrotic nodules in the cavernous bodies following auto-intracavernous injections of moxisylyte compared to papaverine. *Int J Impot Res* **3**:123–8.

Buvat J, Lemaire A, Buvat-Herbaut M (1996). Intravenous pharmacotherapy: comparison of moxisylyte and prostaglandin E_1. *Int J Impot Res* **8**:41–6.

Cavallini C (1991). Minoxidil versus niotroglycerin: a prospective double-blind controlled trial in transcutaneous erection facilitation for organic impotence. *J Urol* **146**:50–3.

Charney DS, Heninger GR (1986). Alpha2-adrenergic and opiate receptor blockade. *Arch Gen Psychiatry* **43**:1037–41.

Charney DS, Heninger GR, Sternberg DE (1982). Assessment of alpha2-adrenergic autoregulator function in humans: effects of oral yohimbine. *Life Sci* **30**:2033–41.

Charney DS, Heninger GR, Redmond Jr DE (1983). Yohimbine induced anxiety and increased noradrenergic function in humans: effects of diazepam and clonidine. *Life Sci* **33**:19–29.

Chen J-K, Hwang TIS, Yang C-R (1992. Comparison of effects following the intracorporeal injection of papaverine and prostaglandin E1. *Br J Urol* **69**:404–7.

Chen RN, Lakin MM, Montague DK, et al (1995). Penile scarring with intracavernous injection therapy using prostaglandin E1: a risk factor analysis. *J Urol* **154**:138–40.

Claes H, Baert L (1989). Transcutaneous nitroglycerin therapy in the treatment of impotence. *Urol Int* **44**:309–12.

Clark JT, Smith ER, Davidson JM (1984). Enhancement of sexual motivation in male rats by yohimbine. *Science* **225**:847–8.

Crossman D, McEwan J, MacDermott J, et al (1987). Human calcitonin gene-related peptide activates adenylate cyclase and releases prostacyclin from human umbilical vein endothelial cells. *Br J Pharmacol* **92**:695–701.

Crowley TJ, Simpson A (1978). Methadone dose and human sexual behavior. *Int J Addict* **13**:285–95.

Danjou P, Alexandre L, Warot D, et al (1988). Assessment of erectogenic properties of apomorphine and yohimbine in man. *Br J Clin Pharmacol* **26**:733–9.

De Groat WC, Booth AM (1993). Neural control of penile erection. In: *The Autonomic Nervous System*, Vol. 6, *Nervous Control of the Urogenital System*, ed CA Maggi, pp. 465–513. Harwood Academic Publishers, London.

Delcour C, Wespes E, Vandenbosch G, et al (1987). The effect of papaverine on arterial and venous hemodynamics of erection. *J Urol* **138**:187–9.

Derouet H, Eckert R, Trautwein W, et al (1994). Muscular cavernous single cell analysis in patients with venoocclusive dysfunction. *Eur Urol* **25**:145–50.

Derry F, Gardner BP, Glass C, et al (1997). Sildenafil (Viagra): a double-blind, placebo-controlled, single-dose, two-way crossover study in men with erectile dysfunction caused by traumatic spinal injury. *J Urol* **157**:181 (abstract 702).

Fabbri A, Janini EA, Gnessi L, et al (1989). Endorphins in male impotence: evidence for naltrexone stimulation of erectile activity in patient therapy. *Psychoneuroendocrinology* **14**:103–11.

Fahrenkrug J (1989). VIP and autonomic neutransmission. *Pharmacol Ther* **45**:515–34.

Feelisch M (1992). Cellular and non-cellular metbolism of organic nitrates to nitric oxide: involvement of enzymic and non-enzymic pathways. In: *The Biology of Nitric Oxide, I. Physiological and clinical aspects*, ed. S Moncada, MA Marletta, JB Hibbs Jr, EA Higgs, pp. 13–17. Portland Press Proceedings, London.

Ferrari M (1974). Effects of papaverine on smooth muscle and their mechanisms. *Pharmacol Res Commun* **6**:97–115.

Foreman MM, Hall JL (1987). Effects of D2 dopaminergic receptor stimulation on male rat sexual behavior. *J Neural Transm* **68**:153–70.

Galitzky J, Rivière D, Tran MA (1990). Pharmacodynamic effects of chronic yohimbine treatment in healthy volunteers. *Eur J Clin Pharmacol* **39**:447–51.

Georgotas A, Forsell TL, Mann JJ, et al (1982). Trazodone hydrochloride: a wide spectrum antidepressant with a unique pharmacological profile. A review of its neurochemical effects, pharmacology, clinical efficacy, and toxicology. *Pharmacotherapy* **2**:255–67.

Gerstenberg TC, Metz P, Ottesen B, et al (1992). Intracavernous self-injection with vasoactive intestinal polypeptide and phentolamine in the management of erectile failure. *J Urol* **147**:1277–9.

Giuliano FA, Rampin O, Benoit G, et al (1995). Neural control of penile erection. *Urol Clin North Am* **22**:747–66.

Giuliano FA, Rampin O, Benoit G, et al (1997). The peripheral pharmacology of erection. *Progrès en Urologie* **7**:24–33.

Gloub M, Zia P, Mastsuno M (1975). Metabolism of prostaglandins A and E1 in man. *J Clin Invest* **56**:1404–10.

Goldberg MR, Robertson D (1983). Yohimbine: a pharmacological probe for study of the α_2-adrenoceptor. *Pharmacol Rev* **35**:143–80.

Goldstein JA (1986). Erectile function and naltrexone. *Ann Intern Med* **105**:799.

Goldstein A, Hansteen RW (1977). Evidence against involvement of endorphine in sexual arousal and orgasm in man. *Arch Gen Psychiatry* **34**:1179–80.

Gregoire A (1992). New treatments for erectile impotence. *Br J Psychiatry* **160**:315–26.

Gwinup G (1988). Oral phentolamine in non-specific erectile insufficency. *Ann Intern Med* **109**:162–3.

Hakenberg O, Wetterauer U, Koppermann U, et al (1990). Systemic pharmacokinetics of papaverine and phentolamine: comparison of intravenous and intracavernous application. *Int J Impot Res* **2** (suppl 2):247–8.

Hashmat AI, Abrahams J, Fani K, et al (1991). A lethal complication of papaverine-induced priapism. *J Urol* **145**:146–7.

Heaton JPW (1989). Synthetic nitrovasodilators are effective, in vitro, in relaxing penile tissue from impotent men: the findings and their implications. *Can J Physiol Pharmacol* **67**:78–81.

Heaton JPW, Morales A, Adams MA, et al (1995). Recovery of erectile function by the oral administration of apomorphine. *Urology* **45**:200–6.

Heaton JPW, Adams MA, Morales A (1997). A therapeutic taxonomy of treatments for erectile dysfunction: an evolutionary imperative. *Int J Impot Res* **9**:115–21.

Hedlund H, Andersson K-E (1985). Contraction and relaxation induced by some prostanoids in isolated human penile erectile tissue and cavernous artery. *J Urol* **134**:1245–50.

Hedlund H, Andersson K-E, Fovaeus M, et al (1989a). Characterization of contraction-mediating prostanoid receptors in human penile erectile tissues. *J Urol* **141**:182–6.

Hedlund H, Andersson K-E, Holmquist F, et al (1989b). Effect of the thromboxane receptor antagonist AH 23848 on human isolated corpus cavernosum. *Int J Impot Res* **1**:19–25.

Hellstrom WJG, Bennett AH, Gesundheit N, et al (1996). A double-blind, placebo-controlled evaluation of the erectile response to transurethral alprostadil. *Urology* **48**:851–6.

Hieble JP, Bylund DB, Clarke DE, et al (1995). International Union of Pharmacology X. Recommendation nomenclature of α_1-adrenoceptors: consensus update. *Pharmacol Rev* **47**:267–70.

Holmquist F, Andersson K-E, Hedlund H (1992). Characterization of inhibitory neurotransmission in the isolated corpus cavernosum from rabbit and man. *J Physiol (London)* **449**:295–311.

Huang PL, Dawson T, Bredt DS, et al (1993). Targeted disruption of the neuronal nitric oxide synthase gene. *Cell* **75**:1273–86.

Imagawa A, Kimura K, Kawanishi Y, et al (1989). Effect of moxisylyte hydrochloride on isolated human penile corpus cavernosum tissue. *Life Sci* **44**:619–23.

Imhof PR, Garnier B, Brunner L (1975). Human pharmacology of orally administered phentolamine. In: *Phentolamine in Heart Failure and Other Cardiac Disorders*, Proceedings of an International Workshop, London, November 1975, ed. SH Taylor, LA Gould, pp. 11–22. Hans Huber Publishers, Berne.

Ishii N, Watanabe H, Irisawa M (1986). Intracavernous injection of prostaglandin E1 for the treatment of erectile impotence. *J Urol* **141**:323–5.

Jacobsen FM (1992). Fluoxetin-induced sexual dysfunction and an open trial of yohimbine. *J Clin Psychiatry* **53**:119–22.

Julien E, Over R (1984). Male sexual arousal with repeated exposure to erotic stimuli. *Arch Sexual Behav* **13**:211–21.

Jünemann K-P (1992). Pharmacotherapy of impotence: where are we going? In: *World Book of Impotence*, ed. TF Lue, pp. 181–8. Smith-Gordon, London.

Jünemann K-P, Alken P (1989). Pharmacotherapy of erectile dysfunction: a review. *Int J Impot Res* **1**:71–93.

Jünemann K-P, Lue TF, Fournier Jr GR, et al (1986). Hemodynamics of papaverine and phentolamine-induced penile erection. *J Urol* **136**:158–61.

Kiely EA, Bloom SR, Williams G (1989). Penile response to intracavernosal vasoactive intestinal polypeptide alone and in combination with other vasoactive agents. *Br J Urol* **64**:191–4.

Kimoto Y, Kessler R, Constantinou CE (1990). Endothelium dependent relaxation of human corpus cavernosum by bradykinin. *J Urol* **144**:1015–17.

Kirkeby H-J, Forman A, Andersson K-E (1990). Comparison of the papaverine effects on isolated human penile circumflex veins and corpus cavernosum. *Int J Impot Res* **2**:49–54.

Krejs GJ (1988). Effect of vasoactive intestinal peptide in man. *Ann N Y Acad Sci* **527**:501–7.

Kunelius P, Häkkinen J, Lukkarinen O (1997). Is high-dose yohimbine hydrochloride effective in the treatment of mixed-type impotence? A prospective, randomized, controlled double-blind crossover study. *Urology* **49**:441–4.

Lal S, Ackman D, Thavundayil JX, et al (1984). Effect of apmorphine, a dopamine receptor agonist, on penile tumescence in normal subjects. *Prog Neuro-Psychopharmacol Biol Psychiatry* **8**:695–9.

Lal S, Laryea E, Thavundayil JX, et al (1987). Apomorphine-induced penile tumescence in impotent patients–preliminary findings. *Prog Neuro-Psychopharmacol Biol Psychiatry* **11**:235–42.

Lal S, Tesfaye Y, Thavundayil JX, et al (1989). Apomorphine: clinical studies on erectile impotence and yawning. *Prog Neuro-Psychopharmacol Biol Psychiatry* **13**:329–39.

Lance RL, Albo M, Costabile RA, et al (1995). Oral trazodone as empirical therapy for erectile dysfunctions: a retrospective review. *Urology* **46**:117–20.

Levin RM, Wein AJ (1980). Adrenergic alpha-receptors outnumber beta-receptors in human penile corpus cavernosum. *Invest Urol* **18**:225–6.

Linet OI, Ogrinc FG (1996). Efficacy and safety of intracavernosal alprostadil in men with erectile dysfunction. *N Engl J Med* **334**:873–7.

Lomas GM, Jarow JP (1992). Risk factors for papaverine-induced priapism. *J Urol* **147**:1280–1.

Longman SD, Hamilton TC (1992). Potassium channel activator drugs: mechanism of action, pharmacological properties, and therapeutic potential. *Med Res Rev* **12**:73–148.

Lue TF and The Sildenafil Study Group (1997). A study of sildenafil (Viagra), a new oral agent for the treatment of male erectile dysfunction. *J Urol* **157**:181 (abstract 701).

McCall JM, Aiken JW, Chidester CG, et al (1983). Pyrimidine and triazine 3-oxide sulfates: a new family of vasodilators. *J Med Chem* **26**:1791–3.

McMahon CG (1996). A pilot study of the role of intracavernous injection of vasoactive intestinal peptide (VIP) and phentolamine mesylate in the treatment of erectile dysfunction. *Int J Impot Res* **8**:233–6.

Martinez-Pineiro L, Lopez-Tello J, Alonso Dorrego JM, et al (1995). Preliminary results of a comparative study with intracavernous sodium nitroprusside and prostaglandin E1 in patients with erectile dysfunction. *J Urol* **153**:1487–90.

Meinhardt W, Schmitz PIM, Kropman RF, et al (1997). Trazodone, a double blind trial for treatment of erectile dysfunction. *Int J Impot Res* **9**:163–5.

Meyhoff HH, Rosenkilde P, Bødker A (1992). Non-invasive management of impotence with transcutaneous nitroglycerin. *Br J Urol* **69**:88–90.

Miller MAW, Morgan RJ (1994). Eicosanoids, erections and erectile dysfunction. *Prostaglandins Leukot Essent Fatty Acids* **51**:1–9.

Mogilnika E, Klimek V (1977). Drugs affecting dopamine neurons and yawning behaviour *Pharmacol Biochem Behav* **31**:303–5.

Molderings GJ, van Ahlen H, Göthert M (1992) Modulation of noradrenaline release in human corpus cavernosum by presynaptic prostaglandin receptors. *Int J Impot Res* **4**:19–26.

Monsma FJ, Shen Y, Ward RP (1993). Cloning and expression of a novel serotonin receptor with high affinity for tricyclic psychotropic drugs. *Mol Pharmacol* **43**:320–7.

Montorsi F, Strambi LF, Guazzoni G, et al (1994). Effect of yohimbine–trazodone on psychogenic impotence: a randomized, double-blind, placebo-controlled study. *Urology* **44**:732–6.

Morales A, Condra M, Owen JA (1987). Is yohimbine effective in the treatment of organic impotence? Results of a controlled trial. *J Urol* **137**:1168–72.

Moreland RB, Traish A, McMillan MA, et al (1995). PGE1 suppresses the induction of collagen synthesis by transforming growth factor-β1 in human corpus cavernosum smooth muscle. *J Urol* **153**:826–34.

Muramatsu I, Ohmura T, Hashimoto S, et al (1995). Functional subclassification of vascular α_1-adrenoceptors. *Pharmacol Commun* **6**:23–8.

Owen JA, Nakatsu SL, Fenemore J, et al (1987). The pharmacokinetics of yohimbine in man. *Eur J Clin Pharmacol* **32**:577–82.

Owen JA, Saunders F, Harris C, et al (1989). Topical nitroglycerin: a potential treatment for impotence. *J Urol* **141**:546–8.

Padma-Nathan H, Bennett AH, Gesundheit N, et al (1995). Treatment of erectile dysfunction by the medicated urethral system for erection (MUSE). *J Urol* **153**:473A.

Padma-Nathan H, Hellstrom WJG, Kaiser FE, et al (1997). Treatment of men with erectile dysfunction with transurethral alprostadil. *N Engl J Med* **336**:1–7.

Palmer JBD, Cuss FM, Warren JB, et al (1986). Effect of infused vasoactive intestinal peptide on airway function in normal subjects. *Thorax* **41**:663–6.

Parr D (1976). Sexual aspects of drug abuse in narcotic addicts. *Br J Addict* **71**:261–8.

Persson K, Garcia-Pascual A, Andersson K-E (1992). Differences in the actions of calcitonin gene-related peptide (CGRP) in pig detrusor and vesical arterial smooth muscle. *Acta Physiol Scand* **143**:45–53.

Pomerantz SM (1991). Quinelorane (LY 163502), a D2 dopamine receptor agonist, acts centrally to facilitate penile erections of male rhesus monkeys. *Pharmacol Biochem Behav* **39**:123–8.

Porst H (1993). Prostaglandin E1 and the nitric oxide donor linsidomine for erectile failure: a diagnostic comparative study of 40 patients. *J Urol* **149**:1280–3.

Porst H (1996). A rationale for prostaglandin E1 in erectile failure: a survey of worldwide experience. *J Urol* **155**:802–15.

Price LH, Charney DS, Heninger GR (1984). Three cases of manic symptoms following yohimbine administration. *Am J Psychiatry* **141**:1267–8.

Price DT, Schwinn DA, Kim JH, et al (1993). Alpha1 adrenergic receptor subtype mRNA expression in human corpus cavernosum. *J Urol* **149**:285A (abstract 287).

Reden J (1990) Molsidomine. *Blood Vessels* **27**:282–94.

Reid K, Morales A, Harris C, et al (1987). Double-blind trial of yohimbine in treatment of psychogenic impotence. *Lancet* **i**:421–3.

Renganathan R, Suranjan B, Kurien T (1997). Comparison of transdermal nitroglycerin and intracavernous injection of papaverine in the treatment of erectile dysfunction in patients with spinal cord injuries. *Spinal Cord* **35**:99–103.

Riley AJ, Goodman RE, Kellet JM, et al (1989). Double blind trial of yohimbine hydrochloride in the treatment of erection inadequacy. *Sex Marital Ther* **4**:17–26.

Rosenkranz B, Winkelmann BR, Parnham MJ (1996). Clinical pharmacokinetics of molsidomine. *Clin Pharmacokinet* **30**:372–84.

Roy AC, Adaikan PG, Sen DK, et al (1989). Prostaglandin 15-hydroxydehydrogenase activity in human penile corpora cavernosa and its significance in prostaglandin-mediated penile erection. *Br J Urol* **64**:180–2.

Roy JB, Petrone RL, Said S (1990). A clinical trial of intracavernous vasoactive intestinal peptide to induce penile erection. *J Urol* **143**:302–4.

Saenz de Tejada I, Ware JC, Blanco R, et al (1991). Pathophysiology of prolonged penile erection associated with trazodone use. *J Urol* **145**:60–4.

Segraves RT, Bari M, Segraves K, et al (1991). Effect of apomorphine on penile tumescence in men with psychogenic impotence. *J Urol* **145**:1174–5.

Seidmon EJ, Samaha Jr AM (1989). The pH analysis of papaverine–phentolamine and prostaglandin E1 for pharmacological erection. *J Urol* **141**:1458–9.

Smith ER, Lee RL, Schnur SL, et al (1987a). Alpha 2-adrenoceptor antagonists and male sexual behaviour: I. mating behaviour. *Physiol Behav* **41**:7–14.

Smith ER, Lee RL, Schnur SL, et al (1987b). Alpha 2-adrenoceptor antagonists and male sexual behavior: II. erectile and ejaculatory reflexes. *Physiol Behav* **41**:15–19.

Sønksen J, Biering Sørensen F (1992).Transcutaneous nitroglycerin in the treatment of erectile dysfunction in spinal cord injured. *Paraplegia* **30**:554–7.

Stackl W (1992). Comment on 'Pharmacotherapy of impotence'. In: *World Book of Impotence*, ed. TF Lue, p. 189. Smith-Gordon, London.

Steers WD (1990). Neural control of penile erection. *Semin Urol* **8**:66–79.

Steers WD, De Groat WC (1989). Effects of m-chlorophenylpiperazine on penile and bladder function in rats. *Am J Physiol* **257**:R1441–9.

Steers WD and the Sildenafil Study Group (1997). Sildenafil (Viagra) is effective in the treatment of severe male erectile dysfunction. 2nd Meeting of the European Society for Impotence Research, Madrid, October 1–4, 1997, abstract 55.

Stief CG, Bernard F, Bosch RJLH, et al (1990). A possible role for calcitonin-gene-related peptide in the regulation of the smooth muscle tone of the bladder and penis. *J Urol* **143**:392–7.

Stief CG, Holmquist F, Allhof EP, et al (1991a). Preliminary report of the effect of the nitric oxide (NO) donor SIN-1 on human cavernous tissue in vivo. *World J Urol* **9**:237–9.

Stief CG, Wetterauer U, Schaebsdau F, et al (1991b). Calcitonin-gene-related peptide: a possible role in human penile erection and its therapeutical application in impotent patients. *J Urol* **146**:1010.

Steif CG, Holmquist F, Djamilian M (1992). Preliminary results with the nitric oxide donor linsidomine chlorhydrate in the treatment of human erectile dysfunction. *J Urol* **148**:1437–40.

Stief CG, Übert S, Truss M (1995). Cyclic nucleotide phosphodiesterase (PDE) isoenzymes in human cavernous smooth muscle: characterization and functional effects of PDE-inhibitors in vitro and in vivo. *Int J Impot Res* Suppl 1:6–7.

Susset JG, Tessier CD, Wincze J, et al (1989). Effect of yohimbine hydrochloride on erectile impotence: a double-blind study. *J Urol* **141**:1360–3.

Talley JD, Crawley IS (1985). Transdermal nitrate, penile erection and spousal headache. *Ann Intern Med* **103**:804.

Tanaka T (1990). Papaverine hydrochloride in peripheral blood and the degree of penile erection. *J Urol* **143**:1135–7.

Tarhan T, Kuyumcuoglu U, Kolsuz A, et al (1996). Effect of intracavernosal sodium nitroprusside in impotence. *Urol Int* **56**:211–14.

Taylor S, Sutherland G, MacKenzie GJ, et al (1965). The circulatory effect of intravenous phentolamine. *Circulation* **31**:741–54.

Traish A, Netsuwan N, Daley J, et al (1995). A heterogenous population of α_1-adrenergic receptors mediates contraction of human corpus cavernosum smooth muscle to norepinephrine. *J Urol* **153**:222–7.

Traish A, Gupta S, Toselli P, et al (1996). Identification of α_1-adrenergic receptor subtypes in human corpus cavernosum tissue and in cultured trabecular smooth muscle cells. *Receptor* **5**:145–57.

Trigo-Rocha F, Hsu GL, Donatucci CF, et al (1993). The role of cyclic adenosine monophosphate, cyclic guanosine monophosphate, endothelium and nonadrenergic, noncholinergic neurotransmission in canine penile erection. *J Urol* **149**:872–7.

Truss MC, Becker AJ, Thon WF (1994a). Intracavernous calcitonin gene-related peptide plus prostaglandin E1: possible alternative to penile implants in selected patients. *Eur Urol* **26**:40–5.

Truss MC, Becker AJ, Djamilian MH, et al (1994b). Role of the nitric oxide donor linsidomine chlorhydrate (SIN-1) in the diagnosis and treatment of erectile dysfunction. *Urology* **44**:553–6.

Turchi P, Canale D, Ducci M, et al (1992). The trandsdermal route in the treatment of male sexual impotence: preliminary data on the use of yohimbine. *Int J Impot Res* **4**:45–50.

Virag R (1982). Intracavernous injection of papaverine for erectile failure. *Lancet* **ii**:938.

Vogel HP, Schiffter R (1983). Hypersexuality – a complication of dopaminergic therapy in Parkinson's disease. *Pharmacopsychiatry* **16**:107–10.

Vogt H-J, Brandl P, Kockott G (1997). Double-blind, placebo-controlled safety and efficacy trial with yohimbine hydrochloride in the treatment of nonorganic erectile dysfunction. *Int J Impot Res* **9**:155–61.

Wagner G, Gerstenberg T (1988). Vasoactive intestinal peptide facilitates normal erection. In *Proceedings of the Sixth Biennial International Symposium for Corpus Cavernosum Revascularization and the Third Biennial World Meeting on Impotence*, Boston, Massachusetts, October 6–9, p. 146.

Wegner HEH, Knispel HH, Klän R, et al (1994). Prostaglandin E1 versus linsidomine chlorhydrate in erectile dysfunction. *Urol Int* **53**:214–16.

Wespes E, Rondeux C, Schulman CC (1989). Effect of phentolamine on venous return in human erection. *Br J Urol* **63**:95–7.

Wildgrube HJ, Ostrowski J, Chamberlain J, et al (1986). 3-Morpholinosydnonimine in healthy volunteers. *Arzneim Forsch (Drug Res)* **36**:1129–33.

Zarrindast M-R, Shokravi S, Samini M (1992). Opposite influences of dopaminergic receptor subtypes on penile erection. *Gen Pharmacol* **23**:671–5.

Zorgniotti AW (1992). "On demand" erection with oral preparations for impotence: 3-(N-(2-imidazoline-2ylmethyl)-p-toluidinol) phenol mesylate. *Int J Impot Res* **4**(suppl 2):A99.

Zorgniotti AW, Lafleur RS (1985). Auto-injection of the corpus cavernosum with a vasoactive drug combination for vasculogenic impotence. *J Urol* **133**:39–41.

8

A unified taxonomy of erectogenic drugs

Jeremy P W Heaton

Introduction

Erectile dysfunction (ED) is common (Feldman et al 1994), underdiagnosed, undertreated and important from the point of view of personal, social and economic impact. We have a good understanding of the complexities of the peripheral neural and penile systems. We have known for many years from many epidemiological (Feldman et al 1994; Lauman et al 1994), clinical and laboratory (Karacan et al 1977; Bauer et al 1978; Thase et al 1988) studies what are the most common associations of ED. We are clear on some processes that actually cause ED with high frequency (Lue et al 1983), but there is still a fundamental problem in defining diagnostic criteria that allow a classification that is clear, universally understood and relevant to predicting clinical outcomes and prognosis. Without this objectivity and reproducibility diagnostic criteria and classification will mean little. Remember, having diagnostic criteria has proved invaluable in evolving meaningful treatment strategies in many common disease entities. We have only to look at cancer diagnosis to see how a good classification system can help in the understanding and management of the disease itself. Within the framework of these classifications the understanding then increases in a logical way. This progress is usually achieved through an iterative cycle of hypothesis testing, trial and observation. The original classifications develop subsets that are more precise and the cycle of investigation and refinement continues.

Treatment classification

The field of treatment for ED is at a watershed in the late 1990s. A vast wealth of new agents is about to enter common use and the field is without a clear usable basis for etiologic diagnosis. So there is little, aside from the art of medicine, to guide the practitioner in choosing appropriate therapy for ED. Little harm may be done with benign treatments by implementing a policy of sequential trial and error. But it is clear that there are different reasons for men to end up with the symptom of erectile failure. It is also clear that the treatments are not equivalent in mechanism, time-course, effect, side-effect, cost and probably in many other respects. It would be unusual, and ultimately naïve, to suggest that a single drug will successfully treat everyone. Therefore there must be a way of matching mankind and medicine.

A rational taxonomy that brings all treatments into a single classification will at least provide some clarity. It should accelerate the ability of prescribers to match patient with therapy. It should lead to a better definition of patients, by reason of their response to drugs within a defined class. It should improve the accuracy of communication, which will facilitate education within the specialties and of the patients and public. Used well, such concepts could improve the design of trials and the comparison of treatments. It will also open the way to helpful diagnostic and etiologic definitions. Such a scheme has been proposed for treatments (Heaton et al 1997) and a simple conceptual key to this is shown in Figure 1 (Heaton, 1998).

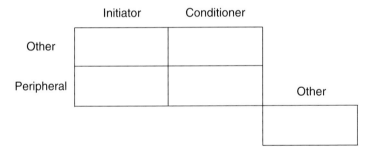

Figure 1
Treatments are placed in this classification on the basis of their intended prime mechanism of action as a treatment for ED. (Copyright of JPW Heaton.)

Defining the man with erectile dysfunction

In the past a single diagnostic group was felt to explain most cases of ED – psychogenic impotence (Hengenvelt 1991). When there is only one known cause there hardly needs to be a classification scheme. Finding that this did not provide any real depth of understanding or open any therapeutic windows, clinicians turned to a new, but potentially treatable, explanation – hormones. Regardless of the biochemical clues, hormones were blamed for erectile difficulties and testosterone was prescribed (Braunstein 1983). Serum testosterone should have been the ideal diagnostic criterion to determine which patients needed this treatment. As we now know, serum values are only helpful in patients with profound, and usually relatively acute, reductions in serum testosterone. Interestingly, we are still not very clear how to interpret subtle hormonal changes, or even which serum value to look at, or how to predict the benefits of treatment with testosterone (Morales et al 1997). Perhaps for these and other reasons the testosterone issue has a life of its own, and testosterone is still frequently and erroneously prescribed for ED as a first-line drug – simple concepts, such as sex hormones, are difficult to overwrite, especially when the real explanations are still blurred.

The penile prosthesis was the first treatment available that actually managed, uniquely, the problem of a penis not rigid enough for intercourse (Bogoras 1936; Scott et al 1973). The issue became how to define which patients should get this treatment. Effective as it is, the placement of a penile prosthesis is an irreversible step, and it is clear that patients with transient or reversible causes of ED should not undergo this treatment without a reasonable assessment. Again, this introduced the need to define the characteristics of a patient population that was suited to a particular form of treatment. Since prostheses were, and are, effective the main requirement was to define a population who really did not get erections – the 'organically' impotent men, for whom there would be no alternative treatment. Nocturnal penile tumescence and rigidity (NPTR) testing appeared to offer a logical division between men who had some endogenous potential for erection and men in whom even night-time erections had disappeared (Marshall et al 1981). At least a negative NPTR (no night-time erection of significance) would document that there were no readily available erections and provide the surgeon and patient with some degree of comfort that definitive, even drastic, measures were justified. From this perspective and the studies of NPTR itself came a hope that NPTR would separate psychogenic from organic ED. These concepts are flawed, as countless authors have pointed out – for instance depressed or sleep-derived patients may not have positive NPTR, but they may be able to have intercourse.

The psychogenic versus organic dichotomy was a frustrating concept to test and verify (Derogatis et al 1976). It held out the promise of radically different populations deserving fundamentally different treatments. Some of the underlying concepts are still useful today, but the labels are too flexible to apply with any degree of precision. The

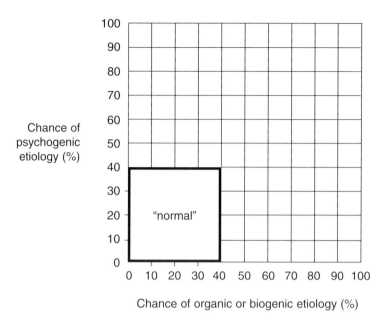

Figure 2
A conceptual representation of the orthogonal relationship of organic and psychogenic factors as they relate to the etiology of erectile dysfunction.

real information about any patients classified into these two catch-alls is contained in exactly how the categories are defined. For instance, in drugs trials any precision of these diagnostic labels is to be found only in the detail of the exclusion criteria. The value of the labels, organic or psychogenic, in the absence of this detail is modest. So this intuitively appealing classification still appears, and may help, but is usually used only as a general reference to a type of patient.

This is not a good forum in which to enter into a full analysis of the issues of organic versus psychogenic classification, but it is instructive to point to why it may not be a reasonable basis for classification as originally proposed. Classifications may work if they are definable and largely mutually exclusive – they have relevance only if they are useful in practical decision-making. Placing organic and psychogenic etiologies at opposite ends of a linear scale offers the hope that a dividing line may be drawn to distinguish one from the other. Lopiccolo has suggested that psychogenic factors and organic, or biogenic, factors could more properly be placed on orthogonal axes (Figure 2). This construct allows that a man, for example, with no recognized medical disease could have the same risk of severe psychologic problems with impact on erectile function as his neighbor who has just had radical extirpative pelvic surgery. It explains graphically why searching for mutual exclusivity in the organic versus psychogenic classifications is unlikely to be a definitive help. None of this explains how to incorporate the organic, biochemical, cellular, molecular or genetic content of psychogenic factors, but then that is a completely different and important discussion. The point here is that organic and psychogenic are convenient constructs that are so difficult to define and apply that, while they may guide the art of practice in ED, they are not useful as classifications.

Classification of drug response

With the advent of intracavernous injection (ICI) therapy whole new possibilities for understanding emerged. In fact ICI came from observation (Virag 1982) and scientific understanding, and spawned a whole new, and very productive, cycle of research and clinical progress that continues today. Lue has been very influential in guiding our thinking about ICI with his intuitively appealing "goal-directed therapy" (Lue 1990). The essence of this approach is to mix patient needs with a choice of effective therapy – make the therapy suit their goals. The fundamental application of this principle can be found in the simple sequence: try ICI; if ICI works, and is acceptable, use it. This test actually classifies patients into ICI responders and non-responders (largely on a pharmacologic basis). Clinical follow-up would subdivide responders into long-term users and non-users. This is the first clear demonstration, in clinical ED management, of a therapeutic agent being used to define a population of men with ED – the therapy-as-classifier.

The implications of this inadvertent and unexpected classification are profound. A man on successful ICI might be offered the equivalent drug by an alternative route. This suggestion arises out of the understanding that a prostaglandin E_1 (PGE_1) ICI responder should also respond to PGE_1 applied in different ways. It also teaches that drugs that are equivalent to PGE_1 should also work. It probably indicates, about the individual, that there is functional cavernosal smooth muscle, good arterial inflow and not too much abnormal cavernous collagen. Probably, other drugs with direct action on vasoconstrictor or vasodilator smooth muscle systems will also work well. In fact, as Lue and others recognized, the simple response of a man to a test injection of PGE_1, even if aided by other stimulants, means that this is a therapy that may be used at home. But it also means a lot more than that – it actually fits the man into a category of "ED that is amenable to ICI therapy." As treatments evolve, without further analysis or instruction, the prescribers will recognize the message in a good response to ICI and use it to direct their patients to try new therapies. The ICI trial classifies ED in a very functional way.

There are many other tests for ED that have been designed with exclusively diagnostic intent, such as dynamic infusion cavernosometry, duplex ultrasound, magnetic resonance imaging (MRI), selective arteriography, etc. These might have provided a basis for diagnostic classification that could be used to select different treatments, but in several years of use no diagnostic criteria have been widely accepted and used. The purely diagnostic approach was less successful than the therapy-as-classifier – the trial of ICI. A few focused diagnostic situations are important. Discrete arterial lesions may be identified and repaired, but these are not common and have success rates that would not justify widespread adoption of this intervention (Sharlip 1991). Similarly, venous leak identification and repair have fallen out of general favor because they too failed to deliver high enough success rates (Lewis 1997), probably because the tests were poorly executed (Hatzichristou et al 1995) and the conceptual understanding of the etiologic process was flawed.

It would not be fair to say that our diagnostic tests have been a total failure. But it is true today that a trial of therapy in an individual provides almost all the information needed for rational therapeutic planning in a majority of patients. As we enter a phase of rapid growth in available therapies we should recognize the utility and simplicity of using therapeutic trials as classifiers and predictors. Hence, a classification based on broad concepts of drug type and action will serve our patients well. Responders within one class will be likely to be responders to equivalent drugs from the same class. Partial successes with a drug from a class given optimally may indicate the need for the adjunctive use of drugs from another class. Clinical trials of the drugs will identify responders, and we will then learn the distinguishing features of these men in the responding group. Looking at these men, their disease and their response in a critical fashion will enable us to design or select alternative or even more specific therapies.

The field of ED should be classified as shown in Figure 1. This classification will allow clinicians to understand the differences and similarities between the new therapies. To use the route of administration as a distinctive characteristic, say, is not enough. For instance, oral drugs will be able to act in many ways in the future to treat many specific defects – that is a poor basis for a therapeutic class. Also, to group drugs simply by their chemical action may not be helpful enough – although it is certainly a valid pharmacologic classification system, and may ultimately be the therapeutic/diagnostic key of choice. For example, phosphodiesterase inhibitors and adrenoceptor blockers act to amplify smooth muscle relaxation in the periphery – until we become sophisticated in understanding the distinct smooth muscle flaws that require one or another treatment specifically, it is enough to know that there is some overlap in their application, although efficacies may or may not be equivalent.

The careful characterization of responders to specific classes of therapy will enable us to determine true etiologic factors. These responders will have characteristics that could be identifiable prospectively, and the emphasis will then shift to the other side of the cycle – classifying patients, not therapies, by known and predictive features. For instance patients may be found to be phosphodiesterase inhibitor-dependent – and for these men their treatment option is obvious.

Before this clean level of understanding emerges we will undoubtedly go through a phase of management that is a simple extension of the "goal-directed" approach: "We have a new medication, try it, if it works that's the one for you." However, individual drugs will not work in everybody. Some agents will be better in some patients than others. Eventually, with a large and pharmacologically sophisticated selection, the right drug for an individual, the one that works best all around, will be selected on the basis of a real etiologic defect that is being targeted for treatment. Think of how sophisticated the actions of anti-neoplastic drugs have become in comparison to their progenitors. This precision is in the future for ED.

This is just the first tentative step in improving classification, and it is possible because of the new expansion in drug availability that we face in the final years of the twentieth century. If a classification can help practitioners formulate strategic therapeutic decisions and improve clinical response rates then it will also teach about mechanisms of dysfunction and direction to look for new therapies. It will lead to diagnostic classifications based on logical trials of therapy, just like those Lue gave us so insightfully a decade ago. This time the diagnostic classifications will be more complex and based on the responses to drugs with sophisticated and known mechanisms of action. By fixing the spotlight on therapeutic classification now, simple treatment alternatives will be obvious for the first of the new agents, and this will progressively allow diagnostic understanding and outcomes information to catch up and eventually put in place a true (and useful) diagnostic classification.

The matrix of treatment strategies

The classification suggested here rests on the identification of two main characteristics (Heaton et al 1997). First, an erection has to be initiated and, once initiated, may be modulated by changes in the systems that are involved in the erection (conditioners). Secondly, the anatomic target of the drug action has critically different implications in many respects: hence the division of agents into those with preponderantly central versus those with peripheral action. Then, in a non-specific category, there are the other treatments that are peculiar to ED, like prostheses and vacuum devices, which need to be accommodated in a special class. These properties naturally suggest the filled matrix of treatments (Figure 3).

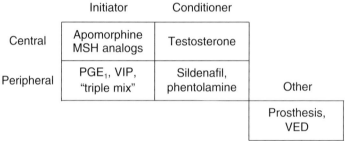

Figure 3
The Matrix of Treatment Strategies (MATS) with representative drugs (as of 1997) entered into the schema. MSH, melanocyte-stimulating hormone; VED, VIP, vasoactive intestinal polypeptide. (Copyright of JPW Heaton)

In this classification the following definitions are suggested – see Table 1.

The putative sites and mechanisms of action of each drug intended for the treatment of ED should be considered as each drug is classified. The specificity of the actions of new drugs will permit a functional classification of ED subtypes based on patient responses. These classifications will be amenable to specific diagnosis, using the therapy-as-classifier principles. The increasing specificity of drugs, and consequently the increasing understanding of patient subtypes, will enable prescribers to target treatments much more closely to the biochemical dysfunctions causing individual ED. As this increase in precision spreads through clinical practice the clinical outcomes will improve and the adverse components of treatment will decrease.

Even now we do not have to place a penile prosthesis in men that respond to PGE_1. We will, in the future, be able to treat some men

Table 1   The functional definitions of the classes identified in the Matrix of Treatment Strategies

Class and name	Definition
I. Central initiator	Compounds that have the main site of action in the CNS to activate neural events that result in coordinated signaling which results in the initiation of a penile erection
II. Peripheral initiator	Compounds that have the main site of action in the periphery to activate events that result in a penile erection
III. Central conditioner	Compounds that act mainly to improve the internal milieu of the CNS so that penile erection is enabled or enhanced, but do not on their own initiate an erection
IV Peripheral conditioner (local or systemic)	Compounds that act mainly to improve the local or systemic internal milieu so that penile erection is enabled or enhanced
V. Other	Other ways of promoting penile rigidity, including devices and surgery

with oral agents targeted, say, to their inability to initiate an erection. Not only will these men not have to be injected; they will take a drug by mouth a few minutes before an erection is required, and by their response we will know how to classify them diagnostically. We will be able logically to select from a range of therapeutic agents once we have a therapeutic classification.

The implications of a system of therapeutic classification

This classification provides tools useful in assessing drugs:

- We will be able to compare agents within logical classes.
- We will be able to select patient populations based on therapeutic response.
- We will be able to select instruments of evaluation appropriate to therapeutic class.

One of the early and intuitive consequences of this understanding is that different standards of rigidity may be appropriate for different classes of therapy. This may be a point to consider in interpreting, or designing, studies of drugs. If you replace cavernous tissue with an inert substitute you should apply a high standard of rigidity, whereas an intervention of lesser invasiveness will be acceptable to patients with standards of rigidity and reliability that are proportionately less impressive. Since there is no standard erection that will satisfy all needs, and one is not likely to be formulated, a single number for 'satisfactory rigidity' is unlikely to have much value across classes.

Since it is likely that there will be differences in the characteristics of patients needing or choosing therapies from the different classes, it is also logical to expect them to have different goals – not only individually but also collectively. Consequently "home-use success" instruments may be helpful to compare drugs within a homogeneous class, but may be much less accurate compared across classes. For example, the target percentage of home-use success (successful intercourse per attempt) for a peripheral initiator requiring injection would probably be higher than that for an oral peripheral conditioner, yet the overall indices of satisfaction for the patients might be equal for each of them.

Truly equivalent comparisons of different agents would be much easier to make within a class than across classes. And, within a class, route of delivery, selectivity and timing of action will have further implications in making effective comparisons.

Central initiators

The factors that act as central initiators which are most familiar to patients and the ED specialist are endogenous: erotic images and ideation, nocturnal penile tumescence (NPT), non-genital touching. Drugs that have been associated with central initiation include apomorphine (Heaton et al 1995), other dopamine agonists, serotonin agonists, oxytocinergic agonists and melanocyte-stimulating hormone (MSH) analogs (Wessells et al 1997). These drugs, in certain circumstances, are also active in peripheral systems, promoting effects via receptors at a range of concentrations usually far above those required for central nervous system (CNS) effects. An agent with a central mode of action takes advantage of the natural amplification that occurs between the CNS and the effector systems in the periphery. These central processes are, however, susceptible to a sensitive balance of excitatory and inhibitory influences. The output from the CNS will be dramatically affected by inhibitory factors such as noxious stimuli, stress and behavioral restrictions. The final erectogenic signaling from the CNS, even if originating with a central initiator, will be modified by these inhibitory factors, and there may be, in parallel, an activation of peripheral erectolytic signaling – for instance, increased sympathetic tone.

Thus drugs in this class produce erections only as well as the peripheral endogenous systems permit. They may specifically treat failures of erectile initiation, but should also be expected to have activity where there is insufficient neural signal to enforce adequate vasodilatation, but where additional vasodilator capacity is available – circumstances now commonly referred to as minor organic disease and "situational stress."

Peripheral initiators

Both patients and specialists are most familiar with peripheral initiators because they were the first approved drugs for ED and because of their pre-eminence in the ED market in the late 1990s. The drugs for peripheral initiation have been chosen because of their known effects in the vasculature in causing vasodilatation. Currently PGE_1 forms the basis of the most common forms of treatment.

The penis is highly accessible to the direct introduction of agents, and so almost anything that will cause vasodilatation has been used for ICI. The drugs cause erections because of their overwhelming effect in relaxing intracavernous smooth muscle, almost, but not entirely, regardless of what neural signals there are. The route of administration is currently by ICI (Linet and Ogrinc 1996) or transurethral (TU) (Padma-Nathan et al 1997), although transdermal strategies are being developed.

These vasoactive agents bring about changes in the function of the penile vasculature, either by interacting directly with the vascular smooth muscle cells (VSMC) or, indirectly, by actions which lead to the release of vasoactive agents from vascular endothelial cells (for instance nitric oxide (NO) (Rajfer et al 1992) and prostacyclin (PGI_2) (Furchgott and Zawadski 1980; Palmer et al 1987)). Whatever the chemical form of the therapy, if it is to be applied in the periphery with the intention of causing an erection then it should be counted in this class (triple therapy (Padma-Nathan 1990); new forms of PGE_1 for ICI; SIN-1 (Stief et al 1992); VIP (Gerstenberg et al 1992); calcitonin gene-related peptide or CGRP; (Stief et al 1991); K^+ channel openers (Spektor et al 1997)).

Drugs in this class should have, as a standard of efficacy, the best erection that the supplying vasculature, blood pressure and penile anatomy can support. In low doses, and in agents with low efficacy (such as phentolamine ICI monotherapy), the effects should be susceptible to modulation by neural erectogenic and erectolytic signals. Drugs in this class may be expected to demonstrate the most robust responses of which the penis is capable, although the lack of pelvic vessel recruitment makes their onset time less impressive than what is possible with a centrally stimulated erection.

Central conditioners

Testosterone (Morales et al 1994) is the clearest example of a drug capable of conditioning CNS components of the erectile cascade. Testosterone has growth and organizational effects in the CNS and also acute effects that are permissive on erectile function. There is some evidence to suggest that there is variable sensitivity to androgenic effects in the CNS-to-penis pathways (Carani et al 1992).

Peripheral conditioners

This is the class of agents and mechanisms that is currently being pursued most vigorously. These agents increase activity of peripheral systems that support or cause erections. There are pharmacologic strategies that can be employed to increase the effect of a normal pro-erectile system. In simple terms a pro-erectile pathway can be enhanced (increasing sensitivity, decreasing neurotransmitter inactivation, etc.) or a balancing or erectolytic pathway can be attenuated.

In subsequent chapters there will be much more detail about the mechanism of action of phosphodiesterase (PDE) inhibitors (PDEI) (Virag et al 1996) – they slow the "degradation" of the active cyclic nucleotide, causing activity to be prolonged. The selectively of action of a PDEI depends on its action on the isoforms of the PDEs responsible for penile erection. Sympatholytic agents reduce general vasoconstrictive α-adrenergic activity (Porst et al 1996) and are mainly dependent on the timing of administration for their selectivity for erectile processes.

These agents depend for their effect on the existence of activity in the erectile system – i.e. an initiated erection. For example, a PDEI significantly decreases the degradation of the cyclic nucleotide only when the cyclic nucleotide system is operating at activities above basal levels. They are therefore the most difficult to standardize from the point of view of assessment. There is no standardized stimulus (to get the process going) and, since the total response will be dependent on both the stimulus and the agent, study design becomes critically important.

Summary

The Matrix of Therapeutic Strategies described here provides a first classification based on relatively clear characterizations. It should be possible to place any drug in its most appropriate class with reasonable reproducibility. Within a class there is a basis for closer comparisons of drug equivalence and a basis for selecting certain evaluative strategies. The lack of overlap between classes, at least in terms of the intended mode of action, suggests that there will be logical combinations of drugs that could be assembled in clinical practice which use suitable agents from each of two or more classes. It is vital that prescribers, and patients, have useful results of good trials of these agents to guide them.

This breadth of choice in therapeutic agents illustrates the multiplicity of mechanisms that determine erectile function and also how interrelated these mechanisms are. Selecting a drug to take advantage of a determining mechanism in erectile function has never before covered such a wide range of possibilities. Across these approaches the playing field is not even – some mechanisms are more potent than others, some drugs have more adverse systemic effects, and some drugs require more invasive delivery strategies than others. No single mechanism can stand out as overwhelming,and no single drug will treat all patients with ED.

References

Bauer GE, Baker J, Hunyor SN, Marshall P (1978). Side-effects of antihypertensive treatment: a placebo-controlled study. *Clin Sci Mol Med* **4** (suppl): 341S–4S.

Bogoras NA (1936). Uber die volle plastiche Weiderherstellung eines rum koitus fahigen Penis (Peniplastica totalis). *Zentralbl Chir* **63**:1271.

Braunstein GD (1983). Endocrine causes of impotence. Optimistic outlook for restoration of potency. *Postgrad Med* **74**:207.

Carani C, Bancroft J, Granata A, et al. (1992). Testosterone and erectile function, nocturnal penile tumescence and rigidity, and erectile response to visual erotic stimuli in hypogonadal and eugonadal men. *Psychoneuroendrocrinology* **17**:647–54.

Derogatis LR, Meyer JK, Dupkin CN (1976). Discrimination of oganic versus psychogenic impotence with the DSFI. *J Sex Marital Ther* **2**:229–40.

Feldman HA, Goldstein I, Hatzichristou DG, et al (1994). Impotence and its medical and psychosocial correlates: Results of the Massachusetts Male Aging Study. *J Urol* **151**:54–61.

Furchgott RF, Zawadzi JV (1980). The obligatory role of endothelial cells in the relaxation of arterial smooth muscle by acetylcholine. *Nature* **288**:373–6.

Gerstenberg TC, Metz P, Ottesen B, et al (1992). Intracavernous self-injection with vasoactive intestinal polypeptide and phentolamine in the management of erectile failure. *J Urol* **147**:1277–9.

Hatzichristou DG, Saenz de Tehada I, Kupferman S, et al (1995). In vivo assessment of trabecular smooth muscle tone, its application in pharmaco-cavernosometry and analysis of intracavernous pressure determinants. *J Urol* **153**:1126.

Heaton JPW (1998). Neural and pharmacological determinants of erection. *Int J Impot Res* in press.

Heaton JPW, Morales A, Adams M, et al (1995). Recovery of erectile function by oral administration of apomorphine. *Urology* **45**:200–3.

Heaton JPW, Adams MA, Morales A (1997). A therapeutic taxonomy of treatments for erectile dysfunction: an evolutionary imperative. *Int J Impot Res* **9**:115–21.

Hengenvelt MW (1991). Erectile disorders: a psychosexological review. In: *Erectile Dysfunction*, eds U Jonas, WF Thon, CG Steif, p. 207 Springer-Verlag, Berlin.

Karacan I, Scott FB, Salis PJ, et al (1977). Nocturnal erections, differential diagnosis of impotence, and diabetes. *Biol Psychiatry* **12**:373–80.

Lauman EO, Gagnon JH, Michael RT, Michaels S (eds) (1994). *The Social Organization of Sexuality*, The University of Chicago Press, Chicago.

Lewis RW (1997). *Venous Surgery for Impotence in Male Infertility and Sexual Dysfunction*, ed. WJG Hellstrom, pp. 503–13. Springer-Verlag, New York.

Linet OL, Ogrinc FG (1996). Efficacy and safety of intracavernousal alprostadil in men with erectile dysfunction. *N Engl J Med* **334**:873–7.

Lue TF (1990). Impotence: A patient's goal-directed approach to treatment. *World J Urol* **8**:67–74.

Lue TF, Takamura T, Schmidt RA, Tanagho EA (1983). Potential preservation of potency after radical prostatectomy. *Urology* **22**:165–7.

Marshall P, Surridge DHC, Delva N (1981). The role of nocturnal penile tumescence in differentiating between organic and psychogenic impotence: The first stage of validation. *Arch Sex Behav* **10**:1–7.

Morales A, Johnson B, Heaton JPW, et al (1994). Oral androgens in the treatment of hypogonadal impotent men. *J Urol* **152**:1115.

Morales A, Johnston B, Heaton JPW, Lundie M (1997). Testosterone supplementation for hypogonadal impotence: Assessment of biochemical measures and therapeutic outcomes. *J Urol* **157**:849–54.

Padma-Nathan H (1990). The efficacy and syngery of polypharmacotherapy in primary and salvage therapy of vasculogenic erectile dysfunction. *Int J Impot Res* **2**(suppl 2):257–8.

Padma-Nathan H, Hellstrom WJG, Kaiser FE, et al (1977). Treatment of men with erectile dysfunction with transurethral alprostadil. *N Engl J Med* **336**:1–7.

Palmer RM, Ferrige AG, Moncada S (1987). Nitric oxide release accounts for the biological activity of endothelium-derived relaxing factor. *Nature* **327**:524–6.

Porst H, Derouet H, Idzikowski M, et al (1996). Oral phentolamine (Vasomax) in erectile dysfunction – results of a German Multicenter-Study in 177 patients. *Int J Impot Res* **8**:117.

Rajfer J, Aronson WJ, Bush PA (1992). Nitric oxide as a mediator of relaxation of the corpus cavernosum in response to nonadrenergic, noncholinergic neurotransmission. *N Engl J Med* **362**:90–4.

Scott FB, Bradley WE, Timm GE (1973). Management of erectile impotence: use of implanatable inflatable prosthesis. *Urology* **2**:80.

Sharlip I (1991). The incredible results of penile vascular surgery. *Int J Impot Res* **3**:16.

Spektor M, Rosenbaum R, Melman A, et al (1997). Further demonstration of the physiological relevance of potassium (K) channels to contraction of human corporal smooth muscle *in vitro*. *J Urol* **157**(4):149.

Stief CG, Wetterauer U, Schaebsdau FH, et al (1991). Calcitonin gene-related peptide: a possible role in human penile erection and its therapeutic application in impotent patients. *J Urol* **146**:1010–14.

Stief CG, Holmquist F, Djamilian M, et al (1992). Preliminary results with the nitric oxide donor linsidomine chlorhydrate in the treatment of human erectile dysfunction. *J Urol* **148**:1437–40.

Thase ME, Reynolds CF III, Jennings JR, et al. (1988). Nocturnal penile tumescence is diminished in depressed men. *Biol Psychiatry* **24**:33.

Virag R (1982). Intracavernous injection of papaverine for erectile failure. *Lancet* **ii**:398.

Virag R, Hodges M, Hollingshead M, et al (1996). Sildenafil (Viagra™) a new oral treatment for erectile dysfunction (ED): an 8 week double-blind, placebo-controlled parallel group study. *Int J Impot Res* **8**:116(A70).

Wessells H, Hansen JG, Fucciarelli K, et al (1997). Melanotropic peptide for the treatment of psychogenic erectile dysfunction: Double blind placebo controlled crossover dosing study. *J Urol* **157**:201.

9

Andropause, sexual endocrinopathies and their treatment

Alvaro Morales

Endocrinological alterations are frequently implicated in the development of male erectile dysfunction (ED). In some conditions, such as diabetes mellitus, the development of microvascular and autonomic and peripheral neuropathy leads to failure of the erectile mechanisms. In others, the suggestion of a causal relationship is purely circumstantial and remains unproven. However, there are two recognized alterations of the hypothalamus–pituitary–gonadal axis clearly associated with the development of ED: hypogonadism and hyperprolactinemia. This chapter will deal exclusively with the therapy of these two conditions. It should be mentioned from the outset that both endocrinopathies are uncommon causes of ED (Nickel et al 1984). But, despite the rarity of hypogonadal ED (HED), there is a pervasive and indiscriminate use of exogenous androgens on men complaining of ED. This is due, in large part, to the availability of medication capable of correcting the biochemical parameters in the serum of impotent men and the deeply ingrained view that androgen supplementation will result in an overall enhancement of sexual performance. Nevertheless, in no other cause of ED do currently available drugs fulfill so well the ideal model of pharmacological treatment as in these two hormonal abnormalities associated with impotence. The stipulations for such ideal treatment are that it should be: (1) condition-specific; (2) effective; (3) usable "on demand"; (4) free of side effects; (5) easy to administer; and (6) affordable (Morales et al 1995).

Despite the apparent immediate availability of effective medication, the situation regarding hormonal therapy – as will be shown below – is not as simple as it first appears.

Hypogonadism and erectile dysfunction

The estimates for either primary or secondary hypogonadism as a cause of impotence vary (Spark et al 1980; Nickel et al 1984), but are in the vicinity of 10%. On the basis of the common experience it is generally believed that hypogonadal impotence should exhibit both (i) a decrease in libido associated with insufficient erectile quality for intromission and (ii) clear evidence of abnormally low levels of serum total testosterone (tT) and free testosterone (fT). Hyperprolactinemia may or may not be present, and the levels of luteinizing hormone (LH) may be normal or elevated. It is recognized that waking erections of adequate quality are preserved in some hypogonadal states, while sleep erections are usually absent. Other features are often added to those criteria (testicular size and the absence of vasculopathy and psychopathology). However, clinical observations by us (Morales et al 1997) and others (Johnson and Jarow 1992) with regard to the futility of serum testosterone (T) and other endocrine markers in the diagnosis and monitoring of ED, even in biochemically hypogonadal men, are forcing us to question this system of patient assessment. The standard criteria should be maintained until better markers of hypogonadism become available. The causal relationship between prolactinemia and impaired sexual performance has not been questioned, since the elevated levels of this hormone appear to correlate well with libido. It is clear that the fundamental problem with hypogonadism is a matter of definition, since there is no question that agonadal (usually for surgical reasons) men benefit greatly from androgen supplementation. In both situations – hypogonadism and hyperprolactinemia – the borderline biochemical abnormalities are the hardest to interpret and the results of their treatment are the most difficult to evaluate.

The majority of patients complaining of impotence who are found, after investigation, to be hypogonadal are men over the age of 55 years. It is well established that there is a progressive androgen decline in the aging man (ADAM), which has been erroneously equated to the menopause in women. Hypoestrogenism leading to menopause is a well-recognized clinical situation, while ADAM and its consequences remain a controversial issue. It is known, however, that in men advancing age is associated with a decrease in both total and free plasma testosterone (T) and an increase in both the plasma levels of sex hormone-binding globulin and the sensitivity of gonadotropins to androgen feedback, as well as a flattening of the circadian variations in plasma T (Vermeulen 1991). It remains to be defined whether the same biochemical criteria (plasma hormone levels) can be applied to the older as to the young male population. To complicate matters, it is not known whether target organ sensitivities to androgens are the same in old as in young men. The implications of these poorly defined issues for therapy are obvious.

Although it is evident that testosterone supplementation for the hypogonadal or agonadal young man is usually mandatory, the situation may be different for the older man. The adverse effects of hypo-testosteronemia include osteoporosis, decrease in lean body mass, lower red cell counts and hemoglobin, and alterations in sexual response, mood, and cognitive functions. There is increasing evidence that some of these abnormalities may be reversed with testosterone supplementation (Tenover 1994).

Gonadal steroids

The central control for the episodic secretion of LH, and the resulting production of gonadal steroids is based on the hypothalamus, through its secretion of gonadotropin-releasing hormone (GnRH). A variety of steroids is of importance in reproductive and sexual function in men. Testosterone, secreted primarily by the Leydig cells of the testicle, is,

Table 1   Classification of male hypogonadism

Hypothalamic–pituitary disorders
Panhypopituitarism
Isolated LH deficiency
LH and follicle-stimulating hormone (FSH) deficiency (Kallmann's syndrome)
Biologically inactive LH

Gonadal abnormalities
Klinefelter's syndrome
Other chromosomal defects
Bilateral anorchia
Leydig cell aplasia
Adult Leydig cell failure
Defects in androgen biosynthesis
ADAM

Defects in androgen action
Complete androgen insensitivity (testicular feminization)
Incomplete androgen sensitivity
    a. Type I
    b. Type II 5α-reductase deficiency

quantitatively, the most important androgen. The testicle also secretes smaller amounts of dehydroepiandrosterone (DHEA), a weaker androgen that is primarily produced by the adrenal gland. Recent studies suggest that DHEA may play a more important role than previously suspected, and may become a significant supplemental androgen in the future (Barbagallo et al 1995). The classification of hypogonadism is shown in Table 1. Most of the conditions listed are rare, and seldom seen while investigating men with ED. However, severe hypogonadism not due to obvious causes (such as bilateral orchidectomy or

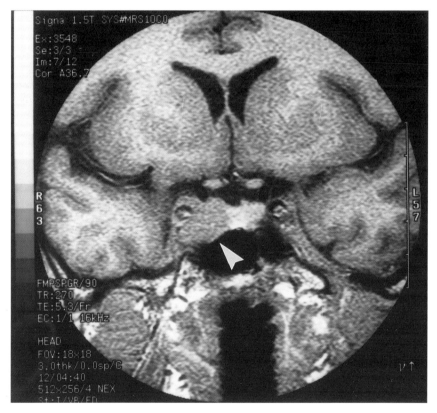

Figure 1
Magnetic resonance imaging scan of the pituitary in a 43-year-old man presenting with a profound decrease in libido. He was hypogonadal and was found to have serum prolactin levels > 300 ng/ml. A 15-mm macroadenoma with minor suprasellar, prepontine, and cavernous sinus extension (white arrow) is clearly visible.

Table 2   Currently available testosterone formulations

Mode	Generic name	Brand name	Recommended dose
Injectable	Testosterone cypionate	Depo-Testosterone PMS-Testosterone	200–300 mg i.m. every 2–4 weeks
	Testosterone enanthate	Delatestryl	200–300 mg i.m. every 2–4 weeks
Oral	Testosterone undecanoate	Andriol	120–160 mg/day in three divided doses
	Fluoxymesterone	Halotestin	10 mg three times daily
	Methyl testosterone	Metandren Virilon	10 mg three times daily
Transdermal	Transdermal testosterone	Androderm	5 mg per day

drugs) requires a thorough evaluation before embarking on a course of supplemental androgen administration. The most common central causes of ED include empty sellar syndrome and hyperprolactinomas (Figure 1). Among the non-iatrogenic causes of hypogonadism the most frequently seen is Klinefelter's syndrome.

Selection of supplemental androgens

Commercially available testosterone preparations and their recommended doses are listed in Table 2. Any of them, when administered appropriately, will invariably result in normal or even supranormal levels of plasma testosterone. This, of course, is not a reliable indication of successful therapy; the outcome should be based, primarily, on the response reported by the patient in regard to improvement in mood and sensation of well-being and on the improvement in sexual parameters such as excitement and performance (Morales et al 1997).

Except for the recommendations of the National Institutes of Health (NIH) Conference on Impotence no practical guidelines exist for the treatment of the hypogonadal impotent man. The recommendations of the NIH Panel are of little use because they failed to provide guidance as to who should benefit from androgen supplementation. In addition, the panel considered acceptable only the injectable esters of testosterone. But there are safe and effective oral and transdermal preparations that are gaining rapid acceptance in the medical community as an alternative to the injectable forms of testosterone. We have developed a set of practical guidelines for exogenous androgen administration. Table 3 shows a summary of the recommendations from this document (Morales et al 1996).

Currently, there is no evidence that supplemental testosterone is of any benefit to eugonadal men. On the contrary, the evidence suggests that men with normal or only marginally low levels of serum testosterone are poor responders to exogenous androgenic steroids. Profound hypogonadism responds best. The practical pros and cons of commonly used preparations are listed in Table 4.

A great deal of concern has been expressed about their effects in a number of metabolic and organ system functions. These include: (1) body composition; (2) bone metabolism; (3) lipid profile; (4) hematological and biochemical parameters; (5) liver function (cholestatic hepatitis and hepatic cancer); and (6) the prostate (promoting of benign prostatic hyperplasia (BPH) and enhancement of carcinoma).

Physicians are particularly aware of these concerns because the various forms of testosterone are prescribed to a population of men who

Table 3   Summary of the clinical practice guidelines for testosterone supplementation in hypogonadic men

1. There must be a clear indication for treatment
2. If an indication exists, no patient is too old for therapy
3. Hypogonadotropic hypogonadism should be thoroughly investigated before treatment
4. Patients > 40 years old should have a digital rectal examination (DRE) and prostate-specific antigen (PSA) determination
5. Mild benign prostatic hyperplasia is a relative contraindication for androgen supplementation but patients with advanced obstructive symptoms are not suitable candidates
6. Known or suspected cancer of the prostate or breast is an absolute contraindication
7. Oil-based testosterone injectables, oral testosterone undecanoate and transdermal preparations are recommended. 17-Alkylated steroids carry a potential for serious toxicity
8. Initially, patients should be followed regularly to rule out adverse effects (ie, lower urinary obstruction and to perform DRE and PSA determination
9. Serum levels of testosterone fluctuate considerably, particularly with the injectable esters. Oral and transdermal routes result in more stable levels
10. Biochemical parameters (eg, serum testosterone) are not reliable indicators of therapeutic results. Patient's self-report is a better and more relevant outcome measure

are usually over 50 years of age, at a stage when alterations of lipid metabolism and effects on the prostate gland may carry serious complications. Early studies have shown that testosterone supplementation in aging males results in an increase in erythopoiesis and lean body mass. More recent studies by Tenover (1992, 1994) have confirmed these findings, but have further shown that patients receiving exogenous testosterone exhibit a significant decline in total cholesterol and low-density lipoprotein cholesterol. Her observations have been further supported by Friedl et al (1990), Marin et al (1992) and Barret-Connor (1992). In addition the recent study of Phillips et al (1994) investigated parameters of sex hormones and their influence in the occurrence of myocardial infarction (MI), and showed that "the correlations found in this study between testosterone and the degree of coronary artery disease and between testosterone and other risk factors for MI raise the possibility that in men hypotesteronemia may be a risk factor for coronary arteriosclerosis." Therefore, the currently available evidence does not support concerns about negative effects on lipid profile for patients receiving exogenous testosterone supplementation.

Urologists frequently express worries about the potential effect of androgen stimulation on the prostate. By now, there is a serious body of information on which to base an opinion on this subject. Experimental evidence has been presented showing that canine prostatic epithelial cells cultured in vitro in the presence or absence of

Table 4   Pros and cons of commonly used preparations in profound hypogonadism

Preparation	Advantages	Disadvantages
Injectable esters (cypionate, enanthate, propionate)	Well tolerated, effective, universally recommended Approximately monthly administration	Intramuscular (i.m.) injection "Roller-coaster" effect Tachyphylaxis
Methyltestosterone	Oral administration	Limited effectiveness Serious liver toxicity
Testosterone undecanoate	Equivalent to intramuscular esters No "roller-coaster" effect Oral administration	Administration 3 times per day Costly
Transdermal testosterone	Easy to use Circadian curve	Daily application Scrotal shaving (for some preparations)

several sex steroids exhibit the same growth pattern regardless of whether steroids are present or not. The same studies demonstrated that the proliferative response was dependent on the time and concentration of serum. Therefore, these investigators (Chevalier et al 1984) concluded that humoral factors other than steroids may be of importance in the activation of epithelial cells leading to the development of prostatic hyperplasia. Short-term clinical studies in aging men treated with injectable testosterone enanthate (100 mg every 3 weeks for 3 months) did not induce a significant increase in prostate size or the amount of post-void residual; but there was a significant increase in the prostate-specific antigen (PSA), which however remained within normal limits (Tenover 1994). The oral undecanoate form of testosterone (TU) has been evaluated in long-term clinical trials. In a controlled study it was found to result in a modest (12%) but statistically significant increase in the gland volume but there were no changes in the values of serum PSA between the readings before, during and after treatment (Marin et al 1992). The discrepancies in findings between these two studies go beyond the differences in the forms of testosterone used. Marine et al treated the patients for a longer period of time, had the PSA samples positioned next to each other in the assay run, and performed the volumetric evaluation of the gland by transrectal ultrasonography. Tenover, on the other hand, determined the PSA values as they were obtained, and the volumetric measures were taken by suprapubic transvesical sonography. Franchi et al (1978), in an 11-month study, found no increase in prostatic size or deterioration of voiding symptoms, but their evaluation was primarily subjective. More recent studies also employing TU help to clarify the picture. Holmang et al (1993) again found no significant increase in serum PSA during 8 months of treatment, while Gooren (1994) documented a mild reduction in urine flow but no increase in prostate size and no evidence of cancer development. An investigation by Bhere et al (1994) has shed a great deal of light on our perception of the role of exogenous testosterone on the prostate gland. In this large and well-designed study hypogonadal men not previously treated with testosterone were compared with age-matched hypogonadic and normal men. The authors concluded that "effective testosterone treatment of hypogonadic men results in prostate volume and prostatic specific antigen levels comparable to age matched normal men. Therefore, testosterone-induced prostate growth should not preclude hypogonadal men from testosterone substitution therapy." These and other studies are reassuring, but not conclusive as to the safety supplemental testosterone for the biological behavior of the gland. Controlled studies with larger cohorts and long periods of treatment and follow-up are mandatory to elucidate these important issues (Vermeulen 1991).

The serious attention given to hepatic toxicity (cholestatic hepatitis and hepatic carcinoma) is based on the well-documented cases in which steroids with a 17α-methyl substituent were employed (Henderson et al 1973; Westaby et al 1977). The short-term (30 days) administration of methylated testosterone is safe but impractical, since these men, normally, require a protracted course of hormonal therapy; in most cases this represents a commitment for life. Conversely, multiple studies have shown that the risk is minimal with the acute or chronic use of the injectable esters or the oral undecanoate preparation (Franchi et al 1978; Holmang et al 1993; Tenover 1994).

Anyone treating men with ED should be familiar with the individual merits and drawbacks of the currently available testosterone preparations when treating hypogonadic patients. The most acceptable to the patients are the oral compounds. Of these, methyl-testosterone requires repeated daily administration, and results in supraphysiological levels of circulating tT with dissociated values of fT (Morales et al 1994). Its major drawbacks include erratic absorption (Wilsen and Griffith 1980) and the previously mentioned hepatic toxicity. The other oral compound is TU, which also requires daily doses at 8-hour intervals, but results in more physiological levels of both serum tT and fT (Morales et al 1997). Its lymphatic absorption requires it to be ingested with meals; this circumvents the first hepatic passage, thus preventing liver toxicity and rapid aromatization. It produces better subjective responses than its methyl counterpart. Both oral forms offer the advantage of stable levels of serum testosterone, thus preventing the ups and downs frequently observed with the injectable esters. In addition, dose titration and adjustment to individual needs are more readily accomplished with oral preparations.

Testosterone patches are relatively new and represent an appealing concept. In a limited study of four patients, McClure et al (1991) reported that their use achieved normal levels of both testosterone and dihydrotestosterone (DHT) and resulted in no hepatic toxicity; there were also no appreciable changes in the lipid profile, although the high-density lipoproteins decreased slightly. This was a short study of 12 weeks. Longer studies using transdermal administration confirm the safety of these preparations (Orwoll et al, 1992). The application of a patch results in a physiological curve of serum testosterone that imitates the circadian serum levels of the hormone. Drawbacks of transdermal testosterone use include the need for daily application – with some formulations to the scrotal skin, where the absorption of the drug is particularly effective. There is also the need to shave the area frequently in order to facilitate its transdermal delivery. More recent preparations do not require scrotal application, but are more frequently associated with significant irritation and blisters from the use of enhancers for transdermal testosterone transport.

Testosterone injectable esters were recommended as the only acceptable form by the panel of the Consensus Conference on impotence (NIH Consensus Conference on Impotence 1993). This view, of course was based on concerns about the toxicity of some oral preparations and disregard for new forms of delivery. The injectable drugs (cypionate, enanthate, or propionate) are generally well tolerated, and remain the gold standard for effectiveness. Drawbacks of these preparations include the need for periodic intramuscular administration (every 2–3 weeks) and the high activity observed in the first 10 days after administration, which is followed by a noticeable decrease towards the end of the cycle (Snyder and Lawrence 1980). Patients and their partners find this "roller-coaster" effect disturbing and unpleasant.

Hyperprolactinemia

Chromophobe adenomas of the pituitary most frequently secrete abnormally high amounts of prolactin (PRL). Most of these tumors are asymptomatic, and nowadays they are frequently discovered during the investigation of a man with ED by the routine measurement of serum PRL levels, although there is a lack of consensus in the literature regarding the value of routine evaluation of serum PRL (Leonard et al 1989; Akpunonu et al 1994). There is agreement, however, on the need to have PRL determinations in men found to be hypogonadal (particularly with hypogonadotropic hypogonadism), especially in men with a main complaint of a marked decreased in libido. The finding of decreased libido is an initial and prominent manifestation of this condition. Galactorrhea is seldom seen in men, while headaches and visual impairment are late manifestations, associated with large tumors. In addition to pituitary tumors there are a number of situations that result in increased PRL secretion. These include: pathologic conditions (chronic renal failure, severe liver disease); drug-induced states (induced by estrogens, dopamine anatagonists, verapamil, or monoamine oxidase inhibitors); and physiological alterations such as intense exercise and stress. In most of these situation the elevations in PRL are modest, seldom reaching the large increases (> 100 ng/ml) noted with prolactinomas. It is not commonly known that there is a heterogeneity in the PRL molecules, and that the macromolecules are biologically inactive. In this regard, an important observation was recently reported by Guay et al (1996) on a group of impotent men found to have elevated serum PRL levels. These men, however, had normal testosterone and gonadotropin levels and negative magnetic resonance imaging (MRI) studies of the pituitary. By specialized separation by column chromatography it was shown that these patients had a predominance of big (60 kDa), big–big (>150 kDa) molecules, which is in contrast to the biologically active small (22 kDa) PRL molecules found in normal individuals. This report emphasizes the need for caution when attributing ED to elevated serum levels of PRL. In Guay's study nocturnal penile tumescence verified the true diagnosis.

Frequently, hyperprolactinemia is associated with low levels of testosterone, and the correction of the pituitary problem may not result in resolution of the sexual dysfunction; supplemental androgens may be necessary (McClure et al 1991). The reverse is also true: testosterone replacement alone is not usually effective until the plasma levels of PRL are within normal range.

Treatment options for hyperprolactinemia

Surgical

Transsphenoidal microsurgery is an effective approach for the treatment of microprolactinomas and often results in long-term remissions, although recurrences of the tumour are likely (Cunnah and Besser 1991). Limited success is reported with this procedure in the treatment of large (>1.5 cm) tumors. Transfrontal craniotomy is rarely employed, and is reserved for patients with major extrasellar extension of the tumor that results in dangerous compression of adjacent structures (the optic chiasma, the internal carotid artery).

Medical

Medical management continues to gain in popularity because of its effectiveness and relatively low risk. It should be mentioned, however, that successful pharmacologic management is limited to a reduction to a normal range of serum PRL levels and resolution of the symptoms. Elimination of the tumor does not occur, since virtually all patients exhibit biochemical and clinical evidence of recurrence following interruption of therapy, even in those cases (> 60%) in which a reduction in tumor size is documented. With the exception of the case of large tumors presenting immediate danger to vital structures, medical therapy is often the preferred initial choice; it is also indicated after incomplete surgical removal of an adenoma.

Dopamine agonists

A number of compounds fall into this category, but only two are used in the treatment of hyperprolactinemia: bromocriptine and pergolide. Bromocriptine is a full agonist at D_2-receptors and a mixed agonist at D_1-receptors, while pergolide, being also a full agonist at D_2-receptors, is ten times more potent than bromocriptine. It is worth mentioning here the effect of another dopamine agonist, apomorphine, on men with a primarily psychogenic ED. Recent studies at our institution have demonstrated it to be an effective erectogenic agent (Heaton et al 1995); however, none of these patients has evidence of hyperprolactinemia, which suggests that dopamine agonists may have a dual effect on erectile function.

Bromocriptine
The drug is administered orally. Because of undesirable side-effects it is best to start with reduced doses such as 1.25 mg once a day, increasing from 2.5 to 10 mg/day in three divided doses. Side-effects common to all dopamine agonists (bromocriptine, pergolide, and apomorphine) include nausea, vomiting, dizziness, and postural hypotension. Side-effects are usually resolved with the continuation of treatment.

Pergolide mesylate
This is used less frequently than bromocriptine in the treatment of hyperprolactinemia. Administration of the drug should be initiated with a single daily dose of 0.05 mg, which is increased progressively to a dose of 1.0–1.5 mg/day in three divided doses. Since pergolide is significantly more active than bromocriptine the progressive increase in dosage should be slower.

Radiotherapy

This modality is restricted to use as an adjuvant to surgery when there is insufficient resolution of the manifestations of the adenoma.

Following the institution of therapy it is important to establish a firm schedule of follow-up, since these tumors are rarely, if ever, completely eliminated. Periodic measures of serum PRL as well as MRI of the sella turcica are indicated. In the presence of a satisfactory bio-chemical response but persistence of the erectile problem or lack of improvement in libido, it is important to ascertain that a concomitant hypogonadism is not present. Patients who have failed to show an improvement when one or both endocrinopathies have been treated deserve a more complete evaluation to rule out the presence of co-morbidity.

Conclusion

The central neuroendocrine interactions and their effect on libido and sexual performance are incompletely understood. Severely hypo-gonadal men promptly lose erectile function during sleep, though many are still able to develop erotic erections, albeit with a significant decrease in sexual interest. Hormonal replacement invariably results in testosterone levels within or above the normal range; however, many of these men experience little improvement in their symptoms. The reasons for this paradoxical response remain to be determined, but clearly reflect the complexity of the human sexual response.

The consequences of aging on sexuality are well recognized. Androgen decline in the aging man, on the other hand, remains an immature field of clinical research, but evidence is rapidly accumu-lating to support the concept that tissue availability of androgens decreases markedly in most men as a consequence of aging, and that this phenomenon translates into significant physical and mental alter-ations. Whether they can be prevented, delayed, or resolved by androgen supplementation remains to be demonstrated. The con-cerns expressed by many about altering a normal process without knowing the consequences in other organ systems are justified. Only through further investigation will these issues be resolved. It is encouraging that the clinical picture is now recognized, and that efforts are directed to the elucidation of the causes and treatment of ADAM.

In February 1998 the 1st World Congress on the Ageing Male took place in Geneva, Switzerland. As a result of this meeting the Geneva Manifesto was developed to promote international multidisciplinary research efforts in this clinical area. Investigators around the world will focus on interventions that may slow the progression of condi-tions such as osteoporosis, cardiovascular disease, Alzheimer's dis-ease, etc by the judicious use of hormonal and other therapies. This is a welcome development with major implications for the next century when over 20% of the world population will be over the age of 65 years.

References

Akpunonu BE, Mutgi AB, Federman BJ, et al (1994). Routine prolactin measurement is not necessary in the initial evaluation of male impotence. *J Gen Intern Med* **9**:336–8.

Barbagallo M, Shan J, PKT, Resnick LM (1995). Effect of dehydroepiandrosterone sulfate on cellular calcium responsiveness to vascular contractility. *Hypertension* **26**:1065–9.

Barret-Connor E (1992). Lower endogenous androgen levels and dyslipidemia in men with non-insulin-dependent diabetes mellitus. *Ann Intern Med* **117**:807.

Bhere HM, Bohmeyer J, Nieschlag E (1994). Prostate volumne in testosterone-treated and untreated hypogondal men in comparison to age-matched controls. *Clin Endocrinol* **40**:341.

Chevalier S, Bleau G, Roberts CD, et al (1984). Non-steroidal serum factors involved in the regulation of the proliferation of canine prostatic epithelial cells in culture. *The Prostate* **5**:503.

Cunnah D, Besser M (1991). Management of prolactinomas. *Clin Endocrinol* **34**:231.

Franchi F, Luisi M, Kicovic PM (1978). Long-term study of testosterone undecanoate in hypogonadal males. *Int J Androl* **1**:270.

Friedl KE, Hannan CJ, Jones RE, et al (1990). High-density lipoprotein cholesterol is not decreased if an aromatizable androgen is administered. *Metabolism* **39**:69.

Gooren LJG (1994). A ten-year safety study of the oral androgen testosterone undecanoate. *J Androl* **15**:212.

Guay AT, Varma S, Sabharwal P, et al (1996). Macroplactinemia causing delay in diagnosis of psychological impotence. *J Clin Endocrinol Metab* **81**:2512–14.

Heaton JPW, Morales A, Adams MA, et al (1995). Recovery of erectile function by the oral administration of apomorphine. *Urology* **45**:200–4.

Henderson JT, Richmond J, Summerling MD (1973). Androgenic–anabolic steroid therapy and hepatocellular carinoma. *Lancet* **i**:934.

Holmang S, Marin P, Lindstedt G, et al (1993). Effect of long-term oral testosterone undecanoate treatment on prostate volume and serum prostate-specific antigen concentration in eugonadal middle-aged men. *The Prostate* **23**:99.

Johnson AR III, Jarow JP III (1992). Is routine endocrine testing for impotent men necessary? *J Urol* **147**:1542–4.

Leonard M, Nickel JC, Morales A (1989). Hyperprolactinemia and impotence. Why, when and how to investigate. *J Urol* **142**:992–5.

McClure RD Oses R, Ernest ML (1991). Hypogonadal impotence treated by transdermal testosterone. *Urology* **37**:224.

Marin P, Holmang S, Jonsson L, et al (1992). The effects of testosterone treatment on body composition and metabolism in middle-aged obese men. *Int J Obesity* **16**:991.

Morales A, Johnston B, Heaton JPW, Clark A (1994). Oral androgens in the treatment of hypogonadal impotent men. *J Urol* **152**:115–18.

Morales A, Heaton JPW, Johnston B, et al (1995). Oral and topical treatment of erectile dysfunction. *Urol Clin North Am* **22**:879–85.

Morales A, Bain J, Ruijs A, et al (1996). Clinical practice guidelines for screening and monitoring male patients receiving testosterone supplementation therapy. *Int J Impotence Res* **8**:95–7.

Morales A, Johnston B, Heaton JPW, et al (1997). Testosterone supplementation for hypogondal impotence: assessment of biochemical measures and therapeutic outcomes. *J Urol* **157**:849–54.

Nickel JC, Morales A, Condra M, et al (1984). Endocrine dysfunction in impotence: incidence, significance and cost-effective screening. *J Urol* **132**:40–4.

NIH Consensus Conference on Impotence (1993). NIH Consensus Development Panel on Impotence. *JAMA* **270**:82–7.

Orwoll E, Oviatt S, Biddle J, et al (1992). Transdermal testosterone supplementation in normal older men. *Abstracts of the 74th Annual Meeting of the Endocrine Society*, p. 319.

Phillips GB, Pinkernell BH, Jing T (1994). The association of hypotestosteronemia with coronary artery disease in men. *Arterioscler Thromb* **14**:701.

Snyder PJ, Lawrence DA (1980). Treatment of male hypogonadism with testosterone enanthate. *J Clin Endocrinol Metab* **51**:1335–41.

Spark RF, White RA, Connolly PB (1980). Impotence is not always psychogenic: newer insights into hypothalamic–pituitary–gonadal dysfunction. *JAMA* **243**:750–5.

Tenover JS (1992). Effects of testosterone supplementation in the aging male. *J Clin Endocrinol Metab* **75**:1092.

Tenover JS (1994). Androgen administration to aging men. *Endocrinol Metab Clin North Am* **23**:877–92.

Vermeulen A. (1991). Clinical review 24: androgens in the aging male. *J Clin Endocrinol Metab* **73**:221–6.

Westaby D, Ogle JD, Paradinas FJ, et al (1977). Liver damage from long term methyltestosterone. *Lancet* **ii**:261–3.

Wilson JD, Griffth JD (1980). The use and misuse of androgens. *Metabolism* **29**:1278.

10

Injectable drugs: advantages and drawbacks

Hartmut Porst

Pharmacological basis (Figures 1 and 2)

Three different neuronal systems are responsible for the nerve supply of the cavernous bodies and the penile vessels. First, sympathetic (adrenergic) nerve fibers terminating in α_1-adrenoceptors of cavernous smooth muscle and α_2-adrenoceptors of penile vessels. At both receptor sites noradrenaline is released, providing an increase of smooth-muscle tone and vasoconstriction. In addition, adrenergic nerve fibers also run to presynaptically located α_2-adrenoceptors at non-adrenergic, non-cholinergic nerve fibers, thereby modulating (inhibiting), after noradrenaline release, non-adrenergically, non-cholinergically mediated erection. Finally, adrenergic nerve fibers also innervate β_2-adrenoceptors, the stimulation of which, after noradrenaline release, leads to a decrease of smooth-muscle tone, and therefore to the initiation of erection (Saenz de Tejada and Moncada 1997). As the ratio of α_1:β_2-adrenoceptors within the cavernous tissue is known to be 10:1 (Levin and Wein 1980), stimulation of the sympathetic nerve system results in an increase of cavernous smooth-muscle tone and prevents erection.

Second, parasympathetic, non-adrenergic, non-cholinergic (so-called peptidergic) nerve fibers synapse at the cavernous smooth muscle, releasing the neurotransmitters vasoactive intestinal polypeptide (VIP) and nitric oxide (NO), leading to a decrease of cavernous and arterial smooth-muscle tone, with subsequent initiation of erection.

Third, parasympathetic cholinergic pathways supplying presynaptic muscarinic receptors of adrenergic nerve endings modulated, (inhibited) by acetylcholine release, the antierectile influences of the sympathetic input. Although muscarinic (cholinergic) receptors were described within the cavernous tissue, their importance for erection

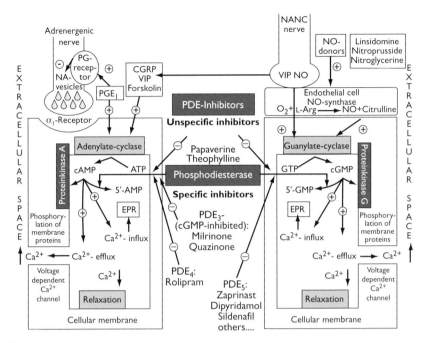

Figure 1
*Smooth-muscle cell. Source: Porst (1996). NANC: non-adrenergic,
non-cholinergic*

seems questionable and remains to be defined (Andersson and
Wagner 1995). Within the smooth-muscle cell three different biochemical mechanisms are principally responsible for initiation and
maintenance of erection.

The cAMP pathway

Stimulation of adenylate cyclase catalyses the formation of cAMP
(adenosine cyclic 3':5'-monophosphate). Substances operating via
this pathway are VIP, calcitonin gene-related peptide (CGRP),
forskolin, prostaglandin E_1 (alprostadil) and E_2 and stimulation of
β_2-receptors.

The cGMP pathway

Stimulation of guanylate cyclase catalyses the formation of cGMP
(guanosine cyclic 3':5'-monophosphate). Substances operating via

this pathway are NO, and therefore all NO donors such as linsidomine (SIN-1), sodium nitroprusside and nitroglycerin.

Phosphodiesterase (PDE) inhibitors

These relatively new agents cause an inhibition of the degradation of cAMP (unspecific: papaverine; specific: the PDE_4 rolipram) or of cGMP (unspecific: papaverine; milrinone, quazinone, specific: the PDE_3 the PDE_5 zaprinast, sildenafil and other substances under investigation), therefore enhancing the maintenance of an erection.

Hyperpolarization

Hyperpolarization of the cell may be induced by cAMP-dependent protein kinases, by cGMP-dependent protein kinases and, independently of these two mechanisms, directly by potassium channel openers (for example, pinacidil, cromakalim, minoxidil, nicorandil and other novel agents under investigation).

All three mechanisms, accumulation of cAMP or cGMP and hyperpolarization mediated by virtue of direct activation of the maxi-K^+ type potassium channels, result in closure of voltage-dependent calcium channels, with subsequent decrease of the concentration of intracellular free calcium and consequent initiation of relaxation of smooth muscle.

Similar effects with decrease of intracellular free calcium followed by relaxation of smooth muscle are achieved by so-called calcium blocking agents, with verapamil, nifedipine and diltiazem being the most well-known representative drugs in this group.

Antierectile, smooth-muscle-contracting agents

Several physiologically produced substances participate in the maintenance of penile flaccidity and therefore contribute to the permanent contractile tone of both the cavernous smooth muscle and the penile arteries. Those agents are some eicosanoids such as $PGF_{2\alpha}$ and thromboxane A_2, prostacyclin (PGI_2) (Andersson and Holmquist 1991), endothelin-1 (Zhao and Christ 1995) and angiotensin II (Kifor et al 1997).

Table 1   Injectable vasoactive drugs for self-injection therapy in erectile dysfunction

Drug	Site of action	Effect
Papaverine	Phosphodiesterase	Inhibition → cAMP ↑, cGMP ↑
	Angiotensin II secretion	Inhibition
PGE$_1$ (alprostadil)	Adenylate cyclase	Stimulation → cAMP ↑
	α_1-Adrenoceptor	Noradrenaline release ↓
	Angiotensin II secretion	Inhibition
VIP	Adenylate cyclase	Stimulation → cAMP ↑
CGRP	Smooth-muscle cell	Relaxation
	Vessels	
NO donors (linsidomine, nitroprusside, nitroglycerin)	NO release: guanylate cyclase	Stimulation → cGMP ↑
α-Adrenoceptor blocker Phentolamine	$\alpha_{1/2}$-Adrenoceptors	Blockade → noradrenaline release ↓
	Potassium channels	Hyperpolarization
	Serotonin receptors	Blockade
Moxisylyte (thymoxamine)	α_1-Adrenoceptors	Blockade → noradrenaline release ↓

In this fashion agents preventing the synthesis or secretion of the aforementioned smooth-muscle contraction-mediating agents or blockers of their receptor sites may decrease the smooth-muscle tone and contribute to the initiation of erection. In animal studies both endothelin receptor antagonists (Whittingham et al 1996) and angiotensin II antagonists such as losartan resulted in a considerable increase of intracavernosal pressure (Kifor et al 1997). In this regard, it was shown in in vitro studies on rabbit corpus cavernosum that the contractile strength of angiotensin II was tenfold higher than its precursor angiotensin I (Park et al 1997). Therefore the contractile effects of angiotensin were also attenuated by captopril, an inhibitor of the angiotensin I-converting enzyme (Park et al 1997).

In conclusion, through their achievement of cavernous smooth-muscle relaxation resulting in initiation and maintenance of penile erection, the various aforementioned substance groups all hold out varying degrees of potential for the pharmacotherapy of erectile dysfunction (Table 1). In what follows those drugs that have gained a considerable importance for self-injection therapy will be described and discussed in detail.

Vasoactive drugs for self-injection therapy

Papaverine

Papaverine, a plant alkaloid (*Papaver somniferum*) contained in crude opium, is assigned to the family of non-selective phosphodiesterase inhibitors. It causes an intracellular increase of both cAMP and cGMP. In human in vitro studies papaverine also suppresses the secretion of endothelial angiotensin II, and thereby prevents angiotensin II-mediated smooth-muscle contraction (Kifor et al 1997). Operating in this fashion, papaverine exhibits considerable relaxant effects on all smooth-muscle cells and was therefore used in the past for ureteral and biliary colic, as well as for vascular spasms. Its potential usefulness for the treatment of erectile dysfunction was described for the first time by Virag (1982). In subsequent years papaverine became a widely used drug for self-injection therapy in erectile dysfunction. With its increasing use a considerable number of side-effects were published in the literature. These side-effects include: priapism (> 6 hours), especially occurring during the in-clinic titration phase, with an average risk of 6% (Porst 1996); the manifestation of local penile fibrotic alterations during the course of self-injection therapy, with an average risk of 5.7% (Porst 1996), ranging in some studies between 10% and 30% (Tullii et al 1989; Virag et al 1994); and in a few cases (1.6%) an elevation of serum liver enzymes (Porst 1996).

Apart from these clinical observations in retrospective studies of self-injection therapy (with papaverine prospective studies are not available), toxic and fibrotic effects of papaverine on the cavernous tissue were proved by several animal studies (Adaikan et al 1990; Aboseif et al 1988) as well as in human in vivo studies (van Ahlen et al 1990 and 1994), though only after intracavernosal papaverine injection. (These detrimental sequelae were, for example, not encountered in the aforementioned studies after intracavernosal injection of PGE_1 (alprostadil).) In the course of my own comprehensive experiences with several vasoactive drugs applied in the clinic for diagnostic purposes, the risk of priapism after papaverine was 5.3% (51/950) compared to 0.3% (299/3362)

Table 2   Efficacy of vasoactive drugs in erectile failure (in office testing)

Drug	Patients	Responders (%)
Papaverine (50 mg)	950	39
Papaverine and phentolamine (50 mg + 2 mg)	249	61
Prostaglandin E_1 (20 μg)	3362	71
SIN-1 (1 mg)	65	15
Moxisylyte (20 mg)	10	10

Table 3   Side-effects of vasoactive drugs

Drug	Dosage	Patients	Side-effects
PGE_1	20 μg	3362	Penile pain: 8.9% (299 patients) Priapism (> 6 h): 0.3% (10 patients) Prolonged erection (2–6 h): 9.2% (309 patients)
Papaverine	50 mg	950	Priapism: 5.3% (51 patients) Injection pain: 85% (808 patients) (glans penis 2–3 min)
Papaverine + phentolamine	50 mg/2 mg	249	Priapism: 5.2% (13 patients) Injection pain: 22% (55 patients) (glans penis 2–3 min)
SIN-1	1 mg	75	Headache/dizziness: 4% (3 patients)
Moxisylyte	20 mg	20	Brief injection pain: 90% (18 patients)

after PGE_1 (Tables 2 and 3). These findings and the relatively low efficacy of papaverine monotherapy make it of historical interest only. Physicians advocating the use of papaverine must keep in mind the greater risk of priapism and fibrotic alterations when compared with PGE_1 therapy and the potential for malpractice law-suits resulting from the occurrence of severe side-effects after papaverine monotherapy. The only argument for the use of papaverine is its considerably lower price, supporting its continuing use especially in the developing and emerging nations.

Combination of papaverine and phentolamine

Phentolamine represents a competitive antagonist of α-adrenoceptors with a similar affinity to α_1- and α_2- subtypes. In addition, serotonin receptor-blocking properties, as well as an influence of phentolamine on the maxi-K^+ channels, are claimed (Andersson et al 1991).

Whereas the injection of phentolamine alone gave rise only to a slight tumescence (Blum et al 1985), the combination of papaverine and phentolamine as proposed for the first time by Zorgniotti and Lefleur (1985), on the one hand, enhanced impressively the efficacy of papaverine monotherapy and, on the other hand, allowed a considerable reduction of the papaverine dosage, thereby lowering the toxic effects. The papaverine and phentolamine combination enjoyed great acceptance worldwide, with reported efficacy rates of up to 72% (Juenemann and Alken 1989). But, as with papaverine monotherapy, with the increasing use of this combination in a growing population of impotent males reports of side-effects piled up in the literature. According to my personal review of the literature on vasoactive drugs in self-injection therapy, the average risk of priapism with the papaverine and phentolamine mixture was 7.8% and the risk of fibrotic changes 12.4% (Tables 4 and 5). In various series the risks of priapisms and fibrosis exceeded 10% and 50% respectively (Girdley et al 1988; Levine et al 1989; Lakin et al 1990). According to a personal diagnostic comparative trial in 249 patients with erectile dysfunction, the efficacy rates after papaverine and phentolamine (50 mg + 2 mg) were 60.6% compared to 72.3% after PGE_2 (20 μg). Priapism occurred in 5.2%, compared to 0% after PGE_1 (Porst 1989). In this comparative trial 11/69 (16%) of the non-responders to PGE_1 converted to responders after papaverine and phentolamine, whereas 40/180 (22%) of the responders to PGE_1 were non-responders to the combination of papaverine and phentolamine. Owing to its higher rate of side-effects the papaverine and phentolamine mixture should be considered a second-choice option for self-injection and reserved for patients in whom PGE_1 fails because of pain or inadequate erection, as was suggested by the American Urological Association (AUA) guidelines panel on erectile dysfunction (Montague et al 1996).

Prostaglandin E_1 (alprostadil)

PGE_1 was first suggested for self-injection therapy by Adaikan and by Ishii at the Second World Meeting on Impotence in Prague in 1986.

Table 4 Efficacy and complications of diagnostic use of vasoactive drugs in erectile failure

Drug	No. of authors	Patients	Dosage (min/max)	Responders (%) (complete erection)	Priapisms (%) >6 hours	Pain
Papaverine	19	2 161	30/110 mg	61 (987/1616)	6.8 (144/2108)	Not stated
	Own series	950	12.5/50 mg	39 (370/950)	5.3 (50/950)	Not stated
Papaverine + phentolamine	13	3 016	15 mg + 1.25 mg 60 mg + 2 mg	68.5 (2065/3016)	6 (73/1210)	Not stated
	Own series	249	15 mg + 1 mg 50 mg + 2 mg	60.6 (151/249)	5.2 (13/249)	Not stated
PGE_1	27	10 353	5/40 µg	72.6 (7519/10 353)	0.25 (26/10 353)	11.5% (881/7637)
	Own series	4 577	5/20 µg	70 (3206/4577)	0.26 (12/4577)	9.2% (422/4577)

Source: Porst (1996). Numbers in parentheses are actual numbers.

Table 5   Complications of self-injection therapy with vasoactive drugs in erectile failure

Drug	No. of authors	Patients	Priapisms >6 hours (%)	Nodules, indurations, fibrosis (%)	Infection (%)	Pain (%)	Hematoma (%)	Elevated liver enzymes (%)
Papaverine	15	1527	7.1 (92/1300)	5.7 (60/1056)	0	4.0 (18/452)	11.4 (98/858)	1.6 (5/314)
Papaverine + phentolamine	22	2263	7.8 (122/1561)	12.4 (228/1843)	1.0 (10/1014)	11.6 (141/1215)	25.6 (250/976)	5.4 (43/799)
PGE$_1$	10	2745	0.36 (10/2745)	0.8 (18/2180)	0	7.2 (40/558)	6.6 (86/1309)	0
	Own series	162	0	1.3 (2/155)	0	1.3 (2/155)	Not stated	0

Source: Porst (1996). Numbers in parentheses are actual numbers.

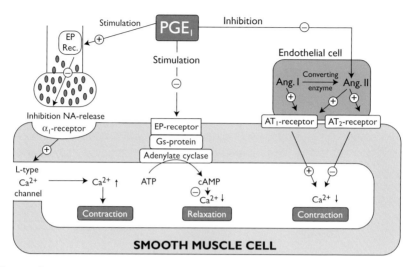

Figure 2
*The impact of alprostadil (PGE₁) on cavernous smooth-muscle
function.*

The publications of Porst (1988) and Stackl et al (1988), both provided evidence on the efficacy, safety and reliability of PGE_1 in representative patient series and prepared the way for its subsequent
worldwide acceptance. The outstanding results with PGE_1 therapy
over the years prompted the AUA clinical guidelines panel on erectile dysfunction to proclaim PGE_1 the first-choice option in self-injection therapy (Montague et al 1996).

The convincing efficacy of alprostadil in erectile dysfunction is
based on several biological activities at different action sites (Figure 2).

Stimulation of adenylate cyclase, mediated via membrane-bound
EP receptors and Gs-proteins, leads to an increase of intracellular
cAMP concentration with intracellular Ca^{2+} depletion and subsequent
relaxation (Porst 1996).

Activation of presynaptic EP receptors of adrenergic nerve fibers by
PGE_1 inhibits the noradrenaline release at α_1-adrenoceptors, resulting
in a decrease of sympathetic input (Molderings et al 1992).

There is also significant suppression of angiotensin II secretion, and
therefore impediment of its muscle contraction-mediating influence
(Kifor et al 1997).

In addition to these features that directly influence the erectile
capacity, several other biological activities are obviously inherent

Table 6 Drop-out rates in self-injection therapy with vasoactive drugs (retrospective studies)

Drug	No. of authors	Patients	Drop-out rate (%)
Papaverine	9	895	46.6 (417/895)
Papaverine + phentolamine	19	2005	45.0 (903/2005)
PGE$_1$	10	2778	37 (608/1641)
	Own series	162	41.3 (67/162)

Source: Porst (1996). Numbers in parentheses are actual numbers.

to PGE$_1$ (Porst 1996): contraction of venous smooth muscle cells in venous capacity vessels; inhibition of platelet aggregation and low-density lipoprotein receptor activity, with subsequent decrease of cholesterol deposition into the arterial wall; antiproliferative activities through its influence on platelet-derived growth factor; and in the gastric system, anti-ulcerative qualities with cytoprotective effects by virtue of the impediment of gastric acid and pepsin secretion.

A retrospective meta-analysis of the literature of vasoactive drugs up to 1996, as well as personal experience with more than 6000 patients, revealed considerable advantages for PGE$_1$ compared to papaverine and the mixture of papaverine and phentolamine with regard to both efficacy and safety, especially in terms of the manifestation of priapisms and penile fibrosis (see Tables 2–6).

Whereas only retrospective studies of papaverine, alone or in combination with phentolamine are available, with both alprostadil–alfadex (Viridal/Edex) and alprostadil sterile powder (Caverject) prospective studies on long-term use and safety for up to 4 years have been conducted, and their results have recently been reported (Porst 1997a, 1997b). The essential results of these studies are as follows.

Efficacy

Of all injections 92–96% were successful at home and resulted in sexual intercourse.

Dosage

In the European Caverject study (evaluable patients: 848) dosages of up to 60 μg were allowed, in the Viridal/Edex studies (evaluable patients: 162) dosages of up to 20 μg. Some 87% of the 848 enrolled patients in the Caverject study applied dosages from 1 to 20 μg, and only 13% of the patients used dosages between 20 and 60 μg. The mean dosages administered in the 4-year-long alprostadil–alfadex study were 13.4 μg at the end of the first year and 12.8 μg at the end of the fourth year. In the 18-month-long study with alprostadil–Caverject no dosage change was reported in 64%, an increase in 21%, and a decrease in 15%. Therefore all these prospective studies provided evidence that no tachyphylaxis occurs during self-injection therapy with alprostadil.

Side-effects

Priapisms > 6 hours with subsequent interruption by antidote-injection. In the European alprostadil–alfadex study 1.2% (2/162) of patients were affected during the initial treatment phase, and in the alprostadil–Caverject study < 1% (8/848) of patients.

Pain

In the alprostadil–alfadex study the reported rate of any pain decreased from 25.9% in the first year to 12.1% in the fourth year. In the alprostadil–Caverject study the average pain rate decreased from 44% during the first 6 months to 16% during the following 12 months. In the majority of patients the reported pain was mild, and corresponded more to a feeling of strong tension than real pain, and therefore did not interfere with pleasure during sexual intercourse. These observations are reflected by the fact that in only 3% of all patients was pain a major reason for the discontinuation of self-injection therapy with alprostadil.

Penile fibrosis

Fibrotic alterations such as nodules, plaques and penile deviations occurred in a total of 11.7% (19/162) in the 4 years of the alprostadil–alfadex trial. After 4 years, in 8 of these 19 patients the fibrotic alterations healed spontaneously; two patients were lost to follow-up; and in only 8/162 patients (4.9%) did the penile fibrotic alterations persist. The average number of injections until the first detection of the fibrotic changes was 60 and the average time until manifestation 12 months. During the course of the trial with alprostadil–Caverject fibrotic alterations were encountered in 4% (34/848) of patients after 6 months and in 5.1% (26/511) during the following 12 months' extension phase. In the US studies with alprostadil–Caverject 7.5% (51/683 men enrolled) developed fibrosis during the 18 months' follow-up (Linet and Ogrinc 1996). The severity of the fibrotic changes was rated as mild in 31 patients, moderate in 19, and severe in one patient. In 33% (17/51) of patients the fibrotic alterations disappeared spontaneously, which means that 5% (34/ 683 patients) suffered from persistent penile fibrotic changes.

Systemic side-effects

In the regular laboratory screenings no deviations of the routine serum values were reported with either alprostadil preparation.

Drop-out rates

In the alprostadil–alfadex study the drop-out rates were 28%, 54%, 61% and 67% for years 1, 2, 3 and 4. In the alprostadil–Caverject study after 18 months of follow-up 384 of 848 patients completed the trial; therefore the drop-out rate totaled 55%.

On the basis of this comprehensive data bank on the long-term use in self-injection therapy, both preparations of alprostadil proved their reliability and safety, with profiles of high efficacy (>90%) and low persistent complications (<7%).

Intracavernous alprostadil versus transurethral alprostadil (MUSE)

A comparison of the efficacy rates (success per application) between the different prospective self-injection trials and transurethral (medicated urethral system for erection or MUSE) studies with alprostadil emphasizes the superiority of intracavernosal alprostadil with a 90–95% home success rate, in contrast to MUSE, with a 51% success rate per application (Padma-Nathan et al 1997; Pryor et al 1997).

A comparative diagnostic study of my own of 103 patients with erectile dysfunction of varied etiology, in whom the efficacy of MUSE up to 1000 µg and PGE_1 up to 20 µg (in three patients up to 40 µg) was assessed, provided overall responder rates of 70% after intracavernosal and 43% after transurethral alprostadil (Porst 1997b). A subdivision of the responders into those with completely rigid and those with incomplete, semirigid erections came to the following conclusions: completely rigid erections: intracavernosal alprostadil 48% (49/103 patients), MUSE 10% (10/103 patients); incompletely rigid erections (partial rigidity requiring additional sexual stimulation): intracavernosal alprostadil 22% (23/103 patients), MUSE 33% (34/103 patients). These data along with the results of the prospective US and European trials with MUSE indicate that, only in the minority of patients, does MUSE provoke completely rigid erections, in contrast to intracavernosal alprostadil. The reported side-effects in this diagnostic trial were: penile/urethral pain 31% after MUSE and 10.6% after intracavernosal alprostadil; pain in testicle or varicose veins in 2.9% each after MUSE; urethral bleeding in 4.8% and blood pressure decrease in 5.8%, with syncope in 1%, after MUSE. No further side-effects were seen after intracavernosal alprostadil. In the European Multicenter Study with MUSE the drop-out rate after 15 months of treatment amounted to 75% (62/249 patients completed the study), which was therefore considerably higher than the reported drop-out rates in self-injection studies with alprostadil, with 55% after 18 months in the European Caverject study and 54% after 2 years or 67% after 4 years in the European alprostadil–alfadex study.

Considering the outcome of the different trials, intracavernosal alprostadil undoubtedly represents a more efficacious and reliable therapeutic option than MUSE for patients suffering from erectile dysfunction, and therefore remains the gold standard.

Drug combinations with alprostadil

Especially in the USA a widespread use and acceptance of the so-called triple drug combination containing PGE_1, papaverine and phentolamine was reported in several publications (Porst 1996).

The combination of alprostadil with the other vasoactive drugs yielded a considerable increase of efficacy (up to more than 90%), but was complicated, on the other hand, by a higher rate of fibrotic penile alterations (Porst 1996).

Whereas the addition of atropine to the Trimix combination of PGE_1, papaverine and phentolamine did not improve the response rates (Sogari et al 1997), the addition of forskolin, a direct adenylate cyclase activator, improved rigidity in 61% of the patients (19/31) with previously poor response to the original Trimix combination (Mulhall et al 1997).

Without any doubt, from the standpoint of improving efficacy alones the use of drug combinations with PGE_1 would seem reasonable, but seen against the background of the common general requests of the national health authorities in the USA and Europe, any official approval of such combinations of several independently vasoactive drugs seems less than likely to be forthcoming.

Moxisylyte (thymoxamine, Erecnos)

Moxisylyte represents predominantly an α_1-adrenoceptor blocking agent, and was the first drug with marketing authorization in France for the treatment of impotence (Bressole et al 1996).

In a placebo-controlled trial in 323 patients with erectile dysfunction of mixed or psychological origin, the responder rates were 11.1% for placebo and 34.9–45.9% for moxisylyte up to 30 mg in in-clinic investigations (Costa et al 1997). In home treatment the success rates were 35% for placebo and 54–71% for moxisylyte. Neither painful erections nor priapisms were observed in this series. In a comparative trial Buvat and Lemaire (1997) have shown that moxisylyte exhibited a considerably lower efficacy rate than papaverine or PGE_1. In the light of these publications and my own limited experience with moxisylyte (see Table 2), this agent represents an erection-facilitating more than an erection-inducing drug, and seems therefore appropriate only for patients with a predominantly psychogenic or neurogenic etiology.

Vasoactive intestinal polypeptide and phentolamine (Invicorp)

VIP stimulates adenylate cyclase, and thereby the formation of cAMP. Injected alone into the cavernous bodies VIP was not able to induce rigid erections sufficient for vaginal penetration (Wagner and Gerstenberg 1987), but, in combination with phentolamine in dosages of 25–30 µg, VIP + 1 mg phentolamine, response rates of 60–70% have been reported (Gerstenberg et al 1992; Buvat and

Lemaire 1997). In the meanwhile several prospective studies with the drug combination of VIP and phentolamine (25 µg/1 mg) were conducted in a total of 718 patients, and efficacy rates of up to 80% in erectile dysfunction of organic etiology were reported at a pre-congress teaching course at the Second Meeting of the European Society for Impotence Research in Madrid, 1–4 October 1997, with minimal side-effects (especially flushing: up to 53%). No priapisms or fibroses were reported. Besides these excellent efficacy and side-effect rates a further major advantage is the delivery of this drug combination in a small convenient autoinjector designed for one-off use with a tiny 29-gauge needle. Recently Invicorp was submitted for official approval both in the USA (FDA) and in Europe, and the company Senetec expects approvals in the course of 1998. Both with respect to its efficacy and side-effects and its convincing autoinjector system the VIP and phentolamine combination will constitute a great enrichment of self-injection therapy.

Calcitonin gene-related peptide and PGE_1

CGRP is known to be a potent vasodilator, and its presence in very close proximity to cavernosal arteries and smooth-muscle cells was demonstrated for the first time by Stief et al (1990). Whereas CGRP injected alone intracavernously failed to induce an erection, combinations of CGRP (5–15 µg) and PGE_1 (20–40 µg) rescued failures of PGE_1 monotherapy (40 µg) in up to 30% of cases (Schwarzer et al 1992). Although this drug combination seemed to be promising, no further clinical phase III studies were launched or pursued by any pharmaceutical company, so that CGRP failed to achieve any further importance in self-injection therapy.

NO donors

Linsidomine (SIN-1)

Linsidomine represents the active metabolite of molsidomin, an antianginal drug used in the oral pharmacotherapy of coronary heart disease. Linsidomine is ranked among NO donors, and generates NO non-enzymatically, with subsequent stimulation of guanylate cyclase and accumulation of cGMP. The implausibly high response rates, with 69% rigid erections to 1 mg linsidomine in 113 patients with erectile dysfunction, reported by Truss et al (1994), were disproved by several other authors, who reported completely rigid erections in only 10–30% after 1 mg linsidomine (Porst 1993; Knispel et al 1995; Buvat and Lemaire 1997). Therefore the NO donor linsidomine was not pursued in prospective phase III studies, and does not currently play any role in self-injection therapy.

Sodium nitroprusside

Sodium nitroprusside, a further NO donor, was investigated in some small series. In the trial of Martinez-Pineiro et al (1994) 12 patients showed a better response rate to 300–400 mg sodium nitroprusside and 21 patients to 20 µg PGE_1. Brock et al (1993) found no response in three patients, but considerable side-effects, with a marked decrease of blood pressure resulting in an early discontinuation of the trial. No further trials with nitroprusside involving significant numbers of patients are published in the literature.

Other vasoactive drugs with potential for self-injection therapy

Several other vasoactive drugs were investigated in in vitro or in vivo animal and/or human studies, and exhibited more or less relaxant activities in cavernous smooth-muscle cells:

- Potassium channel openers: pinacidil, nicorandil, cromakalim and novel agents currently under investigation.
- Calcium antagonists: verapamil, nifedipine and diltiazem.
- Phosphodiesterase inhibitors: milrinone.
- Anti-serotoninergic agents: ketanserin and trazodone.
- Dopamine antagonist: sulpiride.
- Angiotensin II antagonists: losartan and valsartan.
- Endothelin receptor antagonists: bosentan and others.
- Other substances, such as adenosine or histamine.

With none of the aforementioned agents have clinical phase II/III studies been conducted up to now, and therefore no statements are justified on their potential for future use in self-injection therapy.

Technical considerations in self-injection therapy
(Figures 3 and 4)

The major drawback of self-injection therapy is the necessity for needle usage, with a concomitant limited acceptance by patients and partners and therefore, in long-term use, a relatively high drop-out rate. To overcome needlephobia, which is inherent in most patients, several autoinjector devices have been developed (Pescatori 1997) and are currently (Caverject) available, or will be in the near future (Invicorp). In a comparative trial between self-injection devices and common syringe use in self-injection therapy the drop-out rates were 12% as against 36%, indicating that the use of self-injection devices may present one means of reducing drop-out rates (Montorsi et al 1993).

A further factor that may increase the acceptance rate in self-injection therapy is the choice of needle size. In our own comparative trial with 28 experienced self-injecting patients, previously using a 27-gauge needle and subsequently switching to 30-gauge needles, resulted in the outcome that 75% (21 out of 28 patients) preferred the thinner 30 gauge needle: 26 out of 28 patients (93%) confirmed feeling less or no pain in connection with the thinner needle, but 50% stated that the performance of injection was more difficult owing to the higher resistance.

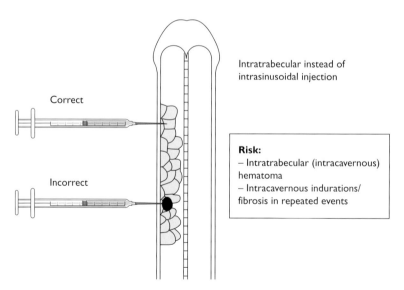

Figure 3
Technical aspects of intracavernous self-injection therapy.

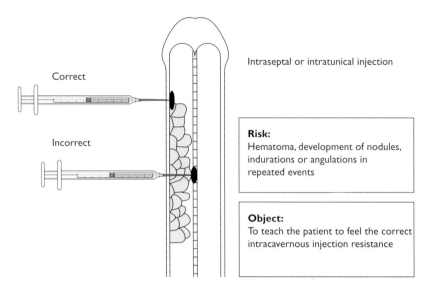

Figure 4
Technical aspects of intracavernous self-injection therapy.

The manifestation of penile fibrotic alterations is considered the most important and frequent side-effect in self-injection therapy. Apart from the drug used (see papaverine), the injection technique seems to play an important role in the prevention of scar formation. The value of induction of the patient by the physician into the correct injection technique should not be underestimated (Figures 3 and 4).

Treatment of drug-induced priapism

On account of the potential risk of irreversible hypoxic tissue damage each priapism lasting longer than 6 hours must be interrupted, and the patient has to be informed in advance by the physician of this necessity (written informed consent). Usually in priapism lasting between 6 and 24 hours the injection of an α-adrenergic agonist is sufficient to induce detumescence. In priapisms >24 hours insertion of a 19-gauge butterfly cannula and evacuation of the entrapped blood, with subsequent injection of an antidote, should be preferred to injection of the antidote alone. Suggested α-adrenergic agonists are adrenaline, ephedrine, noradrenaline, phenylephrine and etilefrine (Nisen and Ruutu 1992; Lee et al 1995; Muruve and Hosking 1996).

Considering the potential impact on the blood pressure and the risk of a hypertensive crisis, etilefrine and phenylephrine carry the lower risk, and are therefore recommended by the most authors. In our own work more than 150 prolonged erections and priapism of up to 38 hours have been successfully treated with etilefrine in dosages between 5 and 15 mg. The rare occurrence of hypertension (>200 mmHg) can be managed by nifedipine SL.

Conclusions

Self-injection therapy with vasoactive drugs laid a cornerstone in the pharmacotherapy of erectile dysfunction. Although facing promising new oral drugs such as sildenafil, apomorphine SL and phentolamine mesylate, or transurethral delivery with MUSE, intracavernous injection therapy will continue to be an important therapeutic option for many patients owing to its unsurpassed efficacy and its high safety profile. In this connection alprostadil and the novel drug combination of VIP and phentolamine represent the agents to be preferred from the standpoints both of efficacy and of safety.

References

Aboseif SR, Breza J, Bosch RJCH, et al (1988). Local and systemic effects of chronic intracavernous injection of papaverine, prostaglandin E_1 and saline in primates. *J Urol* **142**:403–8.

Adaikan PG, Lau LC, Singh G, et al (1990). Long-term intracavernous injection of papaverine and saline are detrimental to the primate cavernosum as compared to PGE_1 – pharmacological and histological evidences. *Int J Impot Res* **2**(suppl 2): 327–8.

van Ahlen H, Piechota HJ, Hermanns M, et al (1990). Metabolic changes in the human corpus cavernosum under vasoactive substances. *Int J Impot Res* **2**(suppl 2): 244.

van Ahlen H, Peskar BA, Sticht G, et al (1994). Pharmacokinetics of vasoactive substances administered into the human corpus cavernosum. *J Urol* **151**: 1227–30.

Andersson KE, Holmquist F (1991). Mechanisms for contraction and relaxation of human penile smooth muscle. *Int J Impot Res* **2**: 209–26.

Andersson KE, Wagner G (1995). Physiology of penile erection. *Physiol Rev* **75**: 191–236.

Andersson KE, Holmquist F, Wagner G (1991). Pharmacology of drugs used for treatment of erectile dysfunction and priapism. *Int J Impot Res* **3**: 155–72.

Blum MD, Bahnson RR, Porter TN, et al (1985). Effect of local alpha-adrenergic blockade on human penile erection. *J Urol* **134**: 479–81.

Bressole F, Costa P, Rouzier-Panis R, et al (1996). Pharmacokinetics of moxisylyte in healthy volunteers after intracavernous injections of increasing doses. *Eur J Pharmacol* **49**: 411–15.

Brock G, Breza J, Lue TF (1993). Intracavernous sodium nitroprusside: inappropriate impotence treatment. *J Urol* **150**: 864–7.

Buvat J, Lemaire A (1997). Intraindividual comparative studies of efficacy, safety and side-effects of different vasoactive drugs in erectile dysfunction. In: *Penile Disorders*, ed H Porst, pp. 191–215. Springer-Verlag, Berlin, Heidelberg, New York.

Costa P, Iacovella JA, Bouvet AA (1997). Efficacy and tolerability of Moxisylyte and placebo injected intracavernously in patients with erectile dysfunction (ED): a multicenter double-blind study. *J Urol* **157**(suppl 203): 790.

Gerstenberg TC, Metz P, Ottesen B, et al (1992). Intracavernous self-injection with vasoactive intestinal polypeptide and phentolamine in the management of erectile failure. *J Urol* **147**: 1277–9.

Girdley FM, Bruskewitz RC, Feyzi J, et al (1988). Intracavernous self-injection for impotence: a long-term therapeutic option? Experience in 78 patients. *J Urol* **140**: 972–4.

Juenemann KP, Alken P (1989). Pharmacotherapy of erectile dysfunction: a review. *Int J Impot Res* **1**: 71–93.

Kifor J, Williams GH, Vickers MA, et al (1997). Tissue angiotensin II as a modulator of erectile function. I. Angiotensin peptide content, secretion and effects in the corpus cavernosum. *J Urol* **157**: 1920–5.

Knispel HH, Wegner HEH, Miller K (1995). Value of nitric oxide donor linsidomine chlorhydrate (SIN-1) in the diagnosis and treatment of erectile dysfunction. *Int J Impot Res* **7**(suppl 1): D26.

Lakin MM, Montague DK, Mendendorp SV, et al (1990). Intracavernous injection therapy – analysis of results and complications. *J Urol* **143**: 1138–41.

Lee M, Cannon B, Sharifi R (1995). Chart for preparation of dilutions of alpha-adrenergic agonists for intracavernous use in treatment of priapism. *J Urol* **153**: 1182–3.

Levin RM, Wein AJ (1980). Adrenergic alpha-receptors outnumber beta-receptors in human penile corpus cavernosum. *Invest Urol* **18**: 225–6.

Levine SB, Althof SE, Turner LA, et al (1989). Side-effects of self-administration of intracavernous papaverine and phentolamine for the treatment of impotence. *J Urol* **141**: 54–7.

Linet OJ, Ogrinc FG (1996). Penile fibrosis during 18 months of intracavernosal therapy with Alprostadil (Caverject™). *Int J Impot Res* **8**(143): D85.

Martinez-Pineiro J, Tello JL, Dorrego JA, et al (1994). Preliminary results of a comparative study with intracavernous sodium nitroprusside and prostaglandin E1 in the diagnosis and treatment of penile erectile dysfunction. *J Urol* **151**: 455A.

Molderings GJ, van Ahlen H, Göthert M (1992). Modulation of noradrenaline release in human corpus cavernosum by presynaptic prostaglandin receptors. *Int J Impot Res* **4**: 19–25.

Montague DK, Barada JH, Belker AM, et al (1996). Clinical guidelines panel on erectile dysfunction: summary report on the treatment of organic erectile dysfunction. *J Urol* **156**: 2007–11.

Montorsi F, Guazzoni G, Bergamaschi F, et al (1993). Intracavernous vasoactive pharmacotherapy: the impact of a new self-injection device. *J Urol* **150**: 1829–32.

Mulhall JP, Daller M, Traish AM, et al (1997). Intracavernosal Forskolin: role in management of vasculogenic impotence resistant to standard 3-agent pharmacotherapy. *J Urol* **158**: 1752–9.

Muruve N, Hosking DH (1996). Intracorporeal phenylephrine in the treatment of priapism. *J Urol* **155**: 141–3.

Nisen HO, Ruutu ML (1992). Etilefrine in the prevention of priapism. *Int J Impot Res* **4**: 187–92.

Padma-Nathan H, Hellstrom WJG, Kaiser FE, et al for the MUSE™ Study Group (1997). Treatment of men with erectile dysfunction with transurethral Alprostadil. *N Engl J Med* **336**: 1–7.

Park JK, Kim SZ, Kim SH, et al (1997). Renin angiotensin system in rabbit corpus cavernosum: functional characterization of angiotensin II receptors. *J Urol* **158**: 653–8.

Pescatori ES (1997). Comparison of self-injection modalities with and without injection devices in erectile dysfunction. In: *Penile Disorders*, ed H Porst, pp. 217–24. Springer-Verlag, Berlin, Heidelberg, New York.

Porst H (1988). Stellenwert von Prostaglandin E_1 (PGE_1) in der Diagnostik der erektilen Dysfunktion im Vergleich zu Papaverin und Papaverin/Phentolamin bei 61 Patienten mit ED. *Urologe* **A27**: 22–6.

Porst H (1989). Prostaglandin E_1 bei erektiler Dysfunktion. *Urologe* **A28**: 94–8.

Porst H (1993). Prostaglandin E1 and the nitric oxide donor linsidomine for erectile failure: a diagnostic comparative study of 40 patients. *J Urol* **149**: 1280–3.

Porst H (1996). Review Article. The rationale for prostaglandin E_1 in erectile failure: a survey of worldwide experience. *J Urol* **155**: 802–15.

Porst H for the European Alprostadil Study Group (1997a). Caverject™ (Alprostadil) in the treatment of erectile dysfunction (ED): an 18 months study. *Abstract book, Second Meeting of the European Society of Impotence Research*, October 1–4, Madrid, **20**: 37.

Porst H (1997b). Transurethral Alprostadil with MUSE™ (Medicated Urethral System for Erection) versus intracavernous Alprostadil – A comparative study in 103 patients with erectile dysfunction. *Int J Impot Res* **9**: 187–92.

Porst H, Buvat J, Meuleman E, et al (1997). Efficacy, safety and psychological impact of a 4-year self-injection therapy of erectile dysfunction (ED) with Alprostadil-Alfadex. *Abstract book, Second Meeting of the European Society of Impotence Research*, October 1–4, Madrid, **18**: 32.

Pryor JP, Abbou CC, Amar E, et al and the European VIVUS-MUSE™ study group (1997). Transurethral Alprostadil for the treatment of chronic erectile dysfunction: A five country experience. *Abstract book, Second Meeting of the European Society of Impotence Research*, October 1–4, Madrid, **25**: 58.

Saenz de Tejada I, Moncada I (1997). Pharmacology of penile smooth muscle. In: *Penile Disorders*, ed H Porst, pp. 125–43. Springer-Verlag, Berlin.

Schwarzer UJ, Hofman R, Pickl U, et al (1992). Calcitonin-gene-related peptide for therapy of erectile impotence. *Int J Impot Res* **4**: 219–22.

Sogari PR, Telöken C, Souto CAV (1997). Atropine role in the pharmacological erection test: study of 228 patients. *J Urol* **158**: 1760–3.

Stackl W, Hasun R, Marberger M (1988). Intracavernous injection of prostaglandin E_1 in impotent men. *J Urol* **140**: 66–8.

Stief CG, Benard F, Bosch RJCH, et al (1990). A possible role for calcitonin gene-related peptide in the regulation of the smooth muscle tone of the bladder and penis. *J Urol* **143**: 392–7.

Truss MC, Becker AJ, Djamilian MH, et al (1994). The role of the nitric oxide donor linsidomine chlorhydrate (SIN-1) in the diagnosis and treatment of erectile dysfunction. *Urology* **44**: 553–6.

Tullii RE, Degni M, Pinto AFC (1989). Fibrosis of the cavernous bodies following intracavernous auto-injection of vasoactive drugs. *Int J Impot Res* **1**: 49–54.

Virag R (1982). Intracavernous injection of papaverine for erectile failure. *Lancet* **ii**: 1938.

Virag R, Nollet F, Greco E, Floresco J (1994). Long-term evaluation of local complications of self-intracavernous injections. *Int J Impot Res* **6**: A37.

Wagner G, Gerstenberg T (1987). Intracavernosal injection of vasoactive intestinal polypeptide (VIP) does not induce erection in man *per se*. *World J Urol* **5**: 171–7.

Whittingham HA, Banting JD, Manabe K, et al (1996). Erectile dysfunction induced by acute NO-synthase blockade is reversed by an endothelin receptor antagonist. *Int J Impot Res* **8**(3): AO6.

Zhao W, Christ GJ (1995). Endothelin-1 as a putative modulator of erectile dysfunction. II. Calcium mobilization in cultured human corporal smooth muscle cells. *J Urol* **154**: 1571–9.

Zorgniotti AW, Lefleur RS (1985). Autoinjection of the corpus cavernosum with a vasoactive drug combination for vasculogenic impotence. *J Urol* **133**: 39–41.

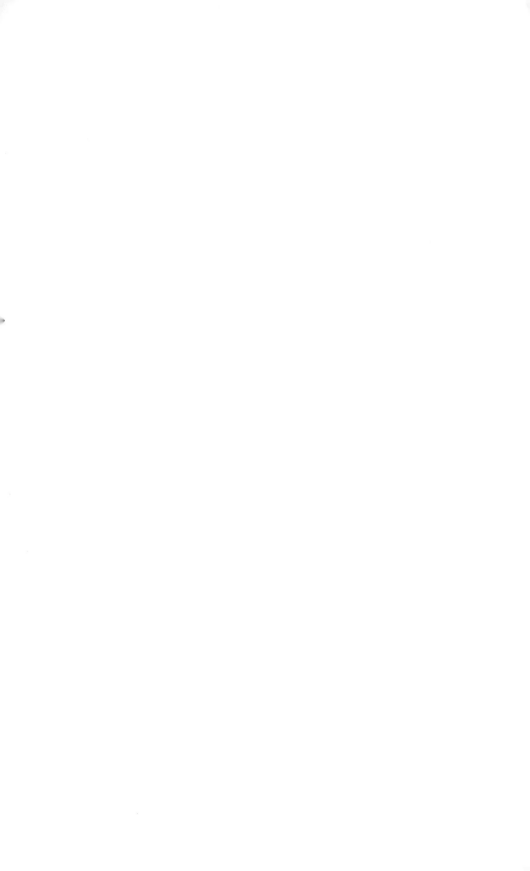

11

Topical administration of erectogenic drugs: is there a role for them in today's therapeutics?

Harin Padma-Nathan

Pharmacologic therapies form the cornerstone of management of erectile dysfunction. Intracavernosal pharmacotherapy by self-injection, to this effect, has become the gold standard of such therapy. However, the long-term utilization of injection therapy is a paradox in view of its efficacy, and reflects in part the need to inject with a needle (Althof et al 1989). The impetus to develop more minimally invasive pharmacologic therapies for the management of erectile dysfunction has led, first, to intraurethral therapy and more recently to topical and oral pharmacologic therapies. The oral therapies promise to become first-line therapies that will dramatically impact on this field from a medical as well as a societal and economic perspective. As the field grows exponentially, intraurethral and topical therapies may play more of a niche role. This chapter will review the current efficacy and safety of intraurethral and topical therapies and project its future role in the field of sexual pharmacotherapy.

Intraurethral pharmacotherapy

Pharmacology and mechanism of drug transfer

The principal pharmacologic agent utilized in intraurethral drug delivery has been alprostadil, the synthetic formulation of prostaglandin E_1. Upon administration to the distal urethra, it is able to elicit hemodynamic alterations in the corpora cavernosa. The drug transfer appears to occur primarily by venous channels that communicate between the corpus spongiosum and the corpora cavernosa. These vascular channels appear to be variable and increase with age. They may also close early in the erection process. The hemodynamic alterations observed following intraurethral administration of alprostadil are primarily an increase in arterial dilatation and flow. This is evidenced by a significant increase in peak systolic velocity (PSV) values determined at the time of color duplex ultrasonography. The PSV values attained following an intraurethral administration of 500 μg MUSE-alprostadil are statistically similar to those seen following a 10 μg injection of alprostadil directly into a corpus cavernosum (Padma-Nathan et al 1994). However, the degree of veno-occlusion, in comparison, is significantly less following intraurethral administration. This is evidenced by the elevated end-diastolic velocity values at the same duplex ultrasonographic examination (Padma-Nathan et al 1994). This is also clinically correlated with the lesser degree of penile rigidity associated with intraurethral administration. Similar hemodynamic effects have been observed with a liposomal encapsulation of alprostadil delivered to the navicular fossa – lyophilized liposomal prostaglandin E_1, LLPGE$_1$ (See et al 1997).

The absorption of alprostadil administered to the distal urethra is rapid, with only 20% of a 100 μg dose remaining after 20 min (VIVUS Inc Pharmacokinetic and Toxicological Data). The transfer of drug to the corpora cavernosa, however, appears to be inconsistent, and this in turn appears to reflect some systemic dispersion and possibly some urothelial metabolism of alprostadil. The total amount of alprostadil found in an ejaculate following administration of the 1000 μg dose appears to be equal to the total prostaglandin level normally in the ejaculate. This increase in prostaglandin appears to be less than the day-to-day variation of prostaglandin within an individual's ejaculate (VIVUS Inc Pharmacokinetic and Toxicological Data). However, nearly 10% of partners report symptoms of vaginitis following intraurethral alprostadil, and thus may be sensitive to this drug when delivered in the ejaculate.

Clinical efficacy and safety

The clinical efficacy and safety of intraurethral alprostadil in the form of the "medicated urethral system for erections", or MUSE, has been established in both clinical reports and regulatory approval (Hellstrom et al 1996; Padma-Nathan et al 1997a). The MUSE formulation of alprostadil is delivered as a semi-solid pellet (3 mm × 1 mm) to the distal 3 cm of the urethra by an applicator following urination. The urine acts as both a lubricant and a diluent for the pellet. In addition to the MUSE system, the previously mentioned lyophilized liposomal (trilaminar membrane-covered spherical drug vehicle) prostaglandin E_1 released in the meatus by a dilute detergent has entered phase II study. The latter has a shelf-life of 3 years and contains 750 µg or 1500 µg per delivery dose. The liposomes are delivered to the distal 1.5 cm of the urethra and a detergent (0.1% polyoxyethylene) is employed to release the alprostadil. It is expected that this second intraurethral approach will result in nearly identical efficacy and safety to that observed with MUSE. The largest clinical trial of intraurethral alprostadil to date utilized the MUSE system and consisted of 1511 men between the ages of 26 and 88 years with complete erectile dysfunction of primarily organic etiology (Padma-Nathan et al 1997a). The men initially underwent an in-office double-blind dose titration with four different doses (125, 250, 500, 100 µg) of MUSE-alprostadil. Nearly 66% (996) of these men had an erection adequate for intercourse. The responders were then randomized to drug at the appropriate dose as determined in the first phase or placebo for a 3-month period of home treatment. The at-home response has been examined from two different perspectives: the percentage of men reporting at least one successful episode of intercourse and the percentage of administrations resulting in successful intercourse. It was observed that, of the 461 men receiving active drug at home, 299 (65%) had successful intercourse at least once. In comparison, only 93 of the 500 men (18.6%) receiving placebo had at least one episode of intercourse ($P < 0.001$). The overall clinical efficacy (in-office and at-home) would thus be 43%. However, only 50.4% of administrations resulted in successful intercourse in those men who were in-office responders. If they responded once at home as well then 69.2% of subsequent administrations were associated with successful intercourse. In contrast nearly 87% of at-home injections with alprostadil sterile powder (Caverject) are associated with successful intercourse (Linet and Ogrinc 1996). In our experience 5–10% of impotent men are able to achieve rigid and consistent erections with intraurethral alprostadil. It is this population that will continue to preserve a role for intraurethral therapy with the advent of oral agents. To date, however, it is not possible to pre-identify them clinically. In patients who are responders, there are significant improvements in quality of life, particularly in the domains of self-esteem and sexual and non-sexual aspects of their relationships to their partners (Padma-Nathan and VIVUS MUSE Study Group 1996).

The long-term safety profile of MUSE-alprostadil was recently reported in 2595 men, with 684 receiving therapy for over 6 months, 265 for over 12 months, 96 for over 18 months and 57 for over 24 months (Spivak et al 1997). This attrition underscores the high dropout rate associated with this form of therapy. Pain, including penile, urethral, testicular and perineal pain, was observed in over 50% of men. Hypotension and synocopy have been observed in 1.2% to near-ly 4% (Hellstrom et al 1996; Padma-Nathan and VIVUS MUSE Study Group 1996; Padma-Nathan et al 1997a; Spivak et al 1997) of men dependent upon the dose. Hypotension, although uncommon, can be associated with serious and potentially life threatening adverse car-diovascular consequences. This therapy should thus be employed with caution in men with such risk profiles and in older men (≥70 years). Minor urethral trauma, prolonged erections and penile fibrosis appear to be rare but not absent. As was previously mentioned, there have also been partner-reported adverse events, with about 10% reporting symptoms of vaginal irritation or vaginitis. The overall safety data indicate that MUSE-alprostadil is well tolerated.

It has become obvious from the clinical experience since its US Food and Drug Administration (FDA) approval that the intraurethral administration of alprostadil for the treatment of erectile dysfunction is, although effective, not sufficiently associated with adequate and consistent penile rigidity to maintain its role as a first-line therapy following the advent of more effective oral pharmacologic agents. An attempt has been made to address this issue by polypharma-cotherapy with the addition of the α-adrenergic antagonist prazosin to alprostadil (Lewis et al 1997). This combination therapy has result-ed in a minimal increase in efficacy, with 68% of patients reporting at least one successful intercourse following in-office response. However, the incidence of hypotension increase dramatically with combination therapy, being observed in up to 9.2%. The develop-ment of a more effective pharmacologic approach is, however, clear-ly the most effective means by which intraurethral therapy will con-tinue to play a role in this field. Alprostadil is an appealing agent for intraurethral administration in comparison to such agents as papaverine, owing to its efficacy at microgram dosages. However, its hyperalgic effects at the doses employed for intraurethral adminis-tration are associated with a high incidence of pain that frequently limits therapy. The next generation of intraurethral agents may include other vasoactive agents, including nitric oxide donors as well as agents such as nitric oxide synthase gene therapy delivered through this novel approach (Rehman et al 1997). A less appealing approach to increasing the drug efficacy of intraurethral alprostadil has been to employ an adjustable penile band (Actis) which appears primarily to effect improved erections by mechanical constriction rather than by improved drug transfer (by increasing the spongiosal pressure and decreasing systemic run-off) (Padma-Nathan et al 1997b). If the latter were possible, the addition of a mechanical device for only a short time following drug application would be bet-ter accepted by patients than the continuous application of such a device throughout the entire sexual episode – thus mimicking the vacuum device experience.

Topical pharmacotherapy

Transdermal/Transglandular corporeal drug delivery

Preliminary trials examining the efficacy of transdermal or transglandular (minoxidil) delivery of nitroglycerin paste (Heaton et al 1990), minoxidil with or without a percutaneous absorption enhancer (2-nonyl-1,3-dioxalane) or capsaicine (Cavallini 1994), papaverine (Kim et al 1995) and prostaglandin E_1 (Kim and McVary 1995) have demonstrated some degree of drug delivery to the corporeal smooth muscle sufficient to elicit Doppler-detected increased arterial inflow and penile tumescence. However, rigid erections have only been produced in the rare spinal cord-injured neurogenic patient. New drug formulations, absorption enhancers, drug carriers and iontophoresis may ultimately make this route of drug delivery clinically efficacious. Currently two proprietary formulations of alprostadil with absorption enhancers are in phase II clinical development. The most rational site of application is the glans penis, and thus this route may be ultimately more efficacious than the intraurethral route, since it bypasses the urothelium. Thus, this form of drug delivery may act to enhance erections in men with mild or moderate erectile dysfunction. However, if effective, it clearly will have a niche, owing to the patient appeal of topical agents. Initial examination of doses up to 4.0 mg prostaglandin are well tolerated by patients and partners, and may produce an erection adequate for intromission in 62% of impotent men previously determined to be excellent responders to intracavernosal injections of low doses of "Trimix" (prostaglandin E_1, papaverine and phentolamine) (Becher et al 1996).

Conclusion

Intraurethral and topical (transglandular) pharmacotherapies appear to be sufficiently efficacious to preserve a role following the advent of effective oral pharmacologic agents. The oral agents alone or in combination are projected to be effective in 70–90% of men with erectile dysfunction, including cases of severe or complete impotence. The second-line pharmacologic step will include injectable, intraurethral and topical agents.

References

Althof SE, Turner LA, Levine SB, et al (1989). Why do so many people drop out from auto-injection therapy for impotence? *J Sex Marital Ther* **15**:121–9.

Becher E, Momesso A, Borghi M, et al (1996). Topical prostaglandin E1 for erectile dysfunction. *J Urol* **155**:741A.

Cavallini G (1994). Minoxidil and capsaicine: an association of transcutaneous active drugs for erection facilitation. *Int J Impot Res* **6**:D71.

Heaton JPW, Morales A, Owen J, et al (1990). Topical glyceryltrinitrate causes measurable penile arterial dilation in impotent men. *J Urol* **43**:729–31.

Hellstrom WJG, Bennett AH, Gesundheit N, et al (1996). A double-blind, placebo-controlled evaluation of the erectile response to transurethral alprostadil. *Urology* **48**:851–6.

Kim ED, McVary KT (1995). Topical prostaglandin E1 for the treatment of erectile dysfunction. *J Urol* **153**:1828–30.

Kim ED, El-Rashidy R, McVary TK (1995). Papaverine topical gel for treatment of erectile dysfunction. *J Urol* **153**:361–5.

Lewis RW, Brendler CB, Burnett Al, et al (1997). A comparison of transurethral alprostadil and alprostadil/prazosin combinations for the treatment of erectile dysfunction (ED). *J Urol* **157**:703A.

Linet OI, Ogrinic FG (1996). Efficacy and safety of intracavernosal alprostadil in men with erectile dysfunction. *N Engl J Med* **334**:873–7.

Padma-Nathan H and the VIVUS MUSE Study Group (1996). Multicenter double-blind, placebo controlled trial of transurethral alprostadil in men with chronic erectile dysfunction. *J Urol* **155**:496A.

Padma-Nathan H, Keller T, Poppiti R, et al (1994). Hemodynamic effects of intraurethral alprostadil: The Medicated Urethral System for Erection (MUSE). *J Urol* **151**:469 (354A).

Padma-Nathan H, Hellstrom WJG, Kaiser FE, et al (1997a). Treatment of men with erectile dysfunction with transurethral alprostadil. *N Engl J Med* **336**:1–7.

Padma-Nathan H, Tam P, Place V, et al (1997b). Improved erectile response to transurethral alprostadil by use of a novel, adjustable penile band. *J Urol* **157**:704A.

Rehman J, Christ G, Melman A, et al (1997). Enhancement of physiologic erectile function with nitric oxide synthase gene therapy. *J Urol* **157**:782A.

See JR, Williams J, Sparkuhl A, et al (1997). Lyophilized liposomal prostaglandin E1 released by a dilute detergent for intrameatal delivery to treat erectile failure. *J Urol* **157**:784A.

Spivak AP, Peterson CA, Cowley C, et al (1997). Long-term safety profile of transurethral alprostadil for the treatment of erectile dysfunction. *J Urol* **157**:792A.

12

Development of an oral drug to treat male erectile dysfunction: from the chemist's bench to the drug store

*Murray C Maytom, Ian H Osterloh,
Pierre A Wicker*

Introduction

The development of new medicines is a long, complex and highly risky process. It generally takes 10–15 years from the start of a discovery project to the regulatory approval of a new pharmacological agent as a prescription medicine. Until the early 1980s the field of erectile dysfunction (ED) was thought to hold little real promise for the introduction of pharmacological treatments. The reports of Virag et al (1982) and Brindley (1983) changed this bleak outlook, and it was recognized that an effective pharmacological treatment of ED was possible through directly influencing the relaxation of the corpus cavernosal smooth-muscle cells. Advances in the cellular biochemistry of this unique biological tissue over the following decade, combined with a variety of innovative drug discovery approaches and careful clinical observation, led to the exciting possibility of the development of the first effective oral agent for the treatment of ED. This chapter reviews the complex considerations and the sequence of events that are required to develop successfully an orally active drug to treat ED.

Within pharmaceutical drug development each stage of the process is shadowed by the risk of failure, and the vast majority of research projects fail to deliver a candidate molecule for clinical testing. Of the 15 000 molecules synthesized by research chemists in the early years after the initiation of new projects, only one will eventually be approved as a medicine. Of the molecules that pass all the early hurdles of pre-clinical development and are actually administered to humans in phase I trials, only one in ten will pass through all the subsequent hurdles and reach the pharmacy shelf. The typical time-frame from initiation of a project to regulatory approval of a new medicine is about 15 years and, of the drugs which are licensed, many will not be successful enough on the market to enable the manufacturers to recoup all the research, development and manufacturing costs. For the very few drugs that succeed, the costs involved are about $US400–500 million. Furthermore, at approval only about one-third of the patent life will remain – some 6 or 7 years on average; in the USA patent-restoration legislation may permit a maximum extension of patent exclusivity for up to 5 years, with a maximum cap of 14 years from marketing approval. It is during this variable period of patent exclusivity that the enormous expense of research and development of both the successful and failed compounds must be recovered. The complex and interrelated processes involved in the research and development of a new medicine are exemplified by the development of an oral agent for the treatment of male erectile dysfunction.

An essential aspect to consider before embarking on a long, risky and expensive project is how the prevalence of the medical condition and the therapeutic options may change during the ensuing 10 years or so of drug development, and how these factors could affect the potential market size at the time the new therapy may be approved. For example, any researchers or pharmaceutical companies currently considering the development of new intracavernosal or intraurethral agents to treat erectile dysfunction must consider the potential impact of the imminent approval of new oral medications. The introduction of oral agents may potentially reduce the number of men willing to accept invasive forms of treatment and hence threaten the long-term viability of such treatment approaches, so that the research and development costs could never be recouped. On the other hand, it is as likely that the availability of oral agents could encourage many more men with ED to seek treatment, and hence the total number of men who might eventually require local forms of treatment could increase. Such scenarios illustrate graphically the considerations that could determine the ultimate ability of research programs to recoup their vast costs, this itself being further determined by the ability of health care systems to pay for new treatments. In summary, the project team must maintain awareness of the changing epidemiological, medical, regulatory, and competitive environment, and must assess the potential to gain regulatory approval to market the new treatment successfully on a global basis in order to recover development costs and maximize the return on investment.

Pharmaceutical drug development could be summarized as the processes of identifying, manufacturing, and testing a new chemical compound to enable it to receive regulatory approval for commercial distribution. Any new medicine that is of high quality, safe, and effective should gain regulatory approval, but the attainment of this objective

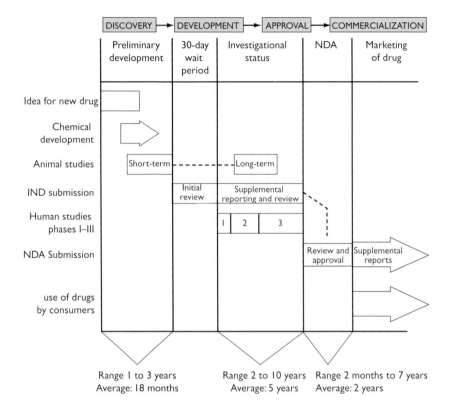

Figure 1
A diagram illustrating key steps involved in the "discovery" and "development" process in the USA.

is complex in the extreme. The discovery and clinical development of any new drug involve a matrix of interactions between discovery biologists and analytical chemists, manufacturing chemists, pharmacokineticists, pharmacists who develop the formulations, toxicologists, and regulatory and marketing groups, as well as clinical groups, working both within the pharmaceutical industry and as independent clinical trialists. These groups work on programs to allow bulk manufacture of drug substance, formulation development, acute and long-term toxicity studies, and clinical studies – all of which need to be managed effectively to allow the research objectives of bringing forward new and innovative products to market to be achieved in the minimal time possible without compromising scientific principles and standards of quality.

Three essential phases occur to develop a chemical compound into a medicine. These phases are the discovery phase, the development phase (which includes both pre- or non-clinical development and clinical development), and finally the regulatory approval and commercialization of the new drug (Figure 1).

The discovery phase

When starting a new project it is necessary to have a clear definition of the disease or condition to be treated and how it impacts on the patient as a whole. With regard to the development of treatments for ED these requirements pose a considerable challenge, as the understanding of the physiological and biochemical processes remains incomplete. The brain centers controlling erection and the neural pathways involved are still only partly defined, and there remains an incomplete understanding of the neurotransmitters involved in tumescence (Ignarro et al 1990). The current belief is that relaxation is possibly a result of the interaction of several endogenous relaxants (Lerner et al 1993).

Not many years ago there was considerable debate as to whether ED had a predominantly psychological or a predominantly organic cause in the majority of sufferers; however, more recently the widespread success of intracorporeal pharmacotherapy has emphasized abnormal corporeal reactivity as probably the most significant etiological factor (Andersson and Wagner 1995; Christ 1995). Organic erectile dysfunction is most frequently attributed to neurogenic and vasculogenic causes; however, there are many organic causes of ED. They encompass the more commonly encountered vascular conditions, such as atherosclerotic arterial insufficiency, and traumatic or post-surgical neurological injuries, as well as diabetes mellitus, which affects the vascular, neurological, and hormonal systems. They also include less common conditions such as multiple sclerosis, hormonal conditions such as hyperprolactinemia, and other vascular abnormalities such as venous incompetence.

In considering which approach to adopt for developing a new compound it is useful to have knowledge of a prototype drug that is known to work on at least part of the biological system; ideally there would already be a pharmacological agent to act as a "lead". Prior to the reports of Virag and Brindley in the early 1980s on the efficacy of self-injection, pharmacotherapy for ED was virtually non-existent. Since that time the most significant advances in the treatment of erectile dysfunction have been the vascular pharmacological approaches, which involve induction of vascular smooth-muscle relaxation of the corpora by direct intrapenile injection of agents such as the α blocker, phentolamine, the prostanoid, prostaglandin (PGE_1), and the nonspecific phosphodiesterase inhibitor, papaverine. Oral medications using similar approaches have not been possible owing to the lack of bioavailability and/or the systemic side-effects of such agents. The challenge has therefore been targeting end-organ responses for oral pharmacological therapy in such a way as either to increase oral bioavailability or to reduce or eliminate systemic side-effects of known compounds that are effective, or more ambitiously to try to identify new mechanisms of action amenable to modification by novel therapeutic compounds.

Basic science advances within the past decade have indicated that relaxation of the smooth-muscle cells of the corpora cavernosa, a requirement for the erectile process, is mediated by the release of nitric oxide from non-adrenergic, non-cholinergic (NANC) nerve endings that supply the corpora (Rajfer et al 1992). Also the discovery that the selective type 5 phosphodiesterase inhibitor, sildenafil, displays a potent pro-erectile effect has highlighted the importance of the intracellular phosphodiesterase enzymes in regulating corporeal smooth-muscle relaxation (Boolell et al 1996a,b; Gingell et al 1996).

Currently research groups within the industry are taking a variety of approaches to developing oral drugs for treating ED. These include peripherally acting oral α blockers (oral phentolamine), and drugs acting centrally to augment pro-erectile pathways (sublingual apomorphine). In further considering which approach to adopt or which prototype to modify, the ideal properties of a drug to treat ED must be considered from the outset. For ED the ideal treatment should be simple to take and use – in other words it should be rapidly effective, so that it can be taken only when required, and ideally the treatment should aim to restore an appropriate erectile response rather than simply induce erections (Foreman and Wernicke 1990). The treatment has to be very reliable in producing an adequate erectile response virtually whenever required – within the limits of the normal male sexual response – and the erection should not persist after sexual activity ceases. Further requirements are that the treatment should be free from unpleasant or dangerous side-effects and, ideally, that it should not interact with other medications routinely used in the patient population. For an oral treatment for ED these requirements translate into an agent that is highly selective for one particular target (membrane receptor or enzyme), which can be formulated in a capsule or tablet, and which is rapidly and consistently absorbed from the gastrointestinal tract to achieve the necessary levels in the target organ for several hours and is then rapidly eliminated. Furthermore, the drug should not interfere with the metabolism of other drugs, and its own route of metabolism and elimination should not be susceptible to modification by other diseases or drug therapies.

As novel compounds are synthesized their biological activity on the target organ system will be determined using appropriate in vivo and in vitro models. For a new treatment of erectile dysfunction appropriate studies might include determining the effect of the agent in relaxing precontracted strips of corpus cavernosum, and/or the ability to enhance centrally induced (apomorphine) or peripherally induced (nitrate or pelvic nerve stimulation) erections in a whole animal (e.g. the dog). The general pharmacology of the more promising compounds will be profiled and the metabolic pathways will be investigated. Usually there will be several different compounds that become the lead at different stages in the project, but many will suffer from deficiencies such as insufficient activity, metabolic instability, etc. The lead compounds are repeatedly tested in in vitro or in vivo animal models and then refined until a compound that reaches the team's targets for selectivity, activity, and biological and pharmacokinetic profile is achieved. This candidate is nominated for further development, including scale-up of manufacture of bulk compound, formulation development and toxicology studies. It usually takes a team of chemists, biologists, and pharmacokineticists several years from the initiation of a project to achieve the milestone of nominating a candidate compound for further development.

Sometimes a discovery project aims to target a receptor subtype or isoenzyme that might play an important role in a variety of disease processes. The project team that discovered sildenafil aimed to develop a highly selective inhibitor of type 5 phosphodiesterase. At the initiation of this research program in the mid-1980s it was believed that this isoenzyme (which regulates cyclic GMP levels) was involved in the control of vascular tone in the systemic circulation. Although it was hypothesized that the compound might also treat erectile dysfunction, the neurotransmitters involved in mediating erection and the distribution of phosphodiesterases in the corpus cavernosum were unknown at the time, and hence sildenafil entered clinical testing in the early 1990s as a potential treatment for angina. However, clinical observations in early human studies and publications on advances in basic science, including the role of NO in mediating erection (Kim et al 1991; Burnett et al 1992), led to a decision to switch the target of development of sildenafil from angina to erectile dysfunction, with dramatic results.

The development phase

The primary objectives of the development phase are to perform the pre- or non-clinical development and the clinical development activities. The non-clinical activities include performing the toxicological studies, and undertaking the formulation and process development required to allow robust mass production of a marketable medicine, while the clinical development activities encompass the many clinical trials, which most crucially must demonstrate efficacy and safety in the selected patient population.

Non-clinical development

Formulation and process development

Although formulations necessary for initial clinical testing in phase I (human volunteer studies) and phase II (pilot studies in patients) can be simple (e.g. powder for dissolving in water) and of limited shelf-life, the eventual needs are for a formulation that can be manufactured reliably and reproducibly on a large scale with good long-term stability. The four principal stages of development are pre-formulation, formulation design, process development, and scale-up. At the pre-formulation stage the drug is usually in very short supply, and hence only a limited evaluation of stability can be undertaken. The drug supplies available need to be channeled into priority activities, such as the toxicology studies. In pre-formulation a knowledge of the effect of temperature, pH, moisture, compatibility with potential formulation components, and other physical and chemical factors of the drug is obtained. It is clear that this knowledge is required for rational selection and development of prototype and eventual commercial formulations. The final outcome of the formulation design stage is the development of the commercial presentation that meets clinical and marketing needs. The object of the process development stage is to translate the laboratory-developed formulation into one that can be routinely manufactured on a large scale and successfully introduced to production. The overall objective if at all possible is to have used a formulation in phase II that probably will require only some slight change in excipient ratio, or addition of dye or shape change to achieve differentiation for commercialization, and to have the commercial presentation (i.e. final color, shape, size) ready for use in all phase III trials.

Toxicology studies

Before administering a new compound to humans, evaluation of potential toxicity is required in at least two animal species. Unless there is a scientific reason not to, toxicity studies are carried out using the same route of administration as that to be used in humans. Internationally accepted guidelines suggest that single-dose studies in two rodent species, repeated-dose studies of up to 14 days' duration in one rodent and one non-rodent species, and tests for detecting genotoxic potential are the minimum requirements for starting "first in man" studies. Reproductive toxicology can be delayed until the drug has passed successfully through phase I clinical studies. Longer-term toxicology studies are also usually required once the duration of dosing to humans increases (i.e. phase IIb or III studies).

Other key toxicology data are generated from the carcinogenicity studies, which are long and expensive and are not normally initiated until after early clinical studies indicate that the compound is well-tolerated and effective. Adverse findings that occur in toxicology studies are often investigated during the ongoing drug development process in mechanistic toxicology studies, but many promising compounds are immediately discontinued from development because of adverse findings during the toxicology program.

Clinical development

The goals of clinical development differ. The key objective in phase I studies is to characterize the safety profile of a drug in a small well-defined population, usually healthy volunteers; extensive pharmacokinetic and pharmacodynamic profiling is also a fundamental component of phase I studies. Phase II studies involve a patient population primarily to establish the effective dose range of the compound, while further extending knowledge of toleration and safety, whereas the larger phase III studies in patients are designed to determine definitively the long-term efficacy, toleration and safety of the compound, and possibly how it compares with leading agents already being prescribed. Ultimately, the clinical development program covered by phases I–III must generate all the data necessary to write the Package Insert (US product document) or Summary of Product Characteristics (European data sheet) that describes the essential information for the prescribing physician. In the USA it is particularly important that there is enough information in the US Package Insert to allow the commercial team to promote and market the new product effectively.

Although there are certain studies that will always be performed (for example, studies to characterize the absorption, distribution, metabolism, and elimination of the drug), there is no predetermined route map for developing an oral drug to treat male erectile dysfunction. The overall strategy must take into account numerous factors, including the mode of administration, the mechanism of action, the kind of patients most likely and least likely to respond to treatment, and the possible side-effects. The various phases of clinical development are further described below.

Phase I volunteer studies

About half the compounds tested in animals will emerge as candidates for testing in humans. The first administration to humans ("first in man" study) is a crucial milestone in the development of any new drug. A prerequisite for approval to conduct such a study includes the accumulation of positive pre-clinical data on the safety and potential efficacy of the drug: the weight of data must convince the project team and an Institutional Review Board (i.e. an independent ethics committee) that the potential benefits of the new medicine outweigh the risks of its administration to normal volunteers or patients when no prior human experience is available. In the USA, before tests can be undertaken in humans, permission to open an IND (Notice of Claimed Investigational Exemption for a New Drug) is required from the Food and Drug Administration (FDA).

In initial phase I studies there are three essential objectives: the first is to assess the tolerability as well as the safety of gradually increasing doses and to define the maximum tolerated dose; the second and third are to obtain basic pharmacokinetic and pharmacodynamic information. These are critical studies, and observations made during this stage will influence the design of later stages. The finding of unacceptable adverse events in volunteer studies will invariably preclude any further development of the drug. With regard to pharmacokinetics (what the body does to the drug), it is essential to know the rate and extent of drug absorption from the gastrointestinal tract for orally administered medications following single and repeated dose administration. In addition, information is gained on accumulation, food effects, and dose proportionality. Hopefully, at tolerated doses, adequate drug concentrations (i.e. levels predicted to be effective from pre-clinical studies) are achieved in the blood, or possibly at the appropriate body site. Pharmacodynamic properties (what the drug does to the body, for example, changes in blood pressure or heart rate) should also be assessed, and the relationship between plasma concentrations of drug and these effects should be defined. The results of these investigations are critical to determining the doses and regimens to be investigated in phase II.

To permit accurate determination of the pharmacokinetics of a drug a sensitive and specific drug assay is required. Furthermore, consideration should be given both to the parent compound and to any circulating metabolites. Examination of the relationship between plasma concentrations of drug and metabolite and the pharmacodynamic end-points can often provide information on the importance of the metabolite in terms of the safety and efficacy profile of the drug. In some instances a metabolite may be identified as being more effective than the parent drug, and this may raise the possibility of developing such a compound directly.

Throughout drug development a variety of other clinical pharmacology studies are performed to investigate metabolism, to evaluate the bioequivalence of new formulations, to investigate adverse events of particular importance, to assess possible interactions with other drugs, and to assess pharmacokinetics in special populations (for example, in the elderly, or in patients with renal or hepatic impairment).

Phase II studies

The primary objectives of the phase II studies are to determine the efficacy, likely dose range and safety of the drug in the selected clinical indications. A phase II program will typically involve several hundred patients. The studies are designed by the project team taking into account the mode of action of the drug, and the knowledge and advice of investigators who have a special interest in the treatment of the disease for which the drug is intended. The trials ultimately identify the most suitable dosage regimen, give an estimate of clinical efficacy in relation to concentration of the drug, and provide information on adverse effects.

In designing a phase II program the project team has to take into account several critical factors. In addition to the mode of action of the drug, other factors that must be considered include the route of administration, the pharmacokinetic and pharmacodynamic profile emerging from the phase I studies, the types of patients most likely and least likely to respond, the objective and subjective efficacy instruments that are available to measure therapeutic effect, the possible side-effects, and the need for any exclusion criteria for safety reasons.

The choice of what efficacy measurements to use in phase II studies will very much depend on the mode of action. Heaton et al (1997) have recently classified treatments for ED into five major classes: (a) central initiators, (b) peripheral initiators, (c) central conditioners, (d) peripheral conditioners, and (e) others. The first pharmacological treatment to receive FDA approval in the USA (intracavernosal prostaglandin E_1, (Caverject) is an example of a peripheral initiator, i.e. an agent that acts directly in the periphery to activate events leading to an erection. Thus an intracavernosal injection of PGE_1 can cause an erection in the absence of any sexual stimulation. Based on this mode of action the efficacy – dose–response relationship – can be evaluated in a clinic setting, using objective methods such as penile plethysmography for the assessment of the hardness and duration of any resulting erection. In a clinic setting the patient and/or a clinician can also palpate the erection to assess whether the erection is sufficiently rigid for sexual intercourse. Indeed, many of the data submitted in support of regulatory approval consisted of the results of dose–response studies performed in a clinic setting. The mode of action also makes PGE_1 injection suitable as an adjunct to assessing the penile vasculature during erection using Doppler ultrasound. Another aspect of the mode of action of this class II type of drug is that the erection does not necessarily subside when the sexual stimulation ceases and/or ejaculation occurs. Thus all patients must undergo careful dose titration in order to avoid the possibility of an unnecessarily high dose leading to prolonged erection or, more rarely, priapism. Such factors must also be considered when designing trials to assess the efficacy of intracavernosal injections administered in the clinic or at home.

In contrast oral sildenafil is of type IV class (i.e. a peripheral conditioner) – it acts to alter local conditions to favor erection during sexual stimulation. Owing to its mode of action as an inhibitor of phosphodiesterase 5, sildenafil will act to restore the erectile response during sexual stimulation, but will have no direct effect in the absence of sexual stimulation. This has profound implications for the design of phase II and III trials – there is no rationale for simply administering a dose of sildenafil and then monitoring penile rigidity in the absence of sexual stimulation. If objective measurements of rigidity (i.e. RigiScan) are required, then some form of sexual stimulation should be administered during the period of monitoring. This stimulation may be visual or vibratory, and should be timed to coincide with peak plasma concentrations of the drug. Such objective techniques are useful to convince researchers and regulatory authorities that drugs do have a pro-erectile effect in men with ED, but the conditions of passively experiencing visual or tactile stimuli are far removed from the normal interactive forms of sexual activity between partners. Therefore the mainstay of efficacy assessments for drugs which act as conditioners must be based on patient and partner reporting of erections during sexual activity at home.

Erectile dysfunction is defined as the inability to attain and/or maintain an erection sufficient for satisfactory sexual performance (National Institutes of Health 1992). In terms of assessing any therapy for erectile dysfunction, it is, however, necessary to go beyond this purely functional definition and consider the wider aspects of male sexual function, which involve not only the aspects of arousal and the erectile response, but also desire or libido, ejaculation, orgasm, and overall satisfaction with sex life and the partner relationship. The reason for needing a broader view is that some or all of the above aspects of male sexual function may be improved or possibly impaired by a therapy intended to treat the erectile disorder.

In outpatient studies of men with ED the various approaches (diary, questionnaire, interview, partner questionnaire, etc.) to measuring drug effect all present problems; however, it is a good starting point to place strong emphasis on the patient's judgment concerning benefit of treatment. Just as establishing the diagnosis of ED is largely reliant on the history of the patient who states he is unable to perform sexually, similarly selecting an appropriate measure of efficacy will ultimately have to rely on self-reported answers to questions on erectile function. Indeed, both diagnosis and therapy evaluation in ED need to be "goal-directed" – i.e. based on patient and partner expectations and their willingness to use a particular therapeutic option (Lue 1990; De Palma 1996). Thus the actual day-to-day experiences of the patients and their feeling of benefit from treatment are ultimately the final guide to the magnitude of response and acceptability of treatment. Considering this reliance on subjective end-points, as well as the recognition of a significant placebo response rate in ED studies, it is essential to use placebo controls in phase II studies to enable valid assessments of drug effect.

The choice of patient and partner self-report instruments is limited. Diaries are often used, and the patient is asked to record the doses taken and describe the results of sexual activity. Data accuracy and compliance with diary completion are likely to be variable. To attempt to minimize this the design of diaries must be kept simple, and clear instructions should always be provided to ensure a good understanding of the questions by the patient or his partner to ensure the collection of accurate data. Diaries can clearly distinguish positive drug effects from placebo, but to our knowledge there are no fully validated diaries available.

Questionnaires to capture information on drug effects within the privacy of the home are generally completed by the patient before treatment and at intervals during treatment. They rely on the ability of the patient to record aspects of his sexual activity over a recall period of a few days to weeks. Questionnaire precision is determined by the number of sexual events evaluated, and too few events may not yield highly reliable data; on the other hand, extending the duration of the study period is restricted by the resultant loss of accurate recall by the patients. Until relatively recently, although a number of male sexual function questionnaires did exist, few were validated and none appeared to be designed with international, multicenter clinical trials of ED in mind. More recently O'Leary et al (1996) developed the Brief Male Sexual Function Inventory, and Rosen et al (1997) published the procedures used to develop and validate the International Index of Erectile Function (IIEF). The latter instrument was used extensively throughout the sildenafil clinical development program, and has been used in trials of phentolamine, but at present there is no instrument that has been endorsed for assessment of efficacy by the FDA or any other regulatory agency. The use of validated sexual function questionnaires can be supplemented by other questions such as asking whether the patient would consider taking the treatment on a long-term basis, and whether he considers his erections to be sufficiently or fully improved with the experimental drug. As experience with these new and validated instruments is gained it is hoped that a common scoring system can be adopted so as to allow classification of the severity of ED in individual patients based on their baseline scores, and to capture the extent of response to therapy by the absolute change in score.

Other factors to consider in the design of phase II trials include the selection of patients. In the relatively early stages of drug development it is usual to investigate efficacy in a relatively restricted population. If the treatment is one considered suitable only for men with predominantly psychogenic or mild organic forms of ED (such as apomorphine), then it may be necessary to undertake a variety of diagnostic tests to exclude inappropriate patients. However, tests such as nocturnal penile plethysmography and Doppler ultrasound are expensive, complex, and sometimes operator-dependent. Moreover, there are no universally agreed criteria to separate normal and abnormal results. Thus the use of such tests should if possible be restricted to trials involving a limited number of patients and centers. Other factors in trial design include the instruction to both the investigators and the patients as to the best use of the drug when considering its pharmacokinetic profile (for example, ensuring that sexual activity is attempted at an appropriate time after administration). Importantly, the power of the study to detect differences in treatments (i.e. between active drug and placebo or between two different doses of active drug) and hence the number of patients per treatment group must be calculated before finalizing the protocol.

To provide a comprehensive assessment of a treatment for ED it is necessary to cover other significant quality-of-life (QoL) consequences of the condition – all too frequently in quantitative research these are overlooked in the drive to establish evidence of safety and efficacy. Within ED the quantification of how the disorder interferes with basic human needs is of paramount importance – it serves to emphasize the rationale for treatment and the relative success of any treatment options tried. The IIEF deliberately focuses on functional erectile ability, but also includes assessments of orgasm, sexual desire, partner relationship, and overall satisfaction with sex life. Instruments that can complement the IIEF by providing insight into the QoL of ED patients and their partners are needed. The approach taken with the sildenafil program was to develop a QoL battery that combined well-established generic instruments (for example, the Medical Outcomes Short Form Health Survey (SF-12), the Psychological General Well Being Index (PGWBI)), and a specific ED instrument (Impact of Erectile Problems Scale). Although comprehensive, this approach was felt to lack the focus that is described in other QoL instruments, where the psychological, emotional, and social impacts of ED are directly and specifically addressed (Wagner et al 1996). A standard battery of instruments that combines both functional and QoL assessment is still awaited.

Phase II is one of the most demanding but satisfying periods of drug development: a variety of trial designs (for instance, flexible dose escalation, fixed dose–dose response, crossover, parallel group) is possible; a variety of efficacy parameters can be measured; and safety must be rigorously monitored. Careful consideration of mode of action and trial design is critical at this stage to allow the potential efficacy of the treatment to be evaluated and to allow selection of appropriate doses to take forward to phase III studies. A detailed discussion of design considerations for dose-finding studies during phase II is beyond the scope of this review, but the dosing regimen (fixed vs flexible dose), the patient population, and the duration of the treatment period must be carefully debated to ensure that the data generated during this phase can be confidently extrapolated to help design the longer phase III trials, which must assess long-term efficacy and safety in the target patient population. Another important consideration with ED drugs is the potential development of tachyphylaxis or tolerance with long-term treatment. This possibility must be carefully discussed in phase II before embarking on long and costly phase III studies, and a compromise involving trials of sufficient duration to identify the possibility of tachyphylaxis but sufficiently short to advance the development program efficiently must be sought. Many drugs spend an excessively long time in phase II, or are progressed to inadequate phase III programs, because the importance of one or more of the features of the drug (kinetics, dynamics, metabolism, toleration) or of trial design (an adequately powered study covering an appropriate dose range) or of the selection of patients has been misjudged or overlooked in the early trials.

Phase III studies

It is not unusual for only one out of four drugs entering phase II to reach phase III. At the end of phase II the efficacy of the new drug and the therapeutic dose range should be established. The most common adverse events will be known. On the basis of the profile to date a draft Package Insert can be prepared. Phase III is still the most costly phase of drug development, and so a decision to proceed will be taken only if the data are encouraging and the commercial prospects for effective promotion and marketing still appear to be good. The main purpose of the phase III program is to generate sufficient short-term and long-term efficacy and safety data to gain regulatory approval. In general, for the development of new medicines, regulatory guidelines require an absolute minimum of 1500 patients to have received the study drug and at least 100 patients to have received treatment at the recommended dose regimen for at least one year. There are no regulatory guidelines for the development of an oral agent to treat ED, but since the condition is not life-threatening the need for a larger clinical safety database can be anticipated.

It is also essential to review whether the trials conducted in phase II and those proposed for phase III meet the regulators' expectations for establishing efficacy. In the USA it is common for an end of phase II conference to be convened with the FDA. In Europe it is now possible to discuss drug development programs with various national authorities of the CPMP (Committee for Proprietary Medicinal Products). On the basis of the knowledge of the drug so far accumulated and discussions with regulatory authorities, it should be possible to design the remainder of the clinical program to ensure that the trial protocols and the data generated will fully meet the requirements of the drug licensing authorities for efficacy and safety evaluation.

Whereas the phase I and II studies may be performed at a limited number of sites, it is often necessary for the phase III program to be performed in Europe, the USA, and other parts of the world. As with phase I and II studies, it is essential that the trials are performed to Good Clinical Practice (GCP). GCP regulations are many and complex, but are essentially designed to protect the rights of the patients and the integrity of the data. Investigators who participate must be carefully selected by the sponsor company. Only those willing to work to GCP standards, with expertise in the disease area and with sufficient facilities and time to conduct the study properly, should be selected. In agreeing to participate in a trial a clinical investigator takes on responsibilities not only to the patients recruited but also to the sponsor company and to the government authorities. These responsibilities include: submission of the protocol to the Institutional Review Board or local ethics committee; security of the drug supplies; obtaining informed consent from the patients; accurately recording and properly storing all the trial information; and prompt reporting (within 24 hours) of serious adverse events. The sponsor company is required to monitor the progress of the trial, and this includes checking the accuracy and completion of the trial case record forms (CRFs) and ensuring that there is no discrepancy between the CRFs and the patients' clinical notes. For trials that are regarded as pivotal it is usual for the FDA to inspect some of the investigator sites during the regulatory review process.

The regulatory and commercialization phase

Regulatory submission and approval

By the end of the phase III program a huge volume of data will have been collected and databased, and this must be carefully reviewed by data managers and clinicians, and analysed by statisticians (in accordance with the requirements of the protocols), and reports must be prepared by medical writers. Summary documentation which describes and interprets the results of the data pooled from all the studies is also prepared. The Package Insert (USA) and the Summary of Product Characteristics (Europe) is finalized. It usually takes at least 6 months from the date of the last visit of the last patient in the last pre-registration trial to the compilation and submission of the dossier to a regulatory authority. The paper submitted may comprise several hundred volumes. Most authorities now expect at least part of the submission to be provided in electronic format as well.

The procedure for the submission and review of regulatory submissions varies throughout the world. In the USA and Europe it will typically take about a year for the authorities to reach a decision as to the approvability of the new treatment. The process may be extended if the authorities request further data or ask for changes to the US Package Insert (or in Europe the Summary of Product Characteristics) which the sponsor company finds unacceptable. Formal hearings may be convened to hear opinions from external experts and to discuss points of difference.

Phase IV studies

Trials undertaken prior to marketing approval may suffer from the limitations of a restricted patient population and limited duration of patient exposure compared with the overall exposure that will occur once a marketing license has been issued. Thus at approval it is known that the new medicine is effective, but its ultimate role and utility as a new treatment (i.e. as first-line or second-line treatment; which subgroup of patients to select or avoid) may not have been entirely defined. Also, at approval all the more common adverse reactions should have been identified and described in the Package Insert, but rarer idiosyncratic reactions are unlikely to have been identified. To overcome these limitations post-marketing or phase IV studies are performed to evaluate the drug in selected populations, generate comparative data versus other agents, investigate new indications and new dosage forms, and monitor the potential for unexpected drug interactions and rare unexpected adverse events. Careful surveillance of safety data from spontaneous reporting of adverse reactions by physicians prescribing the new medicine is also essential.

The marketing of the medicine does not imply an end of research activities – additional information can lead to further uses for the particular compound. There are many medicines that had initially been launched with one, or sometimes two, indications, but for which continuous research and development over subsequent years has led to increased numbers of indications. Alternatively, new safety concerns may arise, and lead to more restrictions on the use of the medicine or even its withdrawal from the market. The development of the new medicine and the expanding knowledge of its properties create a need to disseminate information throughout the medical profession, which again is the responsibility of the marketing arm of the pharmaceutical industry.

Conclusion

Since the late 1940s there has been so much progress in the field of medical therapeutics that there are few medical conditions that are not at least partially amenable to drug therapy. One medical area that appears to have been somewhat neglected is that of sexual dysfunction. Only relatively recently has the treatment of erectile dysfunction been made possible through the use of intracavernosal injection therapy, and until very recently no efficacious oral formulation had yet been identified.

Making drugs into medicines is clearly extremely complex, involving interactions between individuals of often vastly differing scientific backgrounds and disciplines. This chapter has endeavored to introduce the concepts of relevance to clinicians with an interest in ED who may be involved during the clinical development of new drugs. In doing so it is our hope that any potential conceptual gap between the pharmaceutical research industry and independent clinicians can be bridged. As the place of the controlled clinical trial in the pharmaceutical development of new drugs is undisputed, it is important to ensure that a common understanding of processes does exist between the industry professionals and the medical community with whom they collaborate. The inseparability of the scientific collaboration between these groups, and the requirement for clinicians to be involved in the march of progress of pharmaceutical research are encapsulated in the statement made by the former president of the Royal Society of Medicine, Sir George Pickering – "therapeutics is a branch of medicine that by its very nature should be experimental". The alliance between industry and clinicians is indeed not one of convenience, but is rather an essential response to the challenge of continuing to treat disease.

References

Andersson KE, Wagner G (1995). Physiology of penile erection. *Physiol Rev* **75**.

Boolell M, Gepi-Attee S, Gingell JC, Allen MJ (1996a). Sildenafil, a novel effective oral therapy for male erectile dysfunction. *Br J Urol* **78**: 257–61.

Boolell M, Allen MJ, Ballard SA, et al (1996b). An orally effective type 5 cyclic GMP-specific phosphodiesterase inhibitor for the treatment of penile erectile dysfunction. *Int J Impot Res* **8**: 47–52.

Brindley GS (1983). Cavernosal alpha-blockade: a new technique for investigating and treating erectile impotence. *Br J Psychiatry* **143**: 332–7.

Burnett AL, Lowerstein CJ, Bredt DS, Chang TSK, Snyder SH (1992). Nitric oxide: a physiologic mediator of penile erection. *Science* **257**: 401–3.

Christ GJ (1995). The penis as a vascular organ. *Urol Clin North Am* **22**: 727–45.

De Palma RG (1996). New developments in the diagnosis and treatment of impotence. *World J Med* **164**: 54–61.

Foreman MM, Wernicke JF (1990). Approaches for the development of oral drug therapies for erectile dysfunction. *Semin Urol* **8**: 107–12.

Gingell C, Jardin A, Giuliano FA, et al (1996). The efficacy of sildenafil (Viagra™) a new oral treatment for erectile dysfunction, demonstrated by four different methods in a double-blind placebo-controlled, multinational clinical trial. *Eur Urol* **30**(supp 2): Abs 353.

Heaton JPW, Adams MA, Morales A (1992). A therapeutic taxonomy of treatments for erectile dysfunction: an evolutionary imperative. *Int J Impot Res* **9**: 115–21.

Ignarro LJ, Bush PA, Buga GM, Wood KS, Fukuto JM, Rajfer J (1990). Nitric oxide and cyclic GMP formation upon electrical field stimulation cause relaxation of the corpus cavernosal smooth muscle. *Biochem Biophys Res Commun* **170**: 843–50.

Kim N, Azadzoi KM, Goldstein I, Saenz de Tejada I (1991). A nitric oxide-like factor mediates nonadrenergic-noncholinergic neurogenic relaxation of penile corpus cavernosum smooth muscle. *J Clin Invest* **88**: 112–18.

Lerner SE, Melman A, Christ GJ (1993). A review of erectile dysfunction: new insights and more questions. *J Urol* **149**: 1246–55.

Lue TF (1990). Impotence: a patient's goal-directed approach to treatment. *World J Urol* **8**: 1–28.

National Institutes of Health (1992). *NIH Consensus Statement on Impotence.* **10** vol. pp. 1–31, Bethesda, MA:NIH.

O'Leary MP, Fowler FJ, Lenderking WR, Sagnier PP, Guess HA, Barry MJ (1996). A brief male sexual function inventory for urology. *Urology* **46**: 697–706.

Rajfer J, Aronson WJ, Bush PA, Dorey FJ, Ignarro LJ (1992). Nitric oxide as a mediator of the corpus cavernosum in response to non cholinergic, non adrenergic neurotransmission. *N Engl J Med* **326**: 90–4.

Rosen RC, Riley A, Wagner G, Osterloh IH, Kirkpatrick J, Mishra A (1997). The International Index of Erectile Function (IIEF): a multidimensional scale for assessment of erectile function. *Urology* **49**: 822–30.

Virag RB, Ottesen B, Fahrenkrug J, Levy C, Wagner G (1982). Vasoactive intestinal polypeptide release during penile erection in man. *Lancet* **ii**: 1166.

Wagner TH, Patrick DL, McKenna SP, Froese PS (1996). Cross-cultural development of a quality of life measure for men with erectile difficulties. *Quality of Life Res* **5**: 443–9.

13

A new frontier: gene therapy for erectile dysfunction

George J Christ

Introduction

During the past two decades the knowledge gleaned from a combination of basic and clinical studies has resulted in vast improvements in the understanding, diagnosis and treatment of erectile dysfunction. Intracavernous injection therapy, vacuum devices, surgical implantation of prosthetic devices, intraurethral suppositories, and, most recently, oral medications now provide the physician with a therapeutic armamentarium sufficient to correct even the most severe manifestations of organic impotence. In effect, we have reached the point where erectile potency can be effectively restored in every man who possesses the appropriate level of desire and motivation. However, despite their documented efficacy, all available treatment options have significant side-effects. Consequently, there is still much room for improvement, and it is anticipated that the application of the techniques of molecular biology to the study of erectile physiology/dysfunction will open up an entirely new vista of opportunities for the treatment of erectile dysfunction. The goal of this report, therefore, is to review how these new molecular technologies will be likely to affect the diagnosis and treatment of erectile dysfunction, and furthermore, to describe one initial strategy for utilizing gene therapy for this purpose.

Overview of erectile physiology and dysfunction

Detailed knowledge of the mechanistic basis of normal erectile function, as well as of the etiology of erectile dysfunction, is an absolute prerequisite to understanding the relevance of gene therapy. However, the complexities of the physiology and pharmacology of erectile physiology/dysfunction have been previously described (Carrier et al 1993; Andersson and Wagner 1995; Christ 1995), and furthermore are presented in other chapters in this volume. Thus, only the most basic applicable features will be reviewed here.

Briefly, erection is a complex neurovascular event that is analogous to a myriad other hemodynamic events occurring in the human body (Melman and Christ 1997), that is, increased intrapenile blood flow and intracavernous pressure require coordinated vascular smooth-muscle relaxation. In fact, regardless of the initiating stimulus (neuronal, pharmacological, and so on), rapid and syncytial relaxation of the arterial and corporeal smooth muscle is absolutely critical to transmit the systemic blood pressure/flow effectively into the penis. In the presence of a competent flap valve or veno-occlusive mechanism, the increased blood flow and blood pressure result in compression of the venous blood vessels against the walls of the tunica albuginea, effectively trapping blood in the penis and producing axial rigidity.

In the absence of severe vascular disease, relaxation of corporeal vascular smooth muscle is both necessary and sufficient for normal erection. Thus, the tone of the corporeal smooth-muscle cell serves a pivotal role in the entire erectile process. The fact that the pharmacotherapy of erectile dysfunction relies almost exclusively on the use of vasorelaxing agents is further demonstration of "proof of principle" with regard to the clinical relevance of modulation of the degree of corporeal smooth-muscle tone. Taken together, all these observations reflect the fact that a delicate balance between the effects of multiple contracting and relaxing agents on the tone of the corporeal smooth-muscle cell is required for normal erectile capacity. In short, any physiologic alteration that results in a greater degree of corporeal smooth-muscle contraction, or conversely, is associated with a diminution in corporeal smooth muscle relaxation will promote erectile dysfunction. As discussed in detail below, the underlying assumption behind gene therapy is that one can genetically modify a sufficient number of smooth-muscle cells to restore the "normal" endogenous balance between contracting and relaxing factors.

What is gene therapy?

Before answering this question, let's consider an even more fundamental issue: What is "molecular biology"? As reviewed elsewhere (Kendrew 1994) the term seems to have been first used by Warren

Weaver in his 1938 address to the Rockefeller Foundation, where he stated: "Among the studies to which the Foundation is giving support is a relatively new field, which may be called molecular biology . . .". Since 1938 the term "molecular biology" has come to represent many things, but in its most broad definition "molecular biology" relates to the study of the structure and function of biologically important macromolecules, ranging from proteins to RNA and DNA. Thus, "molecular biology" truly exists at the interface of crystallography, biophysics, biochemistry and genetics. Many very sophisticated techniques were developed as tools to assist in the more efficient study of "molecular biology". The recent commercialization and popularization of some of these techniques, such as northern, western and Southern blots, and the polymerase chain reaction, have moved molecular biology to the forefront of scientific thought and development. As might be expected, many subdisciplines of molecular biology have evolved, but for the purposes of this report the terms molecular biology and molecular genetics and all related terms will be used interchangeably.

The rapid technological advances in molecular biology have placed valuable tools in the hands of organ systems physiologists. More specifically, all the tools required for the identification, isolation, sequencing, synthesis, cloning and foreign expression of genes and gene products of interest are now readily commercially available. The availability of these tools permits physiologists/pharmacologists to explore the contribution of individual genes, or sets of genes, to tissue function/homeostasis. Thus, it is not surprising that these cutting edge molecular techniques have provided many new insights into the understanding of human physiology, while simultaneously ushering in a new era in the diagnosis and treatment of human disease. In this light, it was only natural that "molecular biology" would wind its way into the urology clinic.

The application of the tools of molecular biology to the genetic therapy of human disease

Genetic therapy for human disease derives from the application of these techniques to clinical medicine (Anderson 1992; Miller 1992; Roemer and Friedmann 1992; Crystal 1995; Rowen et al 1997). Historically, and not surprisingly, genetic therapies have been utilized to correct diseases/disorders that have an underlying genetic component. In this scenario, the introduction of foreign genetic information

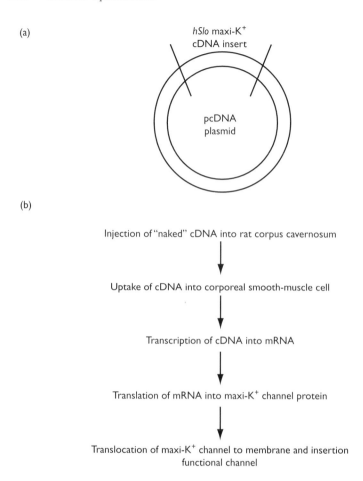

Figure 1

(a) Schematic depiction of the general principles involved in gene therapy for erectile dysfunction. Illustration of a cDNA, referred to as "naked" DNA, that is inserted into a specific region in a double-stranded eukaryotic plasmid DNA. Once injected into the corpora, the plasmid is taken up into the target cell. In this case the target cell is thought to be primarily the corporeal smooth-muscle cell, and the mechanism by which this cellular uptake occurs is not yet entirely clear. The plasmid DNA maintains an episomal profile, that is, the pcDNA/hSlo cDNA complex is never integrated into the host cell genome. As such, the plasmid must, and does, contain all the necessary genetic machinery (i.e. promoter, termination sequence, etc.) to ensure transcription of the hSlo cDNA. (b) A flow chart depicting the series of events leading from intracorporeal injection of "naked" DNA to the expression of a functional potassium channel in the corporeal smooth-muscle cell membrane.

into human cells either restores/supplements defective functions or, conversely, functionally antagonizes the effects of expression of a mutant genetic function. Thus, the term gene therapy has been coined to describe the genetic modification of a population of cells, and is the term that will be used throughout this report.

In short, it is now possible for one to express foreign genes selectively in specific target cells, and thus alter, in a measurable fashion, a desired cellular response. While a detailed description of all the methodologies involved in gene therapy is well beyond the scope of this report, suffice it to say that the identification, isolation, sequencing, synthesis, cloning and foreign expression of genes can now be accomplished in relatively short order, and with great accuracy and fidelity. The goal of this report is to highlight how these strategies will impact on the treatment of erectile dysfunction and, furthermore, to outline one specific application of these technologies to the genetic therapy of erectile dysfunction (Figure 1).

Gene therapy and human cardiovascular disease

Exploration of the potential utility of gene therapy to the treatment of cardiovascular disease can be traced to the beginning of this decade (Nabel et al 1990). Since then, techniques for gene transfer into muscle cells have continued to be developed with the dual purpose of providing insights into myocyte gene regulation, as well as providing novel therapeutic strategies for the treatment of cardiovascular diseases (Nabel et al 1990; Bennett and Schwartz 1995; Chang et al 1995; Finkel and Epstein 1995). The experimental studies conducted thus far have helped delineate the general boundary conditions for the efficiency and persistence of gene transfer into muscle cells and, moreover, have indicated that muscle may be unique in its ability to incorporate and express naked DNA (Miller 1992). In short, the efficiency of transfection rates can vary dramatically depending on the muscle cell type and the vector used, but has been reported to range from transfection rates as low as 0.01% in cardiac myocytes following a single injection of naked DNA (Buttrick 1993; Kass-Eisler et al 1993) to as high as 80% in vascular wall cells using adenovirus-mediated gene transfer techniques (Schulick et al 1995). Meanwhile, incorporation of DNA is thought to be extrachromosomal (i.e. episomal), with persistence of the DNA in cells of the vessel wall reportedly detected for up to 5 months post-transfection (Nabel et al 1990). Overall, such results have to be considered quite exciting and encouraging, given the relatively short time-frame over which these techniques have been applied to the cardiovascular system.

However, despite these initial successes, at least three significant obstacles to the successful clinical treatment of systemic vascular disorders remain. They are: (1) the specificity of gene transfer/incorporation into one vascular bed or vascular cell type, but not another; (2) the efficiency and stability of gene incorporation; that is, what percentage of cells need to be transfected, and for how long? (3) Finding appropriate vectors so that the first two conditions can be met without producing other undesirable side-effects, such as insertional mutagenesis (i.e. such as might be expected with retroviruses (for instance, Rous sarcoma virus, RSV), or immunogenic reactions as a result of employing non-integrating, non-replicating viral vectors such as the adenovirus (Anderson 1992; Miller 1992; Crystal 1995; Finkel and Epstein 1995; Hanania et al 1995).

How can gene therapy be applied to the treatment of erectile dysfunction?

There is currently no compelling evidence either for, or against, a genetic basis for, or a genetic predisposition to, erectile failure. Bearing this in mind, the lack of a documented genetic component to erectile failure still does not necessarily exclude the relevance of a genetic treatment for impotence. While many aspects of erectile dysfunction mimic systemic vascular disease, there is still ample reason to expect that gene therapy will be more immediately successful in the treatment of human erectile dysfunction than might be expected for other cardiovascular disorders, and this will be discussed in detail below. However, as with all other in vivo gene therapy approaches, the potential utility of gene therapy to the treatment of human erectile dysfunction is dependent on the following two primary considerations: (1) What is the likelihood of affecting only the desired cell type(s)? (2) What percentage of target cells must be affected in order to see a physiologically relevant therapeutic effect? In the answers to these two questions lie the two main reasons for suspecting that gene therapy of erectile dysfunction may be inherently more successful than its proposed uses in other, more systemic, cardiovascular disorders, such as atherosclerosis, vasculitis and restenosis after balloon angioplasty (see Nabel et al 1990; Bennett and Schwartz 1995; Chang et al 1995; Finkel and Epstein 1995).

First, it is a well-documented fact that corporeal smooth-muscle cells are interconnected by a ubiquitously distributed population of intercellular channels known as gap-junction proteins (Christ et al

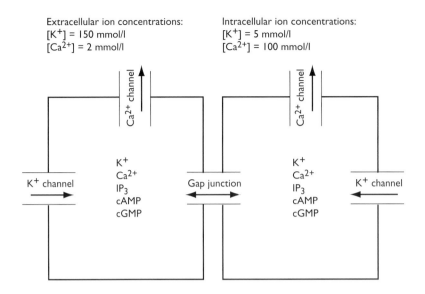

Figure 2

The distribution of ions across the corporeal smooth-muscle cell membrane. The presence of an electrochemical gradient that favors the inward flux of Ca^{2+} and the outward flux of K^+ is very important to the initiation, maintenance and modulation of corporeal smooth-muscle tone. The primary Ca^{2+} channel thought to be present in corporeal smooth muscle is the L-type voltage-dependent Ca^{2+} channel. Any time a Ca^{2+} channel opens, Ca^{2+} move into the corporeal smooth-muscle cell, resulting in cellular depolarization and a transient three- to tenfold increase in the cytosolic intracellular calcium concentration that provides the trigger for smooth-muscle contraction. Furthermore, continuous transmembrane Ca^{2+} flux is an absolute component of sustained corporeal smooth-muscle tone. There are several subtypes of K^+ channel present in corporeal smooth muscle, but, nevertheless, any time a K^+ channel opens, K^+ move out of the cell. Thus, the opening of K^+ channels serves a functionally antagonistic role to that of Ca^{2+} channels, in that the movement of positive charge out of the cell results in cellular hyperpolarization, thus decreasing transmembrane calcium flux in the opposite direction. Also shown are the other second messenger molecules that are known to be important determinants of corporeal smooth-muscle tone. All of these second messengers are freely diffusible through the junctional ion channels (i.e. gap junctions) found between adjacent corporeal smooth-muscle cells. IP_3: inositol triphosphate; cAMP: cyclic adenosine monophosphate; cGMP: cyclic guanosine monophosphate.

Figure 3

Illustration of the neuronal innervation and signal transduction mechanisms that provide the mechanistic basis for rapid and syncytial corporeal smooth-muscle responses. The presence of these extant mechanisms provides a key factor in the ultimate success of gene therapy for the treatment of erectile dysfunction. (a) Schematic depiction of the autonomic effector innervation in corporeal smooth muscle expected on the basis of previous work (see Lerner et al 1993). This schematic diagram depicts the interrelationship of neuronal innervation, gap junctions and the corporeal parenchyma. (b) As the neuronal varicosities course through the corporeal parenchyma, the release of neurotransmitters will result in a graded activation of smooth-muscle cells in direct relation to their proximity to the varicosity. Although not depicted, the cells are interconnected by gap junctions as shown in (a), so that direct activation of cell number 1 would result in intercellular transmission of the information for cellular activation to cells 2, 3 and 4. The anisotropic nature of intercellular diffusion results from the fact that cytoplasmic permeability is approximately one order of magnitude greater than junctional permeability; thus, diffusion along the long axis of the smooth-muscle cell will occur more quickly than diffusion across the width of the cell. (c) How activation of one cell (i.e. cell 1) might lead to recruitment of adjacent, though not directly activated, cells via the passive intercellular spread of second messenger molecules/ions. Such a mechanism is important to permit coordination of corporeal smooth-muscle tone. In this scenario, the cells nearest the activated cell will necessarily "see" much higher concentrations of second messengers than cells that are more distally removed. The sensitivity of the smooth-muscle cells to any given second messenger molecule/ion is thus a very important determinant of the number of smooth-muscle cells recruited by a given stimulus. (d) The predicted intercellular diffusion profiles on the same cells numbered in (c). These intercellular diffusion profiles for junction-permeant second messenger molecules were calculated by mathematical modeling techniques described elsewhere (Christ et al 1994). Briefly, cell 1 is assumed to have some arbitrary, but constant, concentration of second messenger molecules due to persistent receptor activation by an agonist or a neurotransmitter. The arrows in the diffusion profile highlight the differential intercellular second messenger concentrations expected across the junctional membrane of contiguous cells, while the dashed lines depict the anticipated concentration gradients across the width of any given cell. The junctional permeability used for this comparison was 5×10^{-4} cm/s, a junctional permeability characteristic of corporeal smooth-muscle cells expressing conexin 43.

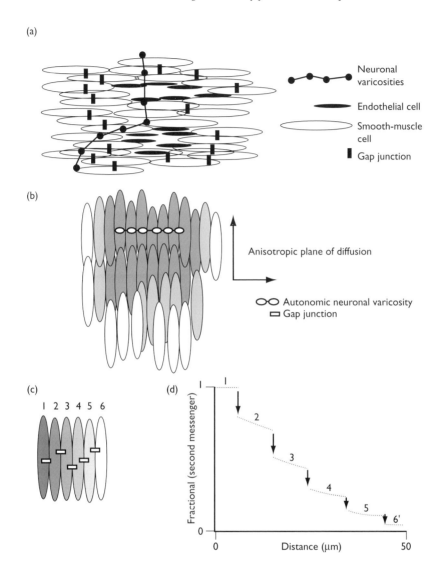

(a)

Neuronal varicosities

Endothelial cell

Smooth-muscle cell

Gap junction

(b)

Anisotropic plane of diffusion

Autonomic neuronal varicosity
Gap junction

(c)

1 2 3 4 5 6

(d)

Fractional (second messenger)

Distance (μm)

1993b; Christ 1995; Brink et al 1996; Christ and Melman 1997), with conexin 43 as the predominant isoform expressed in the human penis. The importance of these intercellular channels to normal erectile function is related to the fact that they provide partial cytoplasmic continuity between adjacent smooth-muscle cells, and thus permit the intercellular exchange of physiologically relevant ions (K^+ and Ca^{2+}) and second messenger molecules (IP_3, cAMP, cGMP) (Figure 2). Gap junctions thus provide the anatomic substrate for coordinating the syncytial contraction and relaxation responses that are a pre-requisite to normal penile erection and detumescence.

More importantly, with respect to the potential success or failure of gene therapy, is the fact that intercellular communication among the smooth-muscle cells permits cells that are not directly activated by a relevant neuronal/hormonal signal to be rapidly, albeit indirectly, recruited into the contraction or relaxation response (Figure 3). In fact, intercellular communication through gap junctions ensures the rapid and syncytial smooth-muscle responses that are required for normal erection and detumescence. Extrapolating to the current discussion, the presence of gap junctions ensures that only a fraction of the corporeal smooth-muscle cells would need to be genetically modified in order to affect rather global changes in corporeal smooth-muscle tone (Figure 3). This fact apparently minimizes the importance of the efficiency of genetic modification of the target cells, and thus obviates the necessity for utilizing more aggressive genetic incorporation strategies that are necessarily dependent on the use of retroviral or adenoviral vectors, with their concomitantly greater potential for side-effects such as insertional mutagenesis or immunological reactions.

A second reason for suspecting that gene therapy will be an attractive therapeutic possibility for the treatment of human erectile dysfunction is the simple fact that, in many men, impotence is likely to be the result of relatively subtle alterations in the balance between contracting and relaxing stimuli and their respective effects on corporeal and arterial smooth-muscle tone (Azadzoi and Saenz de Tejada 1992; Lerner et al 1993; Taub et al 1993; Christ 1995; Adams et al 1997). Thus the goal of gene therapy for erectile dysfunction is relatively straightforward: to restore the normal balance between the effects of contracting and relaxing stimuli on corporeal smooth-muscle cells by altering the degree of expression (for instance, the over-expression) of gene(s) that code(s) for a physiologically relevant protein in the corporeal smooth-muscle cell. One initial strategy for so doing is briefly described below.

Why choose potassium channels as an initial strategy for gene therapy of erectile dysfunction?

As an initial attempt to validate the possibility of genetic therapy for the treatment of human erectile dysfunction, we have conducted

Table 1 Effects of various vasoactive compounds on ion channel activity, membrane potential and corporeal smooth-muscle tone

Agonist	Channel type affected	Putative mechanism	Effect on smooth-muscle tone
		Membrane potential −30 mV (DEPOLARIZED, i.e. contracted)	
ET-1	L-type Ca^{2+} increases →	Voltage or phosphorylation →	Increased tone
PE	K_{Ca} increases →	Ca^{2+} sensitive →	Modulates increase in tone
KCl	K_{ATP} increases →	Decreased ATP →	Modulates increase in tone
TEA	K_{Ca} decreases →	Channel blockade →	Increased tone
Glibenclamide	K_{ATP} decreases →	Channel blockade →	Increased tone
		−40 to −50 mV (RESTING POTENTIAL)	
PGE$_1$	K_{Ca} increases →	Phosphorylation →	Decreased tone
NTG	L-type Ca^{2+} decreases →	Voltage or phosphorylation →	Decreased tone
Pinacidil	K_{ATP} increases →	Increased mean open time →	Decreased tone
		Membrane potential −60 mV (HYPERPOLARIZED, i.e. relaxed)	

ET-1: endothelin-1; PE: phenylephrine; TEA: tetraethylammonium (a relatively non-selective K^+ channel blocker); glibenclamide: a K_{ATP} channel subtype selective blocker; K_{Ca}: the calcium-sensitive maxi-K^+ channel (i.e. *hSlo*); K_{ATP}: the metabolically gated K^+ channel.

Figure 4

The putative mechanistic basis for the ability of increased K^+ channel expression to increase smooth-muscle relaxation. The increased K^+ flux from the smooth-muscle cell is hypothesized to result from the greater number of K^+ channels present on the smooth-muscle cell membrane. Increased K^+ flux would be associated with a greater inhibition of transmembrane Ca^{2+} flux into the smooth-muscle cell, and a corresponding reduction in intracellular calcium levels. Decreased intracellular calcium levels are, in turn, associated with smooth-muscle relaxation.

preclinical studies to examine the effects of over-expression of a potassium (K^+) channel on cavernous nerve-stimulated intracavernous pressure responses in a rat model in vivo. The rationale for the choice of K^+ channels is related to both the ubiquity and the variety of their expression in penile smooth muscle. At least four distinct types of K^+ channels have been identified in human corporeal smooth muscle, and their salient features have been described (Christ et al 1993a; Fan et al 1995). For the purposes of this discussion, we will consider only the most general principles associated with K^+ channels and their function in corporeal smooth muscle. These principles are summarized in Table 1, and illustrated in Figure 4.

K^+ channels are known to play a fundamental role in the physiologic and pathophysiologic regulation of smooth-muscle tone in diverse organ systems (Nelson et al 1990, 1995; Brayden and Nelson 1992; Mayan and Faraci 1993; Nelson 1993; Nelson and Quayle 1995; Fan et al 1995; Ohya et al 1996). K^+ channels modulate smooth-muscle tone by altering membrane potential. The observed K^+ channel-mediated hyperpolarization of smooth muscle is a product of the differential distribution of K^+ ions across the cell membrane, as well as the resting membrane potential (i.e., approximately -50 mV). Specifically, any time a corporeal smooth-muscle K^+ channel opens, K^+ ions will flow down their electrochemical gradient and out of the cell. Thus any intracellular second messenger process that is associated with an increase in K^+ channel activity and/or mean open time will result in increased K^+ ion efflux from the cell interior. Moving positive charge out of the cell results in cellular hyperpolarization.

The corresponding decrease in membrane potential has the additional effect of reducing the activity of L-type voltage-dependent calcium channels (Christ 1995; Christ et al 1997b; Stief et al 1997). Because calcium is also differentially distributed across the cell membrane

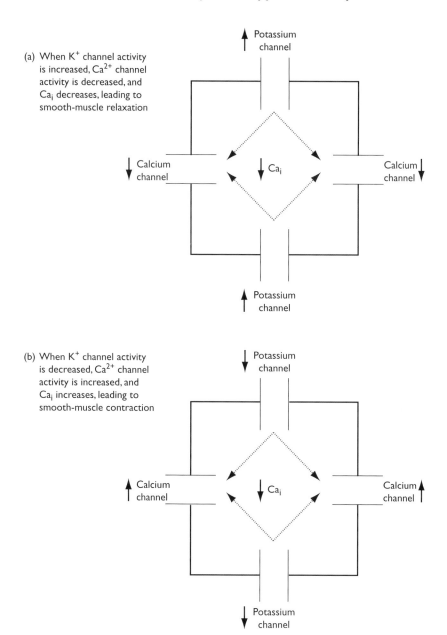

(a) When K$^+$ channel activity is increased, Ca^{2+} channel activity is decreased, and Ca$_i$ decreases, leading to smooth-muscle relaxation

(b) When K$^+$ channel activity is decreased, Ca^{2+} channel activity is increased, and Ca$_i$ increases, leading to smooth-muscle contraction

(Figure 4), a decrease in Ca^{2+} channel activity (i.e. either a decrease in activity or mean open time) is associated with a decrease in calcium ion influx into the smooth muscle. In short, the importance of K$^+$ channels to the modulation of corporeal smooth-muscle tone is related to the important reciprocal interaction that exists between the activity of K^+ channels, their effects on membrane potential, and the subsequent alterations in the activity of voltage-dependent Ca^{2+} channels (see Figure 4 and Table 1).

To take the process one step further, the latter (Ca^{2+} channels) have an important impact on the cytoplasmic intracellular calcium concentration, by virtue of their ability to modulate the flow of calcium ions from the extracellular space into the corporeal smooth-muscle cell (Christ et al 1993a; Zhao and Christ 1995; Noack and Noack 1997). Increases in intracellular calcium levels initially provide the trigger for smooth-muscle contraction and, subsequently, the intracellular calcium concentration remains an important determinant of the degree of smooth-muscle tone (Zhao and Christ 1995; Noack and Noack 1997; Stief et al 1997). In this scenario, the primary importance of K^+ channels to the modulation of corporeal smooth-muscle tone is nominally also a reflection of the critical contribution made by transmembrane calcium flux through voltage-dependent Ca^{2+} channels to the initiation, maintenance and modulation of corporeal smooth-muscle tone.

Given their central role in governing the intracellular calcium concentration, it is not surprising that K^+ channels are a convergence point for the actions elicited by activation of a wide variety of receptor and effector systems that are important to the control of erection in vivo. For example, corporeal smooth-muscle relaxation in response to elevations in intracellular cAMP and cGMP levels are both thought to occur, at least in part, via a phosphorylation-induced increase in K^+ channel activity (i.e. phosphorylation subsequent to activation of a protein kinase; either protein kinase A or G), and thus, cellular hyperpolarization (Chung et al 1991; Tanaguchi et al 1993; Bielefeldt and Jackson 1994; Reinhart and Levitan 1995; Starett et al 1996). In addition, blockade of the flow of K^+ ions through K^+ channels has been shown to augment contractile responses elicited by activation of the α_1-adrenergic receptor with phenylephrine, as well as activation of the endothelin(ET)$_{A/B}$ receptor subtype(s) following addition of endothelin-1 (Christ et al 1997a; Day et al 1997). Taken together, such observations clearly highlight the critical role played by K^+ channels in the modulation of corporeal smooth-muscle tone, and thus, erectile capacity.

For all of the aforementioned reasons, K^+ channels represent a logical first consideration for the genetic therapy of erectile dysfunction. Although there are at least four distinct types of K^+ channel present in human corporeal smooth muscle, the metabolically gated (K_{ATP}) and the calcium-sensitive (i.e. the maxi-K^+) K^+ channel subtypes are clearly the most physiologically relevant. Therefore, as an initial step toward the genetic therapy of human erectile dysfunction, we tested this hypothesis in a well-established rat model (Rehman et al 1997a), using the objective endpoint of nerve-stimulated intracavernous pressure increases as a proximal index of the potential physiological relevance of the proposed gene therapy. As depicted in Figure 5, injection of *hSlo* cDNA (which encodes the α or pore-forming subunit of the human smooth-muscle maxi-K^+ channel; McCobb et al 1995) into the rat corpora resulted in measurable, and physiologically relevant, alterations in penile erection in vivo. Consistent with observations on the longevity of gene therapy in another vascular tissue (Nabel et al 1990), expression of the maxi-K^+ *hSlo* cDNA appeared sustained for 1–4 months post-injection.

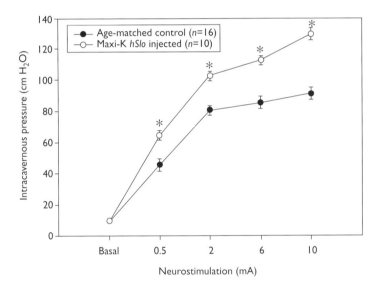

Figure 5

*Comparison of the effects of cavernous nerve-stimulation on intracavernous pressure responses in Sprague–Dawley rats following a single intracorporeal injection of hSlo/pcDNA (o), relative to the responses obtained on age-matched control animals (●) receiving injection of vehicle only. The data are a graphical representation of observations from a previous report (Christ et al, 1997a). Data are expressed as the Mean ± S.E.M., and were obtained on a total of 26 rats as follows: n = 16 for the age-matched control animals and, n = 10 for the hSlo injected animals. * - Significantly different from age-matched control, P<0.05, Student's t test for unpaired samples.*

Why does gene therapy with potassium channels work?

While one preclinical study does not a genetic therapy make, it is still worthwhile to speculate on the mechanistic basis for these compelling in vivo observations. In this regard, it is clear that the injected

(a)

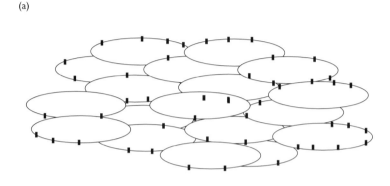

(b)

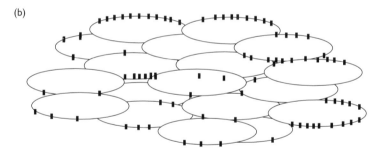

Figure 6
Schematic depiction of the putative rationale for the efficacy of intracorporeal injection of hSlo cDNA on the nerve-stimulated intracavernous pressure response. (a) An arbitrary distribution of potassium channels (dark rectangles on cell membrane) on corporeal smooth-muscle cells. (b) Depiction of an increased expression of K+ channels (again this is entirely arbitrary, as it has not yet been documented) on some fraction of the smooth-muscle cells. The increased K+ channel expression is not expected to be homogeneous, but merely sufficient to provide an increased hyperpolarizing ability to a sufficient number of corporeal smooth-muscle cells to ensure greater relaxation, even for the same stimulus.

hSlo cDNA was probably taken up into all cell types present in the rat corpora. While one cannot unequivocally exclude a role for uptake of the *hSlo* cDNA in the endothelial cell in mediating the observed increases in nerve-stimulated intracavernous pressure, we will confine the current discussion to the much more likely possibility of

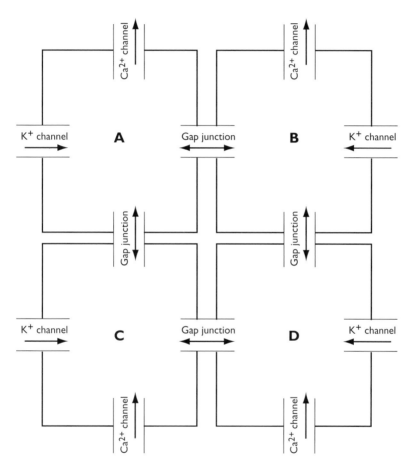

Figure 7
Signal spread through corporeal smooth muscle. A schematic depiction to remind one that corporeal smooth-muscle cells function as a syncytial network. Therefore any alteration in a single cell will have effects on not only the affected cell, but also on adjacent cells via intercellular diffusion through gap junctions. Thus, alterations in K^+ *and* Ca^{2+} *in one cell can be quite easily conveyed to neighboring cells.*

effects resulting from *hSlo* uptake and expression in the corporeal smooth-muscle cell. This seems a reasonable assumption given the fact that the corporeal smooth-muscle cell makes up the vast majority of the corporeal parenchyma and, moreover, that relaxation of the corporeal smooth muscle is both necessary and sufficient for erection.

In the light of such caveats, nominally the mechanistic basis for the increased maxi-K^+ channel activity would then be related to the commensurate augmentation in the hyperpolarizing ability of the corporeal smooth-muscle cells (Figures 4 and 6). Moreover, given the exquisite dependence of sustained corporeal smooth-muscle contraction on continuous transmembrane calcium flux, it stands to reason that the increase in hyperpolarization is associated with a decreased transmembrane calcium flux through L-type voltage-dependent calcium channels, and a corresponding decrease in the free intracellular calcium concentration; ultimately promoting greater corporeal smooth-muscle relaxation (Figure 7). Thus, increasing the expression of the maxi-K^+ channel in some physiologically relevant fraction of corporeal smooth-muscle cells would logically dictate an increased sensitivity of the smooth-muscle cells to the same level of a neural stimulation for relaxation. Certainly, a more precise analysis of the cellular disposition of the *hSlo* cDNA and the resulting expression of the α-subunit of the maxi-K^+ channel, as well as the relative percentage of cells thus affected, is still required in future preclinical studies.

So what does all this mean to the man with erectile dysfunction related to heightened contractility or impaired relaxation of corporeal smooth muscle?

In the light of the multifactorial nature of erectile dysfunction in man, there may in fact be many distinct genetic therapeutic strategies that will be effective in the restoration of erectile potency. For example, it is worth noting that qualitatively similar effects on intracavernous pressure were observed following the intracavernous injection of an inducible form of the nitric oxide synthase (bNOS) enzyme in a rat model (Garban et al 1997). Similar observations were also made following the intracavernous injection of bNOS cDNA in our laboratory (Rehman et al 1997b). Thus, if expression of these or other extrachromosomal genes can be maintained in humans for a period of weeks to months (as the preliminary preclinical data indicate), it is conceivable that a patient could obtain "normal" erections in the absence of any other exogenous manipulation during this time period. Clearly this would be a major advance over all currently available therapies.

The future of gene therapy for erectile dysfunction

In the light of the fact that it is anticipated that the human genome project will provide 70 000–100 000 genes that will be candidates for human gene transfer (Crystal 1995; Rowen et al 1997), the number of options for gene therapy in the future are enormous. As we continue to gain an even greater understanding of all the details concerning the regulation of corporeal and arterial smooth-muscle tone, as well as the manifold alterations that are associated with erectile dysfunction, the techniques of molecular genetics will provide an ever more valuable tool with which to alter erectile capacity more specifically. It is not difficult to envision the day when the genetic therapy of erectile dysfunction can be tailored on an individual patient basis, by matching the genetic therapy to the specific deficit responsible for the compromised erectile capacity.

Acknowledgements

The author gratefully acknowledges the assistance of Ms Masha Spektor with preparation of several figures, and Ms Diane DiTrapani for her excellent secretarial assistance. This work was supported in part by USPHS NIH grants DK46379 & DK42027.

References

Adams MA, Banting JD, Maurice DH, et al (1997). Vascular control mechanisms in penile erection: phylogeny and the inevitability of multiple and overlapping systems. *Int J Impot Res* **9**: 85–91.

Anderson WF (1992). Human gene therapy. *Science* **256**: 808–13.

Andersson K-E, Wagner, G (1995). Physiology of penile erection [Review]. *Physiol Rev* **75**: 191–236.

Azadzoi KM, Saenz de Tejada I (1992). Diabetes mellitus impairs neurogenic and endothelium-dependent relaxation of rabbit corpus cavernosum smooth muscle. *J Urol* **148**: 1587–91.

Bennett MR, Schwartz SM (1995). Antisense therapy for angioplasty restenosis. *Circulation* **92**: 1981–93.

Bielefeldt K, Jackson MB (1994). Phosphorylation and dephosphorylation modulate a Ca^{2+}-activated K^+ channel in rat peptidergic nerve terminals. *J Physiol* **475**: 241–54.

Brayden JE, Nelson MT (1992). Regulation of arterial tone by activation of calcium dependent potassium channels. *Science* **256**: 533.

Brink PR, Ramanan SV, Christ GJ (1996). Human connexin43 gap junction channel gating: evidence for mode shifts and/or heterogeneity. *Am J Physiol* **271**: C321–31.

Buttrick PM, Kaplan ML, Kitsis RN et al (1993) Distinct behaviour of cardiac myosin heavy chain gene constructs in vivo: discordance with in vitro results. *Circ Res* **72**: 1211–17.

Carrier S, Brock G, Kour NW, et al (1993). Pathophysiology of erectile dysfunction. *Urology* **42**: 468–81.

Chang MW, Barr E, Lu MM, et al (1995). Adenovirus-mediated over-expression of the cyclin/cyclin-dependent kinase inhibitor, p21 inhibits vascular smooth muscle cell proliferation and neointima formation in the rat carotid artery model of balloon angioplasty. *J Clin Invest* **96**: 2260–8.

Christ GJ (1995). The penis as a vascular organ: the importance of corporal smooth muscle tone in the control of penile erection. *Urol Clin North Am* **22**: 727–45.

Christ GJ, Melman A (1997). Molecular studies of human corporal smooth muscle: implications for the understanding, diagnosis, and treatment of erectile dysfunction. *Mol Urol* **1**: 45–54.

Christ GJ, Spray DC, Brink PR (1993a). Characterization of K currents in cultured human corporal smooth muscle cells. *J Androl* **14**: 319–28.

Christ GJ, Brink PR, Melman A, et al (1993b). The role of gap junctions and ion channels in the modulation of electrical and chemical signals in human corpus cavernosum smooth muscle. *Int J Impot Res* **5**: 77–96.

Christ GJ, Brink PR, Ramanan SV (1994). Dynamic gap junctional communication: a delimiting model for tissue responses. *Biophys J* **67**: 1335–44.

Christ GJ, Zhao W, Richards S, et al (1997a). Expression and significance of the maxi-K (K_{Ca}) potassium channel subtype in human corporal smooth muscle. *FASEB J* **11**: A197.

Christ GJ, Richards S, Winkler A (1997b). Integrative erectile biology: the role of signal transduction and cell-to-cell communication in coordinating corporal smooth muscle tone and penile erection. *Int J Impot Res* **9**: 69–84.

Crystal RG (1995). Transfer of genes to humans: early lessons and obstacles to success. *Science* **270**: 404–10.

Chung S, Reinhart PH, Martin BL, et al (1991). Protein kinase activity closely associated with a reconstituted calcium-activated potassium channel. *Science* **253**: 560–2.

Day NS, Giraldi A, Zhao W, et al (1997). Expression and function of a putative K_{ATP} channel subtype in human corpus cavernosum smooth muscle. *FASEB J* **11**: A328.

Fan SF, Brink PR, Melman A, et al (1995). An analysis of the Maxi-K^+ (K_{Ca}) channel in cultured human corporal smooth muscle cells. *J Urol* **153**: 818.

Finkel T, Epstein SE (1995). Gene therapy for vascular disease [Review]. *FASEB J* **9**: 843–51.

Garban H, Marquez D, Magee T, et al (1997). Cloning of rat and human inducible penile nitric oxide synthase. Application for gene therapy of erectile dysfunction. *Biol Reprod* **56**: 954–63.

Hanania EG, Kavanagh J, Hortobagyi G, et al (1995). Recent advances in the application of gene therapy to human disease. *Am J Med* **99**: 537–52.

Kass-Eisler A, Falck-Pedersen E, Alvira M, et al (1993). Quantitative determination of adenovirus-mediated gene delivery to rat cardiac myocytes in vitro and in vivo. *Proc Natl Acad Sci USA* **90**: 11498–502.

Kendrew, J (ed) (1994). *The Encyclopedia of Molecular Biology*, p. 664. Blackwell Science, Oxford.

Lerner SE, Melman A, Christ GJ (1993). A review of erectile dysfunction: new insights and more questions. *J Urol* **149**: 1246–55.

McCobb DP, Fowler NL, Featherstone T, et al (1995). Human calcium-activated potassium channel gene expressed in vascular smooth muscle. *Am J Physiol* **269**: H767–77.

Mayan WG, Faraci FM (1993). Responses of cerebral arterioles in diabetic rats to activation of ATP-sensitive potassium channels. *Am J Physiol* **265**: H152–7.

Melman A, Christ GJ (1997). The vascular physiology of penile erection and pharmacotherapy of erectile dysfunction. In: *Cardiovascular Pharmacotherapeutics*, eds WH Frishman, EH Sonnenblick, pp. 1221–9. McGraw-Hill, New York.

Miller AD (1992). Human gene therapy comes of age. *Nature* **357**: 455–60.

Nabel EG, Plautz G, Nabel GJ (1990). Site-specific gene expression in vivo by direct gene transfer into the arterial wall. *Science* **249**: 1285–8.

Nelson MT (1993). Ca^{2+}-activated potassium channels and ATP-sensitive potassium channels as modulators of vascular tone. *Trends Cardiovasc Med* **3**: 54–60.

Nelson MT, Quayle JM (1995). Physiological roles and properties of potassium channels in arterial smooth muscle. *Am J Physiol* **268**: C799–822.

Nelson MT, Patlak HB, Worley JF, et al (1990). Calcium channels, potassium channels, and voltage dependence of arterial smooth muscle tone. *Am J Physiol* **259**: C3–18.

Nelson MT, Cheng H, Rubart M, et al (1995). Relaxation of arterial smooth muscle by calcium sparks. *Science* **270**: 633–7.

Noack T, Noack P (1997). Multiple types of ion channels in cavernous smooth muscle. *World J Urol* **15**: 45–9.

Ohya Y, Setoguchi M, Fuji K, et al (1996). Impaired action of levcromakalim on ATP-sensitive K^+ channels in mesenteric artery cells from hypertensive rats. *Hypertension* **27**: 1234–9.

Rehman J, Chenven E, Brink PR, et al (1997a). Diminished neurogenic-, but not pharmacologic-induced intracavernous pressure responses in the 3 month Streptozotocin (STZ)-diabetic rat. *Am J Physiol* **272**: H1960–71.

Rehman J, Christ GJ, Werber J, et al (1997b). Enhancement of physiologic erectile function with nitric oxide synthase gene therapy. *J Urol* **157**: 201.

Reinhart PH, Levitan IB (1995). Kinase and phosphatase activities intimately associated with a reconstituted calcium-dependent potassium channel. *J Neurosci* **15**: 4572–9.

Roemer K, Friedmann T (1992). Concepts and strategies for human gene therapy. *Eur J Biochem* **208**: 211–25.

Rowen L, Mahairas G, Hood L (1997). Sequencing the human genome. *Science* **278**: 605–7.

Schulick AH, Newman KD, Virmani R, et al (1995). In vivo gene transfer into injured carotid arteries. *Circulation* **91**: 2407–14.

Starrett JE, Dworetzky SI, Gribkoff VK (1996). Modulators of large-conductance calcium-activated potassium (BK) channels as potential therapeutic targets. *Curr Pharmac Des* **2**: 413–28.

Stief CG, Noack T, Andersson K-E (1997). Signal transduction in cavernous smooth muscle. *World J Urol* **15**: 27–31.

Tanaguchi J, Furukawa K-I, Shigekawa M (1993). Maxi-K+ channels are stimulated by cyclic guanosine monophosphate-dependent protein kinase in canine coronary artery smooth muscle cells. *Pflügers Arch* **423**: 167–72.

Taub H, Melman A, Christ GJ (1993). The relationship between contraction and relaxation in human corpus cavernosum smooth muscle. *Urology* **42**: 698–704.

Zhao W, Christ GJ (1995). Endothelin-1 as a putative modulator of erectile dysfunction. II. Calcium mobilization in cultured human corporal smooth muscle cells. *J Urol* **154**: 1571–9.

14

Penile prosthesis in the age of effective pharmacotherapy

Culley C Carson

With the development of less invasive devices and newer pharmacologic approaches to the treatment of erectile dysfunction, the use of surgical therapy, especially penile prostheses or implants, has been scrutinized more skeptically by both patients and physicians. Many believe that the advent of newer oral medications for the treatment of male erectile dysfunction will be effective in most men and no one will choose to undergo penile prosthesis implantation. It is clear, however, that patients with poor penile blood supply or anatomic abnormalities and those who fail conservative treatment will require more aggressive treatment alternatives. The history of surgical implantation for erectile dysfunction was first recorded in the 1930s by Bogoras, who used a tailored section of rib cartilage to recreate the os penis of animals and produce penile rigidity in a reconstructed penis. Unfortunately, the use of this autologous material resulted in partial reabsorption, infection, and extrusion, with the ultimate result of a curved, shortened, non-functional penis. Subsequently, Goodwin and Scott (Goodwin et al 1952) used acrylic splints implanted beneath Buck's fascia to produce erectile rigidity. Similar materials and designs were used by Loeffler and Sayegh in the 1960s with little acceptance and few successes (Kim and Carson 1993). Beheri changed the course of penile prosthesis implantation by using synthetic rod implants placed directly into the corpora cavernosa (Kim and Carson 1993). The placement of rods in the corpora cavernosa heralded the modern age of penile prosthesis implantation by producing an erect penis that was more physiologic, less painful, and less likely to erode than previously designed devices. Because of inadequate materials, fear of infection, and poor public acceptance, however, these devices were not widely used. The space program in the 1960s resulted in the development of silicone rubber for human implantation (Habal 1984). These materials were first used for penile prosthesis implantation in the 1960s, when Pearman reported successful silicone rod implants beneath Buck's fascia in 126 patients in 1972 (Kim and Carson 1993).

The forerunners of current designs of penile prosthesis began in the early 1970s with the contributions of Small et al and Scott et al (Kim and Carson 1993). Each of these investigators reported unique designs of penile implants constructed of silicone elastomer and placed in the corpora cavernosa, with early reports of excellent physiologic erectile function and satisfactory patient tolerance.

The semirigid rod, non-inflatable penis prostheses designed by Small, Carrion, and Gordon have been modified in a variety of fashions to make them more physiologically adapted and positionable, but the basic design characteristics continue to be those of a silicone elastomer semirigid cylinder. The original Small–Carrion–Gordon prostheses contained a silicone sponge in the center of each prosthetic cylinder to increase its flexibility, while subsequent devices designed by Jonas and Jacobi (1980) contained a central silver wire helical twisted core to increase rigidity and improve positionability of the prosthesis when not in use. Current semirigid rod prostheses utilize these design characteristics (Table 1).

In 1973, Scott, Bradley and Timm first reported the use of inflatable penile prostheses to produce penile rigidity and satisfactory penile flaccidity when the prosthesis is not in use (Kim and Carson 1993). These prostheses, initially constructed of four parts, including an inflation pump separate and distinct from the deflation pump, were subsequently replaced by a three-piece inflatable penile prosthesis consisting of a reservoir containing activation fluid, an inflation/deflation pump placed in the scrotum, and two inflatable cylinders placed in the corpora cavernosa of the penis. These inflatable prostheses have been refined, redesigned, and perfected over the past two decades and are currently manufactured by American Medical Systems and Mentor Corporation.

Indications for prosthesis implantation

Currently available penile prosthetic devices are designed to provide penile shaft rigidity and permit satisfactory erection for vaginal penetration. These devices are indicated primarily in patients with erectile dysfunction or deformity that precludes adequate sexual activity and who do not respond to or are not candidates for pharmacologic or less invasive treatment options. Occasionally penile prosthetic devices are implanted to enhance the ability to maintain condom catheter placement in patients who are paraplegic or quadriplegic. Before the introduction of effective pharmacologic agents for the treatment of erectile dysfunction, the majority of patients implanted with penile prostheses were diabetics, principally in the younger age group. Since these usually have normal vascular supply to the corpora cavernosa, they are more effectively treated with pharmacologic agents; the majority of patients now implanted with penile prostheses have the diagnosis of severe vascular disease or penile deformity. These latter patients are most commonly those who have failed to respond to other forms of therapy, including pharmacologic manipulation, vacuum constriction devices, venous ligation, and other forms of non-prosthetic treatment. Occasionally, patients who are psychologically impotent and who do not respond well to more conservative treatment modalities will undergo penile prosthesis implantation. These devices, when properly implanted in carefully selected patients, improve the quality of life of the patients and relationships with their sexual partners. The National Institutes of Health (NIH) Consensus Conference on Impotence published in December 1992 suggested that the treatment of erectile dysfunction should being with the least invasive, least morbid treatment, including vacuum constriction devices, pharmacologic manipulation, and intracavernosal injections, followed by penile prostheses in patients who fail to respond to these treatments or find them unsatisfactory (NIH 1992). Today, the less invasive alternatives have multiplied, and include the medicated urethral system for erection (MUSE), venous controller rings, and a variety of oral agents for use immediately before coitus.

Current penile prostheses

Penile prostheses available to the implanting surgeon can be grouped according to the design of the device into semirigid rod prostheses, mechanical prostheses, single-component hydraulic devices, and multi-component inflatable devices, which last include both two-piece and three-piece designs.

Semirigid rod penile prostheses

Since Small, Carrion and Gordon described their adjustable penile prosthesis and its results in 1975, a variety of semirigid rod penile prosthesis designs have been developed. This device design is the

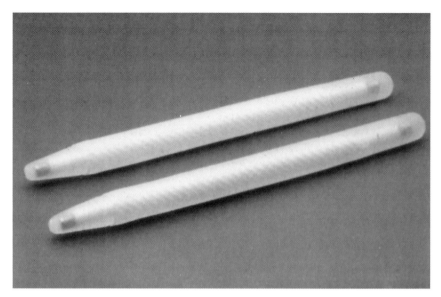

(a)

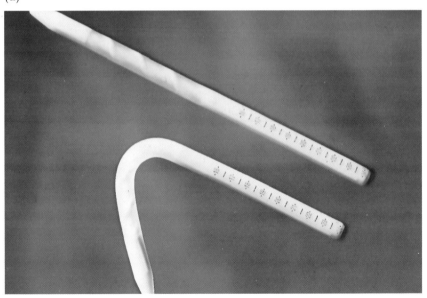

(b)

Figure 1

Semirigid rod prostheses: (a) Aco-Form Malleable Penile Prosthesis. (Courtesy of Mentor Corporation, Santa Barbara, CA.) (b) AMS 650 Malleable Penile Prosthesis. (Courtesy of American Medical Systems Inc., Minnetonka, MN. Medical illustration by Michael Schenk.)

most extensively used for penile prosthetic implantation. Design changes have been created to improve concealment. The first of these modifications was developed by Finney (1977). His flexi-rod prosthesis contained a 5 cm flexible segment of rod to allow a "hinge" at the base of the penis. A subsequent design change described by Jonas and Jacobi (1980) embodied a braided silver wire embedded in the core of the prosthesis to enhance positionability. Subsequent similar designs by American Medical Systems, in the shape of the adjustable penile prosthesis AMS 600 and its successor AMS 650, are also designed with a silicone cylinder containing stainless steel wires in a helical configuration wrapped in a synthetic fabric (Moul and McCloud 1986; Carson 1993a); (Figure 1b). Wires are capped at the ends with stainless steel and there is an eye for the passage of a suture to facilitate pull-through insertion. They further improved the design by placing an external silicone jacket around the prosthesis, allowing a 13 mm diameter with the jacket in place and an 11 mm diameter with the jacket removed. Prosthetic length is varied by placement of 1, 2, or 3 cm rear tip extenders to adjust the three base lengths of 12, 16, and 20 cm to a range of 12–26 cm.

The Mentor Corporation also has a competing adjustable prosthesis. The Mentor adjustable prosthesis consists of a silicone elastomer cylinder with an inner double-coiled silver wire contained in a Teflon sheath. Rather than rear tip extenders the rods can be trimmed proximally and are available in 9.5, 11, and 13 mm diameters. Following trimming, a silicone cap is applied to the trimmed portion. The Acu-Form prosthesis (Acu-Form Malleable Penile Prosthesis also available from the Mentor Corporation, is similar to the Mentor adjustable, but contains no internal silver wire (Figure 1a). It can also be trimmed, with proximal cap devices to cover the trimmed areas.

Mechanical penile prostheses

Recently, a subgroup of penile prosthetic devices was designed for improved concealability. These are mechanical devices designed by Dacomed (Mulcahy et al 1990) (Figure 2). The original Omniphase prosthesis has given way to the Duraphase Penile Prosthesis. Each of these prostheses consists of two cylinders, each comprising a distal tip, a proximal tip, and central body portion in 10 and 20 mm diameters. Distal segments are available in 1–7 cm lengths and proximal segments are available in 2–7 cm lengths. The middle or body portion is 13 cm in length. The newer Duraphase Penile Prosthesis consists of a row of polysulfone cylinders that fit together in a ball and socket

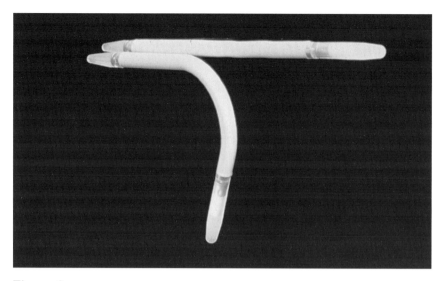

Figure 2
*Dura-II mechanical penile prosthesis. (Courtesy of Dacomed
Corporation, Madison, WI.)*

fashion, articulating with each other. A stainless steel cable runs
through these cylinders and is stabilized at both ends. The body of the
device is covered with a polytetrafluoroethylene (PTFE) covering and
an outer silicone layer. The sturdy cable of the Duraphase prosthesis
has decreased the mechanical malfunction experienced with the
Omniphase. This design enhances the flaccid-phase positioning and
concealability of the penis. Implantation is by the same approaches as
with other semirigid rod penile prostheses. While cable breakage
continues to be a potential complication, the design improvement
over Omniphase prosthesis has made this a reliable alternative to
semirigid rod penile prostheses (Mulcahy 1993).

Single-piece hydraulic penile prostheses

These self-contained inflatable prostheses provide improved concealability in comparison with semirigid rod prostheses; however, their
inflation and deflation mechanism provides a less physiologically satisfactory result than do the multiple-component prosthetic devices
(Thrasher 1993). Currently the only available hydraulic penile prosthesis is the Dynaflex prosthesis from the American Medical Systems,

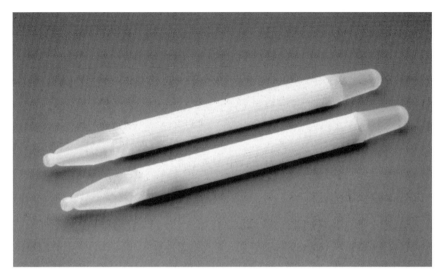

Figure 3
Dynaflex single-piece inflatable prosthesis. (Courtesy of American Medical Systems Inc., Minnetonka, MN. Medical illustration by Michael Schenk.)

replacing the previously available Hydroflex (Figure 3). The Surgitek Flexi-Flate II prostheses are no longer available for implantation. The Dynaflex prosthesis consists of two cylinders placed intracavernosally in a fashion similar to the placement of semirigid rod penile prostheses. Each cylinder contains a pump, reservoir, and inflation chamber to allow inflation and deflation of the device. The pump of these devices is located at the distal portion of the cylinder. The Dynaflex penile prostheses contain a reservoir located in the proximal segment of the cylinder. The pump is palpated just proximal to the glans penis and pressure on each cylinder inflates the prosthesis. Deflation is performed by deflection of the prosthesis increasing pressure on the internal release valve for 10 seconds followed by deflation of the central hydraulic portion. This built-in 10-second delay avoids deflation during coitus. Because these devices are self-contained, only a small amount of fluid is actually moved between inflation and deflation cycles, and deflation flaccidity is poor compared with that of two- and three-piece inflatable penile prostheses. Similarly, the erect state does not result in significant girth expansion, and these prostheses inflate to a size of semirigid rod prostheses. Thus, these prostheses may be more accurately termed "hydraulic hinge" prostheses. The AMS Dynaflex prosthesis is available in 11 and 13 mm widths with lengths of 13, 16, 19, and 22 cm modified by 1 cm and 2 cm rear tip extenders for increased versatility. These prostheses have had few reported mechanical malfunctions (Thrasher 1993).

Inflatable penile prostheses

The original inflatable penile prosthesis design of Scott has now been extended and modified to include the original three-piece prosthesis and more recent two-piece prosthesis designs.

Three piece inflatable penile prostheses

The three-piece penile prostheses are currently available from American Medical Systems Inc. and the Mentor Corporation. These devices are similar in design and function as well as reliability (Woodworth et al 1991; Montague and Lakin 1992; Garber 1994). Each of these prostheses consists of a fluid-containing reservoir with 65 ml or 100 ml volume (AMS) or 40 or 125 ml volume (Mentor). Tubing connects this reservoir to a scrotally placed pump for activation and deflation of the device. The Mentor and AMS pumps are similar in function but different in shape. The pump connects to two inflatable cylinders placed in the corpora cavernosa of the penis. Length modification using 1, 2, and 3 cm rear tip extenders is provided for with each company's prosthesis. These rear tip extenders allow direct, perpendicular exit of the input tubing from the corporotomy incision. AMS cylinders are available as 700 CX, 700 Ultrex, or 700 CXM (Figure 4a). The CX cylinders, which allow controlled expansion, are available in lengths of 12, 15, 18, and 21 cm, and have controlled expansion to 18 mm in diameter. The CX cylinders are constructed of an inner layer of silicone elastomer, a middle layer of controlled-expansion woven fabric, and an outer covering of silicone to prevent tissue adherence. In addition to the standard measurement cylinders, the 700 CX is available in a smaller-diameter, 700 CXM device, and 12, 14, 16, and 18 cm lengths with a diameter of 9.5 mm deflated and 14.2 mm inflated. The standard CX cylinders have a diameter of 12 mm deflated and 18 mm inflated. The Ultrex cylinders differ from the CX cylinders in expanding in length to an increase of approximately 20% (Montague and Lakin 1993). Cylinder lengths and rear tip extenders are the same as for the CX cylinder; however, the cylinder's construction differs in the insertion of a middle layer of fabric that expands longitudinally. The Ultrex cylinders are available for independent connection or preconnected to the pump in penoscrotal and infrapubic implantation lengths as the Ultrex-Plus prosthesis.

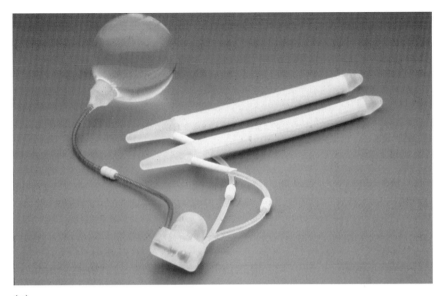

(a)

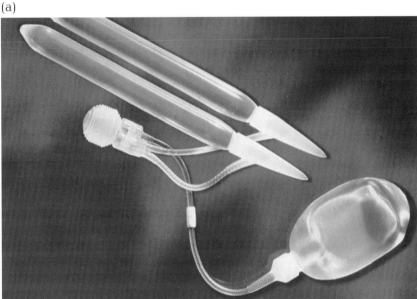

(b)

Figure 4
Multiple-component inflatable penile prostheses: (a) AMS 700 Ultrex-Plus Penile Prosthesis. (Courtesy of American Medical Systems Inc., Minnetonka, MN. Medical illustration by Michael Schenk. (b) Alpha-1 Penile Prosthesis. (Courtesy of Mentor Corporation, Santa Barbara, CA.)

The Mentor three-piece prosthesis is called the Mentor Alpha-1 (Figure 4b). Its design is similar to that of the AMS prosthesis, but its cylinders are constructed of Bioflex, a polyurethane polymer (Goldstein et al 1993). As in the Ultrex-Plus, the pump is attached to the cylinders, and only a single connection between pump and reservoir is necessary. Cylinder lengths available are 12, 14, 16, 18, 20, and 22 cm, with rear tip extenders of 1, 2, and 3 cm. Reservoir sizes include 60, 75, and 100 ml volumes, with tubing lengths available for infrapubic and penoscrotal implantation.

Two-piece inflatable penile prostheses

Recent modifications of inflatable penile prostheses have incorporated a pump and reservoir into a single unit. These two-piece inflatable penile prostheses are available from AMS and Mentor (George et al 1995). These prostheses simplified inflatable penile prosthesis implantation by decreasing the number of parts in an effort to improve reliability without sacrificing the advantages achieved with the inflatable penile prosthesis. The elimination of the reservoir component has simplified implantation and eliminated the difficulty of dissection in patients with previous extensive abdominal surgery. The improved ease of implantation, however, is at the cost of less fluid transfer, a poorer erection, and a flaccid penis. The cylinders of the Ambicor (AMS) two-piece prosthesis are similar to those of the Dynaflex prosthesis (Figure 5a). These cylinders consist of a proximal reservoir and a pump reservoir placed in the scrotum. The proximal reservoir is designed to increase the amount of fluid changing position to enhance inflation and deflation of the prosthesis. The Mentor GFS and Mark II prostheses consist of a single pump reservoir with a capacity of approximately 20–25 ml and cylinders constructed of Bioflex material like those in the Mentor three-piece prosthesis (Figure 5b). Cylinders are sized with rear tip extenders as previously described in the Dynaflex and Mentor Alpha-1 prosthetic devices.

Prosthesis selection

The optimal penile prostheses for each patient must be selected on the basis of the patient's individual needs and anatomy and the etiology of his impotence. While the multiple-component inflatable penile prostheses are the most physiologically satisfactory, these devices

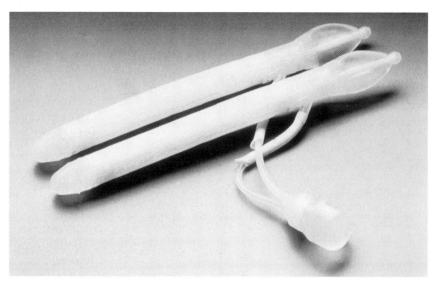

(a)

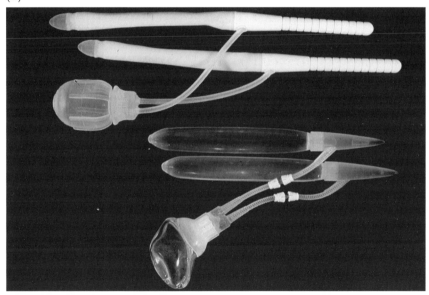

(b)

Figure 5

Two-piece inflatable penile prostheses: (a) Ambicor Inflatable Penile Prosthesis. (Courtesy of American Medical Systems Inc., Minnetonka, MN. Medical illustration by Michael Schenk. (b) Mark II Inflatable Penile Prosthesis. (Courtesy of Mentor Corporation, Santa Barbara, CA.)

may not be appropriate in patients with limited manual dexterity or severe corpus cavernosum fibrosis, or for those patients concerned with mechanical malfunction. It is most important to discuss the advantages and disadvantages of each prosthesis category with the patient and with his sexual partner if possible. Most patients choose an inflatable prosthesis because of a desire for a more natural flaccid penis and an increase in penile girth during erection. Because the mechanical malfunction rate of the inflatable penile prosthesis has declined to an acceptable level over the past decade, patients choosing manually adjustable penile prostheses have declined over the past few years. Any patient discussion, however, should include other possible forms of treatment for erectile dysfunction as well as the complications of penile prosthetic implantation, such as infection, mechanical malfunction, extrusion, and postoperative pain. In carefully selected patients with good surgical results, patient satisfaction exceeds 90%.

Surgical implantation

Penile prostheses can be surgically implanted through a variety of surgical approaches. Initially, malleable penile prostheses were implanted perineally; however, this approach has been largely abandoned because of its complexity and the attendant morbidity. Most semirigid rod and self-contained inflatable penile prostheses are now implanted through a dorsal subcoronal approach, while inflatable penile prostheses are implanted through infrapubic or penoscrotal incisions. Semirigid rod and self-contained inflatable penile prostheses can also be implanted through dorsal penile shaft, ventral penile shaft, penoscrotal, or suprapubic approaches. Once the incision has been considered and carried out, however, the principles of penile prosthesis implantation are similar for all incisions. The infrapubic incision for the implantation of inflatable penile prostheses has the advantage of minimal postoperative scarring and an excellent cosmetic result. Surgical exposure for both surgeon and assistant is excellent. Furthermore, revision of inflatable penile prostheses is facilitated with the infrapubic approach. Reservoir placement is under direct vision and careful dissection beneath the rectus sheath in patients with previous abdominal surgery permits safer reservoir placement. The penoscrotal approach is preferred by many implanters, and has the advantage of an easier approach to the corpora cavernosa and a minimal scar on the scrotum. The disadvantage is the blind placement of the fluid reservoir. With the placement of any prosthetic device, however, careful surgical technique, attention to minimal dissection, and exquisite sterile technique must be maintained to minimize the possibility of postoperative infection. Because perioperative infection is disastrous, frequent irrigation of the surgical wound with antibiotic solution containing bacitracin and an aminoglycoside antibiotic agent is mandatory, and limiting operating room traffic, operating time, and postoperative bleeding will decrease perioperative infections. A careful 10-minute preoperative surgical field preparation using antibiotic solutions is critical.

The infrapubic incision is of a horizontal type in slim patients and at the low midline in more obese patients. Once the skin incision is carried out, careful dissection is performed to expose the corpora cavernosa bilaterally. The tissue between the corpora cavernosa is preserved to avoid the midline neurovascular bundle and the small sensory nerves that run in this area. Unless significant phimosis or redundant foreskin is present, circumcision is usually not necessary, since infection rates are increased with this combined procedure (Fallon and Ghanem 1989). Once the corpora cavernosa have been identified through any of the previously described incisions, Buck's facia is dissected free, and the tunica albuginea is exposed and secured with stay sutures. Longitudinal incisions are carried out between the stay sutures and the corpora cavernosa opened. Once the spongy tissue of the corpora cavernosa is identified, scissor dissection is used to initiate the tunnels both proximally and distally in the corpora cavernosa and to direct subsequent dilatation. Dilatation is carried out proximally and distally using Hegar or Brooks dilators, carefully directing the dilatation instruments in the corpus cavernosum and avoiding crossing into the contralateral corpus. Dilatation must be performed proximally and distally to dilate the corpora completely to the ischial tuberosities and into the area just below the glans penis distally. In patients with significant corpus cavernosum fibrosis from priapism or previous prosthesis implantation, the use of the Roselló cavernotomes may be helpful. Inadequate dilatation results in the placement of an excessively short penile prosthesis cylinder and migration of that prosthesis postoperatively, with a resultant inadequate support for the glans penis, making vaginal penetration uncomfortable. Only aggressive proximal and distal dilatation, however, may perforate the corpora cavernosa, resulting in subsequent prosthesis extrusion. The fibrotic corpora cavernosa can also be incised using an Otis urethrotome for the incision, though care must be taken to avoid the inferior quadrant of the corpus cavernosum in order to preserve the urethra.

Once adequate corpora dilatation is complete, careful sizing must be carried out to fit the individual patient appropriately. The Furlow insertion tool is an excellent device for this purpose.

Cylinders must be chosen that will lie flat in the corpus cavernosum without kinking, but will fill the dilated corpus completely.
Once the appropriate size and rear tip extenders are chosen, the
prosthesis is placed using a suture in the distal-most portion of the
cylinder and a Keith needle with the Furlow insertion tool or a
Dilamezensert device. The cylinders are then placed in the corpora cavernosa and the corporotomy incisions are closed with interrupted sutures, which best placed before cylinder placement so as
to limited the possibility of puncture resultant upon cylinder placement. Pouches are then created beneath the rectus muscle and
within the right scrotum using sharp and blunt dissection for the
reservoir and pump respectively. Once these components are in
place, input tubing is tailored, the reservoir is filled, and the tubes
are connected with non-suture-connecting devices available from
AMS or Mentor. While the two-piece prosthetic pumps are somewhat larger than the three-piece pumps, little difficulty has been
associated with this increase in size in patients with normal-size
scrotums. Once tubing connections have been completed, inflation
and deflation of the device should be carried out to evaluate
penile shape, cylinder position, and adequacy of size and length.
Changes in size or position should be carried out if necessary.
Thorough antibiotic irrigation of all components of the device is
then performed and wound closure is carried out. A suction drain
can be placed in those patients with some corporeal bleeding after
prosthesis placement. A subcuticular skin closure will facilitate
early hospital discharge and decrease postoperative wound infection. A Foley catheter may be placed for 24 hours for urine
drainage as necessary.

The penoscrotal approach is begun with a Foley catheter placement and incision at the penoscrotal junction over the urethra.
Dissection is continued to isolate the corpora cavernosa lateral to the
urethra. Dilatation and measurement are as described above.
Reservoir placement is through the inguinal canal with a blunt clamp
or reservoir carrier. The pump is placed either in the midline of the
scrotum or lateral to the testes. Skin closure is critical to enhance
healing, and multiple layers should be used if possible.

Perioperative care

Antibiotic treatment is critical in diminishing the incidence of perioperative infection and prosthesis removal (Carson 1989). An initial

perioperative dose of an antibiotic agent effective against the most common infectious pathogens should be administered 1–2 hours prior to surgery and continued for 48 hours postoperatively (Walters et al 1992). Choice of an aminoglycoside with a first-generation cephalosporin, a cephalosporin alone, vancomycin, or a fluoro-quinolone is appropriate for prophylaxis against the most common infections–those with *Staphylococcus epidermidis* (Licht et al 1995). Patients may be discharged for 7 days of continued antibiotic therapy. The penile prosthesis remains deflated for 4 weeks while healing occurs. Before activation, the patient is advised to retract the pump into his scrotum on a daily basis, and tight underwear and athletic supports are to be avoided to maintain pump position. A return office visit for activation of the device is carried out once discomfort has resolved. Patients are advised to inflate and deflate the device on a daily basis for 4 weeks to allow tissue expansion around the prosthesis. Most patients can then begin to use their device immediately.

Postoperative complications

The most worrisome postoperative complication is postoperative infection. Fortunately, this complication occurs in fewer than 10% of all patients. Perioperative prosthetic infections can, however, occur at any time in the postoperative period in patients with penile or other prosthetic devices. Patients continue to be at risk for hematogenously seeded infections from gastrointestinal, dental, or urologic manipulations, as well as from remote infections. Patients must be counseled to request antibiotic coverage if remote infections occur (Carson and Robertson 1988). Most periprosthetic infections are caused by Gram-positive organisms such as *Staphylococcus epidermidis*, but Gram-negative organisms such as *Escherichia coli* and *Pseudomonas* are also possible pathogens (Fallon and Ghanem 1989; Licht et al 1995). Severe gangrenous infections with a combination of Gram-negative and anaerobic organisms have also been identified, and result in significant disability and tissue loss (McClellan and Masih 1985; Walther et al 1987; Bejny et al 1993). Patients at increased risk for perioperative infections include diabetics, patients undergoing penile straightening procedures or circumcision with prosthetic implantation, patients with urinary tract bacterial colonization, and immunocompromised patients such as post-transplant patients (Walther et al

1987; Radmoski and Hershorn 1992). While these patients are at increased risk, the risk of infection continues to be less than 10%, and is in most cases quite acceptable (Carson 1993b). Spinal cord injury patients have also been reported to have a specially increased risk of infections, with rates reported as high as 15% (Fallon and Ghanem 1989). Because of a decrease in sensation, an increased risk of extrusion of semirigid prostheses has been reported in this group of patients. Diabetics with poor control may be evaluated with glycated hemoglobin studies prior to surgery to enhance diabetic control before prosthesis implantation and, perhaps, decrease the possibility of infection (Bishop et al 1992). Recent results of a large study, however, have demonstrated that glycated hemoglobin is a poor predictor of periprosthetic infection risk. Appropriate treatment of periprosthetic infections requires early and immediate identification, with institution of parenteral antibiotic therapy and early prosthesis removal (Montague 1987). Conservative treatment would dictate a healing period of 3–6 months followed by repeat prosthesis implantation. Satisfactory results with prosthesis removal and a 5–7 day course of antibiotic irrigation, followed by prosthesis replacement, has been reported for selected patients (Mulcahy and Steidle 1989; Teloken et al 1992; Fishman 1993; Fishman et al 1997). Reports have also suggested that immediate replacement of the prosthesis following intraoperative irrigation may be successful (Furlow and Goldwasser 1987; Brant et al 1996). Several reviews of the problem of penile prosthesis infection and its treatment have been published (Montague 1987; Carson 1989, 1993).

The most common complication of penile prosthesis function is mechanical malfunction (Carson 1983, 1993c; Merrill 1989). Mechanical malfunction has declined from rates as high as 61% to levels below 5% since the 1970s (Woodworth et al 1991; Bertero and Goldstein 1993; Lewis 1995). Aneurysmal dilatation of inflatable cylinders, both AMS and Mentor, tube kinking, reservoir leakage, and pump malfunction have been limited by device modifications (Seinkohl and Leach 1991; Woodworth et al 1991; Bertero and Goldstein 1993; Garber 1995). Fluid leakage, however, continues to be a problem in many inflatable penile prostheses. These mechanical malfunctions require replacement of the leaking portion of the inflatable part of the prosthesis (Lewis and McLauren 1993). If a non-functioning prosthesis has been in place for more than 4 years, however, we usually replace the entire device in order to reduce the risk of further mechanical malfunction.

Semirigid rod penile prostheses are associated with few mechanical problems, and the most common complication associated with these prostheses is cylinder erosion through skin or urethra (Carson

1993). Prosthesis fracture or breakage has been reported, and patients may return 6–8 months post-implantation with complaints of decreased rigidity of their semirigid rod, indicating fracture of the central prosthetic cylinder's wires (Agastin et al 1986). These wire fractures cannot usually be appreciated radiographically unless the prosthesis is put on stretch once it has been explanted. Replacement of these devices is indicated when patients note decreased rigidity. Prosthesis extrusion or erosion is most common in diabetics and spinal cord injury patients, especially those requiring urinary management with catheter placement of condom collection.

Penile prosthesis implantation for special conditions

Corpus cavernosum fibrosis

The implantation of penile prostheses in patients with severe corporal fibrosis from priapism, intracavernosal injection therapy, or previous explantation of an infected implant can be treated with a semirigid rod or an inflatable penile prosthesis. Frequently, however, reconstruction of the corpus cavernosum or straightening of significant penile curvature may be necessary to provide a satisfactorily functioning penile prosthesis (Kabalin 1984). Techniques to deal with this severe corpus cavernosum fibrosis include resection of scarring and placement of Dacron or PTFE patch grafts once the prosthesis has been placed (Seftel et al 1992). Use of the Roselló–Barbra cavernotome, the Otis urethrotome, and sharp dissection of corpus cavernosum fibrosis may be necessary to place the prosthesis adequately (Fishman 1993; Knoll 1995). In cases of weakening of the proximal distal portions of the corpora cavernosa as a result of infection or priapism, a wind sock reinforcement of the crura or the distal corpus cavernosum may be necessary (Hershorn and Ordorica 1995) (Figure 6). With severe fibrosis, the smaller 700 CXM (AMS) or semirigid rod cylinders may be necessary to overcome corporeal resistance (Kabalin 1984; Knoll et al 1995).

Peyronie's disease

Implantation of penile prostheses for Peyronie's disease usually provides excellent results, with correction of both curvature and erectile dysfunction (Carson et al 1983; Habal 1984). Penile prosthesis

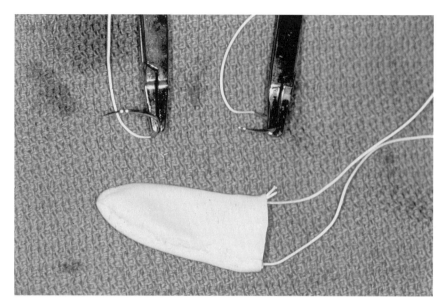

Figure 6
Windsock created from PTFE patch graft with PTFE suture for reinforcement of proximal or distal corpus cavernosum.

implantation for Peyronie's disease is reserved for those patients in whom erections are poor or for whom previous surgical procedures have been inadequate to restore erectile function. A prosthesis is placed initially and, if curvature is minimal, no further manipulation may be necessary. If curvature continues, molding of the penis may be carried out in a fashion described by Wilson and Delk (1994, 1995). Alternatively, the area of curvature may be exposed, the neurovascular bundle elevated, and the area of curvature incised. This incision is best carried out with electrocautery, and has been reported safely performed with both AMS and Mentor penile prostheses (Carson et al 1983; Eigner et al 1991; Kulaksizogla et al 1995). If the resulting defect in the corpus cavernosum is large, a patch graft of Dacron or Gortex may be used to reinforce the corpus cavernosum. If choosing AMS penile prostheses, penile straightening is best carried out using the AMS 700 CX cylinders, since the controlled expansion will preclude aneurysmal dilatation through the defect in the corpus cavernosum. Excellent results have also been reported in patients implanted with semirigid rod penile prostheses, but a recent report suggests that higher satisfaction rates are achieved with inflatable devices (Montorsi et al 1993).

Spinal cord injury patients

Because of the effectiveness of pharmacotherapy, penile prostheses are used less frequently in patients with spinal cord injury. As these patients have increased incidence of infection and erosion, care must be taken in placing penile prostheses (Carossier and Fam 1984). Inflatable prostheses are preferred in patients not requiring condom catheter drainage, since the decreased pressure of the inflatable prosthesis when deflated will reduce extrusion and revision rates. Because patients using intermittent self-catheterization have an increased possibility of catheter injury and cylinder erosion, Mulcahy and Steidle (1989) have recommended alternative urinary diversion techniques with perineal urethrostomy or suprapubic catheter placement in spinal cord injury patients implanted with semirigid rod penile prostheses.

Conclusion

Despite the introduction of newer conservative methods for producing erectile function and innovative precoital oral agents, many men will not respond to these treatment schemes and will require surgical implantation of a penile prosthesis. The excellent mechanical function rate among modern prostheses as well as the high reported patient satisfaction rate continue to recommend these devices. The implantation of penile prostheses is a commonly performed and successful procedure in most urological centers. Knowledge of the types of prostheses available, their advantages, disadvantages, and implantation techniques is necessary for skilled prosthetic management of erectile impotence. Careful discussion of types of prostheses available and their advantages and disadvantages, providing a choice of devices available, optimizes patient and partner satisfaction. Patients should be allowed to choose a prosthesis from each of the classifications of currently available devices. With careful patient selection, prosthesis choice, and currently available reliable prosthetic devices, the urologist can expect excellent patient/partner satisfaction with low morbidity.

References

Agastin EH, Farrer JH, Raz S (1986). Fracture of semirigid rod prosthesis: a rare complication. *J Urol* **135**:376–7.

Bejny DE, Perito PE, Lustgarten M, et al. (1993). Gangrene of the penis after implantation of penile prothesis: cases reports, treatment recommendations and review of the literature. *J Urol* **150**:190–1.

Bertero EB, Goldstein I (1993). Inflatable penile prosthesis: experience with the Mentor Alpha-1. *Probl Urol* **7**:334–41.

Bishop JR, Moul JW, Saihelnik SA, et al. (1992). Use of glycosylated hemoglobin to identify diabetics at high risk for penile preprosthetic infections. *J Urol* **147**:386–8.

Brant MD, Ludlow JK, Mulcahy JJ (1996). The prosthesis salvage operation: immediate replacement of the infected penile prosthesis. *J Urol* **155**:155–7.

Carossier AB, Fam BA (1984). Indication and results of semirigid rod penile prostheses in spinal cord injury patients: long term follow-up. *J Urol* **131**:59–64.

Carson CC (1983). Inflatable penile prosthesis: experience with 100 patients. *South Med J* **76**:1139–45.

Carson CC (1989). Infections in genitourinary prostheses. *Urol Clin North Am* **116**:139–52.

Carson CC (1993a). Implantation of semirigid rod penile prostheses. *Atlas of Urol Rnn A* **1**:61–70.

Carson CC (1993b). Management of penile prosthesis infection. *Probl Urol* **7**:368–80.

Carson CC (1993c). Current status of penile prosthesis surgery. *Probl Urol* **7**:289–97.

Carson CC, Robertson CN (1988). Late hematogenous infection of penile prosthesis. *J Urol* **139**:112–16.

Carson CC, Hodge GB, Anderson EE (1983). Penile prosthesis and Peyronie's disease. *Br J Urol* **55**:417–21.

Eigner EB, Kabolin JN, Kessler R (1991). Penile implants and treatment of Peyronie's disease. *J Urol* **145**:69–74.

Fallon B, Ghanem H (1989). Infected penile prostheses: incidence and outcomes. *Int J Impot Res* **1**:175–86.

Finney RP (1977). New hinged silicone penile implant. *J Urol* **118**:585–92.

Fishman IJ (1993). Corporeal reconstruction for penile prosthesis implantation. *Probl Urol* **7**:350–67.

Fishman IJ, Scott FB, Selim AM (1987) Rescue procedure: an alternative to complete removal for treatment of infected penile prosthesis. *J Urol* **137**:202–8.

Furlow WL, Goldwasser B (1987). Salvage of the eroded inflatable penile prosthesis: a new concept. *J Urol* **138**:312–18.

Garber BB (1994). Mentor Alpha-1 inflatable penile prosthesis: patient satisfaction and device reliability. *Urology* **43**:214–17.

Garber BB (1995). Mentor Alpha-1 inflatable penile prosthesis cylinder aneurysm: an unusual complication. *Int J Impot Res* **7**:13–16.

George VK, Erkham S, Dhabawal CB (1995). Follow-up with Mentor 2-Piece inflatable penile prosthesis. *Int J Impot Res* **7**:17–21.

Goldstein I, Bertero EB, Kaufman JM, et al (1993). Early experience with the first preconnected 3-piece inflatable penile prosthesis: Mentor Alpha-1. *J Urol* **150**:184–8.

Goodwin WE, Scardino PL, Scott WW (1981). Penile prosthesis for impotence: please report. *J Urol* **126**:409–10.

Habal MB (1984). The biological basis for the clinical application of the silicones. *Arch Surg* **119**:843–51.

Hershorn S, Ordorica RC (1995). Penile prosthesis insertion with corporeal reconstruction with synthetic vasculograft material. *J Urol* **154**:80–4.

Jonas U, Jacobi GH (1980). Silicone silver penile prosthesis: prescription, operative approach and results. *J Urol* **123**:865–74.

Kabalin JN (1984). Corporeal fibrosis as a result of priapism prohibited function of self-contained inflatable penile prosthesis. *Urology* **43**:401–3.

Kim JH, Carson CC (1993). History of urologic prostheses for impotence. *Probl Urol* **7**:283–8.

Knoll LD (1995). Use of penile prosthetic implants in patients with penile fibrosis. *Urol Clin North Am* **22**:857–63.

Knoll LD, Furlow WL, Benson RC, Bilhartz DL (1995). Management of nondilatable cavernous fibrosis with the use of downsized inflatable penile prosthesis. *J Urol* **153**:366–7.

Kulaksizogla H, Hakim LS, Hamill B, et al (1995). The first guide to safe electrocautery use with Bioflex inflatable penile cylinders. *J Urol* **153**:360A.

Lewis RW (1995). Long term results of penile prosthetic implants. *Urol Clin North Am* **22**:847–56.

Lewis RW, McLauren R (1993). Re-operation for penile prosthesis implantation. *Probl Urol* **7**:381–401.

Licht MR, Montague DK, Angermeir KW, et al (1995). Cultures from genitourinary prostheses at reoperation: questioning the role of *Staphylococcus epidermidis* in periprosthetic infection. *J Urol* **139**:112–16.

McClellan DS, Masih BK (1985). Gangrene of the penis as a complication of penile prosthesis. *J Urol* **133**:862–5.

McLaren RH, Barrett BM (1992). Patient/partner satisfaction with the AMS 700 penile prosthesis. *J Urol* **147**:62–5.

Merrill DC (1989). Mentor inflatable penile prosthesis. *Urol Clin North Am* **16**:51–64.

Montague DK (1987). Periprosthetic infections. *J Urol* **138**:68–74.

Montague DK, Lakin MM (1992). Early experience with a controlled girth and length expanding cylinder of an American Medical Systems Ultrex penile prosthesis: *J Urol* **148**:1444–6.

Montague DK, Lakin MM (1993). Inflatable penile prosthesis: the AMS experience. *Probl Urol* **7**:328–33.

Montorsi F, Guazzoni G, Bergamaschi F, et al (1993). Patient/partner satisfaction with semirigid penile prosthesis for Peyronie's disease: a five year follow-up study. *J Urol* **150**:1819–21.

Moul JH, McCloud DG (1986). Experience with AMS 600 Malleable Penile Prosthesis. *J Urol* **135**:929–32.

Mulcahy JJ (1993). Mechanical penile prostheses. *Probl Urol* **7**:311–16.

Mulcahy JJ, Steidle CP (1989). Erosion of penile prosthesis: a complication of urethral catheterization. *J Urol* **142**:736–9.

Mulcahy JJ, Krane RJ, Lloyd LK, et al (1990). Duraphase penile prosthesis results in clinical trials of 63 patients. *J Urol* **143**:518–24.

NIH (National Institutes of Health) (1992). *Consensus Statement: Impotence,* Vol. 10, No. 4, December 7–9.

Radomski SB, Hershorn S (1992). Risks factors associated with penile prosthesis infection. *J Urol* **147**:383–5.

Seftel AD, Oats RD, Goldstein I (1992). Use of polytetrafluoroethylene tube graft as a circumferential neotunica during placement of a penile prosthesis. *J Urol* **148**:1531–3.

Seinkohl WB, Leach GE (1991). Mechanical complications associated with Mentor inflatable penile prosthesis. *Urology* **38**:32–6.

Steege JF, Stout AL, Carson CC (1986). Patient satisfaction in small carry-on penile implant recipients: study of 52 patients. *Arch Sex Behav* **15**:393–5.

Teloken C, Souto JC, DaRos C, et al (1992). Prosthetic penile infection: rescue procedure with Rifamycin. *J Urol* **148**:1905–6.

Thrasher JB (1993). Self-contained inflatable prostheses. *Prob Urol* **7**:317–27.

Walters FP, Neal DE, Rege AB, George WJ, Ricci MJ, Hellstrom WJ (1992). Cavernous tissue antibiotic levels in penile prosthesis surgery. *J Urol* **147**:1282–4.

Walther PJ, Andriani RT, Mhaggi MI, Carson CC (1987). Fournier's fascia gangrene: a complication of prosthetic penile implantation in a renal transplant patient. *J Urol* **137**:299–304.

Wilson SK, Delk JR (1994). A new treatment for Peyronie's disease: modeling the penis over an inflatable penile prosthesis. *J Urol* **152**:1121–3.

Wilson SK, Delk JR (1995). Inflatable penile implant infection: predisposing factors and treatment suggestions. *J Urol* **153**:659–61.

Woodworth BW, Carson CC, Webster GD (1991). Inflatable penile prosthesis: effect of device modification on functional longevity. *Urology* **38**:533–41.

15

The forgotten dysfunction: a pharmacological approach to premature ejaculation

Martyn A Vickers, Jr

Introduction

The degree of psychic trauma associated with premature ejaculation (PE) and the frequency of this malady are significant reasons for health care providers to possess a working knowledge of this "forgotten dysfunction." The normal intravaginal ejaculatory latency time (IVELT) (length of time between repetitive insertion of the rigid penis into the vagina and ejaculation) of the functionally active, rigid penis in a receptive vagina is controversial. In Kinsey's opinion premature ejaculation does not exist, since all male upper Mammalia ejaculate almost immediately after entering the vagina (Kinsey et al 1948). With the advent of sexual openness, performance assessment and women's liberation, the man who commonly ejaculates rapidly upon vaginal entry will be likely to experience the open hostility of his sexual partner as well as the threatened or actual termination of their relationship. Frequently, the rapid ejaculator becomes anxious, sexually insecure and isolated. Several self-report studies of "normal" men reveal a prevalence rate of PE of 30–40% (Frank et al 1978; Reading and Wiest 1984).

This chapter will review the physiology of ejaculation, provide a brief overview of the traditional psychoanalytic and behavioral therapies for premature ejaculation, explore the most recent pharmacological treatments, present a physiological basis for studies with new classes of drugs, and, finally, propose practical treatment alternatives.

Functional anatomy

The ejaculatory process consists of two sequential reflex mechanisms. The first is triggered by stimulation of penile skin touch and/or vibratory

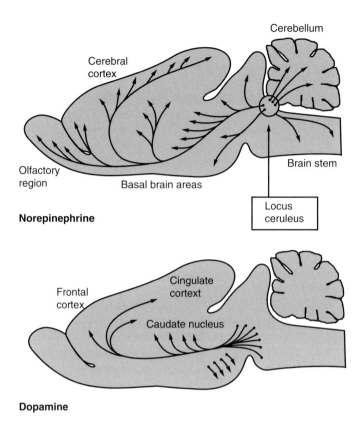

Norepinephrine

Dopamine

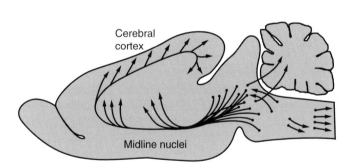

Serotonin

Figure 1
The three neurohormonal systems that have been mapped in the rat brain: a norepinephrine system, a dopamine system and a serotonin system. (Adapted from Kelly, JP, after Cooper, Bloom, and Roth, in Kandel and Schwartz 1985.)

receptors. This stimulus is translated into impulses that are transmitted along the pudendal nerve fibers to the sacral cord and ultimately to the limbic lobe. The limbic/hypothalamic system controls emotional behavior, motivational drive, and visceral physiological homeostasis (body temperature, hunger, sexual reflex). This system sits in the middle of the brain and has neural communications with the cerebral cortex, the cerebellum, the brain-stem nuclei and the spinal cord. Studies of rat brains have revealed that the limbic system is chemically linked with these structures by four neurotransmitters, three of which are amines and one an amino acid. The amines are norepinephine (an excitatory hormone),

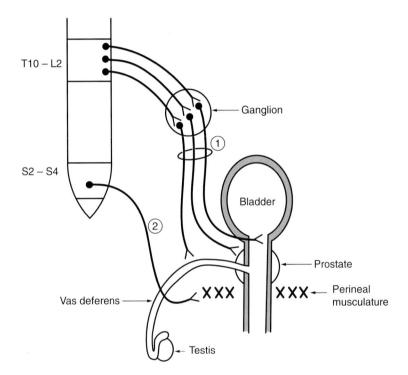

Figure 2
Nerves involved with emission and ejaculation. Sympathetic nerves, from T10 to L2 levels, innervate the vas deferens and prostate, and contraction results in emission. These nerves also innervate the bladder neck, contraction of which results in bladder neck closure. Somatic nerve fibers, specifically the pudendal nerve from S2 to S4, innervate the pelvic floor (perineal musculature), contraction of which results in the forceful ejaculation through the urethra. (From Benson and McDonnell 1983.)

dopamine (an excitatory or inhibitory hormone depending on the area of the brain) and serotonin (an inhibitory hormone). The area of major central activity of these transmitters has been mapped in detail in the rat brain and is illustrated in Figure 1 (Guyton 1991). The fourth neurotransmitter, γ-aminobutyric acid (GABA), is an inhibitory neurohormone, secreted in many areas of the brain and spinal cord. During intercourse, the incoming tactile signals probably cause a significant increase in the level of these neurohormones, which, in turn, results in activation of the sympathetic nervous system. The involved preganglionic sympathetic nerves originate in the spinal cord and pass into the T10–L2 paraspinal sympathetic ganglia (emission center) (Buch 1994). From this center postganglionic efferent sympathetic fibers arise which convey impulses to the vas deferens, the prostate, the seminal vesicles, and the bladder neck. The ultimate result is a discharge of seminal fluid into the posterior urethra.

The second reflex is triggered by the urethral proprioceptive sensation of the seminal emission. These impulses are transmitted to the sacral S2–4 cord (ejaculatory center) and, from there, efferent fibres of pudendal preganglionic parasympathetic nerves carry signals to ganglia adjacent to their end organs. From there the signals pass along the short postganglionic fibers and finally cause the release of neurotransmitters that result in depolarization of the bulbocavernous and perineal muscles and their rhythmic contraction. The final result is propulsion of the seminal fluid through and from the anterior urethra.

The sympathetic and parasympathetic nerve fibers secrete either acetylcholine or norepinephrine. All preganglionic neurons secrete acetylcholine in both the sympathetic and parasympathetic nervous systems. The postganglionic neurons of the parasympathetic system also secrete acetylcholine. Most postganglionic sympathetic neurons secrete norepinephrine (Figure 2).

The temporal aspects of ejaculation

A survey of couples who have a pleasurable sex life has revealed that their duration of intercourse IVELT ranged between 4 and 7 minutes. Surprisingly, Masters and Johnson's definition of premature ejaculation is devoid of a time parameter, but is rather based on the pleasuring of both partners. It states that this condition exists when there is persistent or recurrent ejaculation with minimal sexual stimulation or before, upon or shortly after vaginal penetration, and before the person and/or his partner desire it

(Masters and Johnson 1970). In theory, intercourse could last only 1 minute, yet pleasure both partners and not be considered premature.

In fact, rapid ejaculation is rarely pleasurable to either sexual partner. The woman's climax may be denied because she does not experience adequate vaginal stimulation, in addition to direct clitoral stimulation. The man's full sexual pleasure is also denied. Typically, he experiences an exponential increase in sexual excitement. However, the pleasurable time spent in the "plateau" stage of sexual arousal is shortened by an involuntary ejaculation (Figure 3).

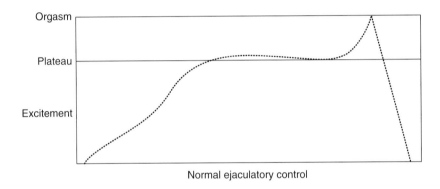

Normal ejaculatory control

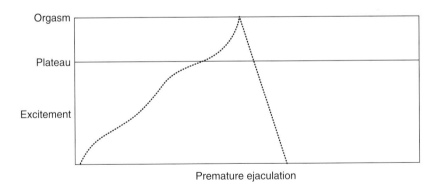

Premature ejaculation

Figure 3
Comparison of the sexual excitement, plateau, and orgasm stages of the sexual response cycle of normal men and men with inadequate ejaculatory control (Kaplan 1989).

Classification of premature ejaculation

Premature ejaculation can be divided into two main types – *primary* when the condition is consistently present from the first coital experience, and *secondary* when satisfactory sexual performance, often for many years, preceded its onset.

Another clinical approach is to subclassify PE into two groups based on cause – *organic* (i.e. spinal cord injury, multiple sclerosis, withdrawal from opiates) or *psychopathological* (i.e. disturbed relationships, high levels of anxiety, anti-sexual childhood messages, a troubled family environment, a demanding partner).

Entry criteria for referenced treatment protocols

The references studies in this chapter, which have evaluated the effect of drugs on premature ejaculation, have selected an IVELT of less than *2 minutes* as a criterion for entry. The vast majority of PE patients participating in pharmacological protocols have had *primary PE without an obvious organic cause*.

Treatment

Psychoanalytic and behavioral therapy

Psychoanalytic therapy has been based on several psychodynamic assumptions. Initially, it was theorized that excessive, unresolved narcissism was manifested in adulthood by PE (Ellis 1936). Subsequent studies, however, did not support this concept. Kaplan suggested it could be the result of unconscious, deep-seated hatred of women. By ejaculating quickly, the man both symbolically soils the woman and robs her of her sexual pleasure (Kaplan 1974). The same author in 1989 suggested that most men with PE do not have discernible neuroses or personality disorders (Kaplan 1989). The ultimate argument against Freudian-based theories is the fact that psychoanalytic therapy has not been effective.

For the past 20 years, behavioral therapy has been commonly used to treat PE. Its pioneers reasoned that by following a "cookbook" set of exercises early, abnormal sexual conditioning (Masters and Johnson) or performance anxiety (Kaplan) could be reversed. The first technique ("stop–start") involved interrupting love-making when ejaculation was felt to be imminent (Semans 1956). In the Masters and Johnson's squeeze technique the partner was instructed to squeeze the penis with her hand hard enough to make him partially lose his erection when he was close to ejaculating (Masters and Johnson 1970). These treatments are empirical, and the proposed underlying psychic abnormalities have never been confirmed. There are no published studies that have compared the early conditioning experiences of men with PE versus men without PE. Anxiety was thought to induce PE through activation of the sympathetic nervous system or by flooding the premature ejaculator's mind with distracting thoughts. Ejaculation sneaks up on the man, so that he is unable to delay it. Again there are no research data to support this theory, only clinical impressions. The early reported success rates for behavioral therapy ("stop–start" technique) of greater than 90% have not been experienced in clinical trials by practising sex therapists (62%) (Kilmann et al 1986). Furthermore, almost all of the post-therapy gains were lost at the 3-year follow-up (DeAmicis et al 1985).

Kaplan subsequently combined behavioral techniques with insight therapy. Psychiatric intervention was used to assist the couple in understanding and resolving interpersonal conflicts as they arose during their behavioral exercises. She reported "virtually universal success with this method and the benefits appear to be permanent in most patients" (Kaplan 1974).

Pharmacological therapy

Topical anesthetics

Several studies have compared the neural circuitry of PE patients and age-matched controls. The findings suggest that patients with psychogenic premature ejaculation have an abnormal autonomic reflex. The various abnormalities that have been detected include a lower penile vibratory threshold, a shorter bulbocavernous (BC) latency time, higher BC evoked potentials, or a greater mean amplitude of dorsal nerve and glans penis somatosensory evoked potentials (Vignoli 1978; Colpi et al 1986; Xin et al 1996, 1997). These abnormalities provide a rational basis for the use of topical anesthetics. In a phase I study, 11 men applied a prilocaine–lidocaine cream to the glans and shaft of the penis: five patients graded the result as excellent and reported an IVELT of 5–10 minutes (Berkovitch et al 1995). In a second study, SS-cream, a topical agent containing nine oriental herbs including ginseng, was used in a double-blind clinical trial involving 43 PE patients (Xin et al 1994). Several lidocaine creams of various strengths were used as the controls. With the lidocaine, five patients reported an increase of IVELT of up to 10–30 seconds. With the SS-cream, 40 patients reported a mean increase of IVELT of 11.3 minutes. The only reported side-effect with the SS-cream was a "transient heat sensation" in the penis.

Oral agents

Oral pharmacological therapy for the treatment of PE has two origins: (1) the reports of adverse outcomes (delayed ejaculation or inability to ejaculate) in the case of various psychotropic agents, and (2) an understanding of the neurotransmitters involved in the ejaculatory reflex. Subsequently performed studies, some of which were double-blind, randomized, placebo-controlled trials, have confirmed or suggested the efficacy of these agents in the treatment of "non-organic" premature ejaculation. The sites and mechanisms of action of many of these drugs have been defined in animals.

Adrenergic antagonists

Shilon reasoned that since sympathectomy was known to cause disturbances in ejaculation, and norepinephrine was the final neurotransmitter in the ejaculatory reflex arc, perhaps an α-adrenergic blocker drug (phenoxybenzamine) would delay ejaculation. Phenoxybenzamine hydrochloride 10–30 mg was administered for 3 weeks to nine patients with PE in a trial that was neither randomized nor placebo controlled (Shilon et al 1984): six patients reported a delay in ejaculation. IVELTs were not provided. All patients experienced a dry ejaculate. A majority of the wives were "satisfied" with therapy. The author highly recommended this regimen for temporary use in cases of PE in men who do not wish to procreate. A second phase I study was performed in 15 patients, using 10–20 mg/day: 12 patients noted a reduced ejaculatory volume and eight patients had an increase in IVELT, with a mean of 10 minutes (Beretta et al 1986).

GABA

Gamma-aminobutyric acid is a neurohormone that inhibits or dampens neural pathways, including the α-adrenergic outflow. Animal studies have demonstrated that anxiolytics (sedatives) that increase GABA activity delay ejaculation (Fernandez-Guasti et al 1991). Drugs that antagonize GABAergic neurotransmission cause a drastic short-ening of the ejaculatory latency time (Fernandez-Guasti et al 1986). A review of adverse outcomes with the benzodiazepine anxiolytics (chlordiazepoxide, lorazepam, alprazolam) reveals a very low inci-dence (<10%) of ejaculatory delay. A retrospective study was per-formed on 100 male veterans with post-traumatic stress disorder (PTSD) who were treated with benzodiazepines (Fossey et al 1994): 42% of the 42 patients receiving clonazepam complained of erectile dysfunction. None of the 84 patients receiving diazepam, the nine patients receiving alprazolam, or the eight patients receiving lorazepam complained of sexual dysfunction during treatment. At the time of writing, a literature search has failed to discover any pub-lished controlled studies in which this class of drugs has been used to treat PE. Perhaps this would be a worthwhile endeavor.

Serotonin re-uptake inhibitors

Non-selective   The tricyclics are non-selective blockers of the re-uptake of serotonin (5-hydroxytryptamine or 5-HT) and norepineph-rine. This action results in an increase in the levels of serotonin in the brain. The higher levels of serotonin inhibit the ejaculatory reflex cen-ter. The tricyclic that has been most extensively studied for use in the treatment of PE is clomipramine. The initial double-blind, placebo-con-trolled study produced equivocal results (Goodman 1980). A subse-quent study showed a significantly higher percentage of satisfactory performances with the drug than with the placebo, and maintenance of the beneficial effect after the drug was replaced by the placebo (Girgis et al 1982). More than 10 years later, there was renewed interest in using this drug in PE patients. Two double-blind, randomized, place-bo-controlled, crossover studies were performed with doses ranging from 25 to 50 mg (Althof et al 1995; Haensel et al 1996). Using 25 mg, the mean intravaginal latency time increased from 1 min to 3.4 min in one study, and from 2 min to more than 8 min in the second; 50 mg increased the latency time from 1 min to more than 7 min. The side-effects commonly reported were dry mouth (anticholinergic), fatigue, dizziness, and altered sensation (antihistaminic). Vaginal latency times returned to baseline following the discontinuation of the drugs.

Selective Serotonin Re-uptake Inhibitors (SSRIs).   When compared to the tricyclics, the SSRIs have a significantly lower incidence of anti-cholinergic side-effects but a higher incidence of gastrointestinal adverse events (nausea, vomiting) (Rickels and Schweizer 1990). (The initial adverse outcome reports indicated that the SSRIs delayed or prevented ejaculation). In the rat model, SSRIs inhibited ejaculation by influencing serotonergic receptors in the nucleus paragigantocellularis, located in the brain stem (Yells et al 1994).

The efficacy of several SSRIs (fluoxetine, paroxetine, and sertraline) in the treatment of patients with PE has been evaluated by controlled studies.

Fluoxetine.   A phase I trial, using fluoxetine 20 mg titrated to 60 mg a day, noted that the median IVELT increased from 1 to 9.6 min (Lee et al 1996); 36% of the patients experienced GI discomfort. In a double-blind, placebo-controlled, parallel groups design, 14 married men with PE who received fluoxetine 20–40 mg experienced an increase in IVELT, after 4 weeks of therapy, from 25 seconds to more than 6 minutes (Kara et al 1996). Two patients discontinued the medication because of nausea.

Paroxetine.   Waldinger treated 14 PE men with 20–40 mg paroxetine in a double-blind, randomized, placebo-controlled manner (Waldinger et al 1994). At 3 weeks, the mean IVELT increased from 30 seconds to 7.5 minutes, and by 6 weeks it increased to 10 minutes. Most patients had fatigue and bursts of frequent intense yawning. A subsequent dose–response study, based on the outcomes of 27 men with PE, demonstrated that 20 mg may be considered "an adequate treatment" (Waldinger et al 1997). Interestingly, very little improvement was noted during the first week of therapy. A second investigator, in a phase I design, evaluated the benefit of a 2-month course of 20 mg paroxetine, taken at bedtime, in 32 men with PE (Ludovico et al 1996). The IVELT increased by "about" 15–20 minutes. The delay time to achieve this outcome was 14 days, and PE reappeared in 90% of the patients within 2–3 weeks after cessation of the drug.

Sertraline.   The final SSRI that has been used in controlled studies in men with PE is sertraline: 52 patients participated in a randomized, placebo-controlled, 8-week study using doses of 50–200 mg per day until the IVELT has been maximized or dose-limiting adverse experiences emerged (Mendels et al 1995). The drug was taken at the evening meal. The mean final daily dose was 121 mg, with the IVELT increasing from 1 minute to 4.30 minutes. There was return to baseline IVELT after stoppage of the medication. Diarrhea (23%), dry mouth (15%) and fatigue (15%) were the most commonly experienced side-effects.

Dopamine blocker

Dopamine is the immediate chemical precursor of norepinephrine. In the rat model, subcutaneous administration of L-dopamine (L-dopa) to sexually experienced male rats decreased the number of penile intromissions taken to reach ejaculation (Paglietti et al 1978). Apomorphine, a dopamine agonist, had a similar effect. Most antipsychotic agents, including the phenothiazines [thioridazine and chlorpromazine], and the heterocyclic compounds [pimozide] have a high affinity for dopamine-2 receptors. All these drugs have been reported to delay ejaculation (Singh 1961; Greenberg 1971; Ananth 1982). In a case report, thioridazine was successfully used in the treatment of PE in a 51-year-old depressed man (Singh 1963). There are no published, controlled studies using dopamine blockers specifically to treat PE, perhaps owing to the magnitude and frequency of their adverse effects (extrapyramidal reactions and sedation).

Smooth muscle relaxants

Intracavernosally injected papaverine hydrochloride in combination with phentolamine mesylate has been successfully used to induce functional penile rigidity for more than 10 years. One investigator studied its efficiency in the treatment of PE (Fein 1990). The study was a phase I design. In the eight study patients, the mixture prolonged penile rigidity, but not IVELTs.

Practical treatment alternatives

At the present time, the treatment of patients with PE will likely be determined by their point of entry into the health care system. The PE patient who encounters a skilled mental health provider, who has a genuine desire to help patients with premature ejaculation and a working knowledge of behavioral and insight therapy, will receive and very likely benefit from non-pharmacological treatment. Long-term follow-up of this therapy is difficult to find in peer-reviewed literature.

Many patients are hesitant to seek out a mental health provider. They believe that their PE has an organic cause and they want a quick fix. These patients present at their primary care provider's office and are frequently referred to a urologist. How should these patients be treated? Today, we have a variety of drugs that have been proven efficacious in the treatment of PE through double-blind, randomized,

Table 1 A synopsis of the clinical trials of the various drugs used to treat premature ejaculation

Drug	Dosage (mg)	Number of patients	Percentage with delay	IVELT (min)	Adverse effects
Topical anesthetics					
Prilocaine–lidocaine	Cream	11	46	5–10	Loss of vaginal sensitivity
SS	Cream	43	93	11.3	Heat sensation in the penis
Alpha-blockers					
Phenoxybenzamine	10–30	9	66	Delayed	Dry ejaculate
Phenoxybenzamine	10–20	15	53	10	Reduced ejaculatory volume
Tricyclics					
Clomipramine	25	15	Mean	3.4	Dry mouth, altered sensation
Clomipramine	25	8	Mean	8.0	Dry mouth, fatigue
Clomipramine	50	15	Mean	7.0	Dry mouth, constipation, altered sensation, dizziness
SSRIs					
Fluoxetine	20–60	11	Mean	9.6	Nausea, indigestion, tingling in extremities
Fluoxetine	20–40	14	Mean	6.0	Nausea, indigestion, insomnia
Paroxetine	20–40	14	Mean	7.5	Fatigue, intense yawning
Paroxetine	20–40	27	Mean	5.0	Fatigue, yawning, dry mouth
Sertraline	50–200	52	Mean	4.3	Diarrhea, dry mouth, fatigue

placebo-controlled trials (Table 1). These include the tricyclic clomipramine and a variety of SSRIs. Any of these drugs may be tried initially on the day of anticipated intercourse. If this approach fails to delay ejaculation, then a daily dosage may be suggested. For the patient who fails to respond to any one treatment, a combination of behavioral techniques and a tricyclic or SSRI drug may be suggested. Alpha-blockers are an option for patients who do not mind a decrease in or absence of ejaculate. Remember that most studies found that PE returned shortly after discontinuance of the drug.

The topical anesthetics may be considered for a select subgroup of PE patients who do not want to take pills and are not disturbed by a decrease in the sensitivity of their penises.

The words of Dr Kaplan – "Naturally, when prematurity is relieved in the setting of individual and marital pathology, cure of the symptom still leaves the couple with their other difficulties" – are a gentle reminder that, if conflicts are present, referral to a mental health provider may be of benefit to the patient (Kaplan 1974).

References

Althof S, Levine S, Corty E, et al (1995). A double-blind crossover trial of clomipramine for rapid ejaculation in 15 couples. *J Clin Psychiatry* **56**:402–7.

Ananth J (1982). Impotence associated with pimozide. *Am J Psychiatry* **139**:1374.

Benson GS, McDonnell J (1983). Erection, emission and ejaculation: physiologic mechanisms. In: *Infertility in the Male*, eds L Lipshultz, SS Howard, p. 181. Churchill Livingstone, New York.

Beretta G, Chelo E, Fanciullacci F, et al (1986). Effect of an alpha-blocking agent (Phenoxybenzamine) in the management of premature ejaculation. *Acta Eur Fertil* **127**:43–5.

Berkovitch M, Keresteci AG, Koren G (1995). Efficacy of prilocaine–lidocaine cream in the treatment of premature ejaculation. *J Urol* **154**:1360–61.

Buch J (1994). Disorders of ejaculation. In: *Impotence*, ed. A Bennett, pp. 186–9. WB Saunders, Philadelphia.

Colpi G, Fanciullacci F, Beretta G, et al (1986). Evoked sacral potentials in subjects with true premature ejaculation. *Andrologia* **18**:583–6.

DeAmicis L, Goldberg D, LoPiccolo J, et al (1985). Clinical follow-up of couples treated for sexual dysfunction. *Arch Sex Behav* **14**:467–89.

Ellis H (1936). *Studies in the Psychology of Sex*. Random House, New York.

Fein R (1990). Intracavernous medication for treatment of premature ejaculation. *Urology* **45**:301–3.

Fernandez-Guasti A, Larsson K, Beyer C (1986).GABAergic control of masculine sexual. Behavior. *Pharmacol Biochem Behav.* **24**:1065–70.

Fernandez-Guasti A, Roldan-Roldan G, Larsson K (1991). Anxiolytics reverse the acceleration of ejaculation resulting from enforced intercopulatory intervals in rats. *Behav Neurosci* **150**:230-40.

Fossey M, Hamner M (1994). Clonazepam-related sexual dysfunction in male veterans with PTSD. *Anxiety* **1**:233–6.

Frank E, Anderson C, Rubinstein D (1978). Frequency of sexual dysfunction in "normal" couples. *N Engl J Med* **299**:111–13.

Girgis S, El-Haggar S, El-Hermouzy S (1982). A double-blind trial of clomipramine in premature ejaculation. *Andrologia* **14**:364–8.

Goodman R (1980). An assessment of clomipramine (anafranil) in the treatment of premature ejaculation. *J Int Med Res* **3**:53–9.

Greenberg H (1971). Inhibition of ejaculation by chlorpromazine. *J Nerv Ment Dis* **152**:364–6.

Guyton AC (1991). *Textbook of Medical Physiology*. WB Saunders, Philadelphia.

Haensel S, Rowland D, Kallan K (1996). Clomipramine and sexual function in men with premature ejaculation and controls. *J Urol* **156**:1310–15.

Kandel ER and Schwartz JH (eds) (1985). *Principles of Neural Science*, 2nd edn. Elsevier, New York.

Kaplan H (1974). *The New Sex Therapy*. Brunner/Mazel, New York.

Kaplan H (1989). *PE: How to overcome premature ejaculation*. Brunner/Mazel, New York.

Kara H, Aydin S, Agargun M, et al (1996). The efficacy of fluoxetine in the treatment of premature ejaculation: a double-blind placebo controlled study. *J Urol* **156**:1631–2.

Kilmann P, Boland J, Noton S, et al (1986). Perspectives of sex therapy outcome: a survey of AASECT providers. *J Sex Marital Ther* **12**:116–38.

Kinsey AC, Pomeroy WB, Martin CE (1948). *Sexual Behavior in the Human Male*. WB Saunders, Philadelphia.

Lee H, Song D, Kim C, et al (1996). An open clinical trial of fluoxetine in the treatment of premature ejaculation. *J Clin Psychopharmacol* **16**:379–82.

Ludovico G, Corvasce A, Pagliarulo G, et al (1996). Paroxetin in the treatment of premature ejaculation. *Br J Urol* **77**:881–2.

Masters W, Johnson V (1970). *Human Sexual Inadequacy*. J & A Churchill, London.

Mendels J, Camera A, Sikes C (1995). Sertraline treatment for premature ejaculation. *J Clin Psychopharmacol* **15**:341–6.

Paglietti E, Pellegrini B, Mereu G, et al (1978). Apomorphine and L-DOPA lower ejaculation threshold in the male rat. *Physiol Behav* **20**:559–62.

Reading A, Wiest W (1984). An analysis of self-reported sexual behavior in a sample of normal makes. *Arch Sex Behav* **13**:69–83.

Rickels K, Schweizer E (1990). Clinical overview of serotonin reuptake inhibitors. *J Clin Psychiatry* **51**(12, suppl B):9–12.

Semans J (1956). Premature ejaculation: a new approach. *South Med J* **49**:353–8.

Shilon M, Paz G, Homonnai Z (1984). The use of phenoxybenzamine treatment in premature ejaculation. *Fertil Steril* **42**:659–61.

Singh H (1961). A case of inhibition of ejaculation as a side effect of Melleril. *Am J Psychiatry* **117**:1041–2.

Singh E (1963). Therapeutic use of thioridazine in premature ejaculation. *Am J Psychiatry* **119**:891.

Vignoli G (1978). Premature ejaculation: new electrophysiologic approach. *Urology* **11**:81–2.

Waldinger M, Hengeveld M, Zwinderman A (1994) Paroxetine treatment of premature ejaculation: a double-blind, randomized, placebo-controlled study. *Am J Psychiatry* **151**:1377–9.

Waldinger M, Hengeveld M, Zwinderman A (1997). Ejaculation-retarding properties of paroxetine in patients with primary premature ejaculation: a double-blind, randomized, dose-response study. *Br J Urol* **79**:592–5.

Xin Z, Seong D, Choi H (1994). A double blind clinical trial of SS-cream on premature ejaculation. *Int J Impot Res* **6**(1):D73.

Xin Z, Chung WS, Choi YD et al (1996). Penile sensitivity in patients with primary premature ejaculation. *J Urol* **156**:978–81.

Xin Z, Choi Y, Rha K, et al (1997). Somatosensory evoked potentials in patients with primary premature ejaculation. *J Urol* **158**:451–5.

Yells D, Prendergast M, Hendricks S, et al (1994). Fluoxetine induced inhibition of make rat copulatory behavior: modification by lesions of the nucleus paragigantocellularis. *Pharmacol Biochem Behav* **49**:121–7.

16

Medical and surgical treatment of Peyronie's disease

John P Pryor and David J Ralph

The aetiology of Peyronie's disease remains obscure even though the pathological changes are well described. The process commences with an inflammatory infiltrate beneath the tunica albuginea and is accompanied by increased fibroblast activity with collagen deposition. Maturation of the collagen leads to the formation of a fibrous plaque, and this is associated with the symptoms of the disease. No curative treatment is available, but fortunately many patients have little in the way of symptoms, and reassurance – particularly that the palpable lump is not cancer – is all that is necessary. Treatment is indicated when the penile pain – and indication of early disease – or deformity is troublesome. Surgery to correct the erectile deformity should only be performed once the disease process has stabilized – usually 12 months after the onset. Some patients also suffer from an impaired erection. The cause of this should be assessed before embarking on any surgical option.

Conservative treatment

The inflammatory exudate in early (painful) Peyronie's disease consists of T lymphocytes and macrophages, which activate the cytokine network to initiate fibrogenesis. Tamoxifen has been shown to increase the secretion of transforming growth factor-β (TGF-β) from human fibroblasts in vitro, and it should inhibit the inflammatory response (Colletta et al 1990). It had been used successfully in the treatment of desmoid tumours (Kinzbrunner et al 1983; Waddel et al 1983), and was therefore used in Peyronie's disease with encouraging results (Ralph et al 1992a). Thirty-six men were treated with tamoxifen, 20 mg twice daily for 3 months. There was some improvement in 20 (55%) of the 36 patients and there was no deterioration in any patient. There was a significantly greater improvement with patients in the earlier stages of the disease (at less than 4 months since the onset). A small biopsy was taken from the plaque in 12 men with painful Peyronie's disease. An excellent response to tamoxifen was found in six of the eight men in whom an acute inflammatory infiltrate was observed, but no improvement occurred in those without an inflammatory response. It is desirable to conduct a double-blind study to assess the benefits of tamoxifen further; but this has not proved to be possible. At the present time we think that it is worthwhile trying tamoxifen for 6 weeks in any patient with painful Peyronie's disease. The nature of Peyronie's disease remains somewhat obscure and, although others have also found tamoxifen to be useful in this condition (Alberti 1996), it may be that its benefit derives from its action on the processes of atherosclerosis or autoimmunity (Grainger and Metcalfe 1996).

Colchicine may decrease collagen synthesis and induce collagenase, and was found to be useful in fibromatosis (Dominguez-Malagon et al 1992). In a series of 24 men with Peyronie's disease, it was found to produce an improvement in plaque size in 12 and an improvement in pain in seven of the nine patients in whom pain was present (Akkus et al 1994). No further reports are available on this treatment. Gelbert et al (1993) injected collagenase directly into the Peyronie's plaque and, in a prospective, double-blind, randomized controlled trial in 49 men, found a significant benefit over placebo ($p = 0.007$) although there was little improvement in the erectile deformity. Levine et al (1994) injected the calcium channel-blocking agent verapamil into the plaque, on the basis that calcium channel blockers alter the metabolism of fibroblasts to inhibit collagen formation. In a study of 14 men, 12 completed the 6-month course of treatment, and the pain improved in 10 of the 11 men in whom it was present, while the deformity improved in five (42%). The improvement in pain always has to be observed against the natural history of the disease.

Duncan et al (1991) showed that interferons are all capable during in vitro culture of inhibiting fibroblast proliferation and collagen production as well as increasing the production of collagenase by Peyronie's tissue. Benson et al (1991) and Judge and Wisniewski (1997) reported favourable clinical results, but in another study there was improvement in only 1 of 25 patients (Wegner et al 1995) in the initial study, and the authors concluded that interferons were ineffective (Wegner et al 1997).

The new methods of treatment all attempt to interfere with fibroblast activity, and might be expected to be useful during the early stages of disease. Their efficacy has to be seen against the natural history of the disease and the knowledge that discomfort on erection rarely persists beyond 6 months (Williams and Thomas 1970; Gelbert et al 1990). Vitamin E is the traditional treatment of choice for Peyronie's disease. It is easy to take, cheap, free of side-effects and better than placebo for treating the pain (Pryor and Farell 1983). p-Aminobenzoate (Potaba) is more expensive, unpleasant to take, has more side-effects and needs to be taken for 12 months (Shah et al 1983; Ludwig 1991). This allows time for the disease to stabilize, and patients with persisting symptoms may then be candidates for surgery. Beneficial results of low-dosage radiotherapy are still being reported (Viljoen et al 1993; Rodrigues et al 1995), but it is probably best avoided in men under the age of 60 years. It has also been reported as the cause of extensive penile fibrosis (Hall et al 1995).

One should mention the use of steroids: either systemically, by local injection, or by transdermal application. Beneficial results have been reported, but have not been found to be reproducible and have been discarded.

Surgical management of Peyronie's disease

Indications for surgery

Surgical intervention is only undertaken once the disease process has stabilized. This is usually one year after the onset; pain on erection has usually subsided and the deformity has been constant for 6 months. The operation should only be performed when the deformity makes penetration difficult or impossible or when there is an associated erectile deficiency due to vasculogenic factors. All the various operations will be discussed, but in general terms the choice rests between a Nesbit-type procedure, the implantation of a penile prosthesis and possibly, in the much shortened penis, a Lue procedure. It is meddlesome to operate just because there is a lump or a minor erectile deformity.

In those men in whom there is an appreciable element of erectile dysfunction it is important to make an assessment of its aetiology. Intracavernosal injection in combination with colour Doppler duplex evaluation and/or cavernometry may yield valuable information (Gasior et al 1990; Ralph et al 1992b; Jordan and Angermeier 1993;

Lopez and Jarow 1993; Montorsi et al 1994; Weidner et al 1997). The erectile defect may be due to psychological causes, an arterial deficit or veno-occlusive dysfunction through abnormal venous drainage at the site of the plaque, deficient elasticity (Akkus et al 1997) in the tunica albuginea, or corporeal muscle dysfunction. In many patients there is a combination of factors, and correction of the deformity should be performed only in those men with an adequate erectile capacity.

Plaque excision and dermal graft

The surgical management of Peyronie's disease was unsuccessful until Devine and Horton (1974) in the USA and Byström et al (1972b) in Scandinavia described the operation of plaque excision and dermal graft replacement of the defect in the tunica albuginea. Byström et al (1972a) reported that despite good results the late results were disappointing, with only 6 of 17 men having a good result after 10 years. Personal experience (Pryor and Fitzpatrick 1979) and a subsequent review of the literature (Pryor 1987) confirmed that many patients had poor results with this operation. This has been confirmed in a recent large series of 418 men treated by plaque excision and a dermal graft operation (Austoni et al 1995). It was found that 17% of patients required further surgery for curvature and that 20% of patients had significant impairment of erection. Erectile dysfunction following plaque excision is due to a combination of factors ranging from damage to the underlying erectile tissue adherent to the plaque, to loss of compliance of the dermal graft, with new venous channels forming to give veno-occlusive dysfunction (Dalkin and Carter 1991) and a deterioration of the underlying aetiological factors. It is now recognized that the histological changes of Peyronie's disease are not confined to the plaque, but may also be seen in the normal tunica albuginea excised during the Nesbit procedure (Iacono et al 1993; Anafarta et al 1994). It is for these reasons that we consider plaque excision and grafting to be an obsolete operation.

The Nesbit procedure

Reed Nesbit (1965) described the correction of erectile deformities due to congenital abnormalities by shortening the opposite side of the penis using plication or the excision of an ellipse of tunica albuginea.

The technique was applied to Peyronie's disease with good initial success (Pryor and Fitzpatrick 1979), and in 359 men operated upon between 1977 and 1992, 295 (82%) had good results and were able to have intercourse (Ralph et al 1995). Operative treatment is only performed when the disease has stabilized – usually at least a year after its onset – and the deformity makes intercourse difficult or impossible.

The operation is performed through a circumglandular incision – circumcising the man if necessary in order to prevent a secondary phimosis. An artificial erection is induced by injecting saline from a rapid transfusion apparatus, and no tourniquet is used, as it sometimes makes for inaccurate assessment of the bend. It is also essential to observe the bend at the time of full erection, otherwise the deformity may be underestimated. The site of maximum bend is marked with a stay suture. Buck's fascia is incised longitudinally and dissected medially to bare the tunica albuginea. This technique permits elevation of the corpus spongiosum ventrally, or the dorsal vascular bundle and the nerves, without appreciable damage. The Nesbit ellipse is marked out opposite the site of maximum deformity and, for every 10 mm of bend, the ellipse is 1 mm wide. In a retrospective study it was found that the mean width of the ellipse was 7 mm and the angle of deformity was 68° (Ralph et al 1995). When in doubt it is possible to apply two Alliss forceps to the tunica albuginea (when the penis is flaccid) and then inflate the penis to check the correction. The ellipse is excised with minimum disturbance to the underlying muscle of the corpus cavernosum and the defect closed with 0 polydioxanone sutures with the knots on the inside. Finally an artificial erection is induced to check that the penis has been straightened.

The results of the Nesbit technique are very satisfactory (Table 1). Some of the poor initial results in the period 1977–83 have been eliminated by preoperative assessment with intracavernous drugs, either alone or combined with colour Doppler ultrasound examination (Ralph et al 1992b). A literature review confirmed the favourable results (Pryor 1987), as have more recent studies (Sulaiman and Gingell 1994; Poulsen and Kirkeby 1995).

Table 1   Results of the Nesbit procedure for Peyronie's disease

	1977–92	*1977–84*	*1985–92*
Excellent result	237 (66%)	101 (58%)	136 (73%)
Satisfactory result	58 (16%)	27 (16%)	31 (17%)
Poor result	64 (18%)	46 (26%)	18 (10%)
Number of men	359	174	185

Table 2   Cause of failure of the Nesbit procedure for Peyronie's disease

Deformity (>30°)	
Surgical error	3
Suture failure	8
Progression of disease	20
Impaired erection	9
Penile shortening (>2 cm)	19[*]
Previous Nesbit	3
Progression of disease	3
Postoperative infection	3

Number of patients = 237.
[*]15 patients were able to have intercourse.

Table 3   Plaque incision and graft replacement of the tunica albuginea in the surgical treatment of Peyronie's disease

Authors	Year	Number of men	Graft technique
Sampaio et al	1992	7	Dura
Brock et al	1993	18	Vein
Faerber and Konnak	1993	9	Dacron
Moriel et al	1994	10	Vein
Ganabathi et al	1995	16	Goretex
Gelbert	1995	30	Temporalis fascia
Kim and McVary	1995	7	Laser and vein
Krishnamurti	1995	17	Pedicled dermal flap
Rigaud and Berger	1995	5	Dermal graft

A variety of corporoplasties that may be regarded as variants of the Nesbit procedure has been introduced; these usually give good results (Yachia 1990; Saissine et al 1994; Geertsen et al 1996; Licht and Lewis 1997; Rehman et al 1997). Some authors favour a simple plication technique (Klevmark et al 1994; Nooter et al 1994), but the problem with this procedure is that the correction is dependent upon the strength of the suture material, and this probably accounts for the unfavourable results of some authors (Poulsen and Kirkeby 1995) and the late failure in others (as high as 24% in one series (Nooter et al 1994)).

The causes of failure of the Nesbit procedure, including patients referred from elsewhere, are shown in Table 2. The alleged drawback of the Nesbit procedure is penile shortening. In Peyronie's disease the penis is shortened by scar tissue, and the operation straightens the penis by shortening the unaffected side. In reality the shortening is rarely troublesome, and was only more than 2 cm in 17 of 359 men, and intercourse was possible in 15 of these (Anafarta et al 1994). The past 5 years have seen attempts to lengthen the penis by incising the fibrous plaque (Table 3) and covering the defect with a graft that does not contract. Dorsal penile, or saphenous, vein would seem to be the simplest method, but, in the uncircumcised man, the pedicle dermal graft of Krishnamurti (Ganabathi et al 1995) is a good alternative. These procedures would seem to have a role to play in those men with an already shortened penis, but longer-term follow-up is still required. Early recurrence of deformity (Table 2) after the Nesbit procedure is due to the sutures cutting out, whereas poor results stemming from the use of absorbable sutures occur after 3 months. Recurrent deformity due to progression of the disease is not usually apparent for 9–15 months.

Implantation of a penile prosthesis

In those men where there is an appreciable element of vasculogenic impotence it is sensible to implant a penile prosthesis. These have always given excellent results (Pryor 1987) provided that the men have a realistic expectation from the operation. The plaque may cause some narrowing of the corpus cavernosal space, but this seldom makes for difficulties. A malleable prosthesis usually corrects the deformity, but with an inflatable prosthesis it may be necessary to incise the plaque. Operative moulding of the penis (Wilson and Delk 1994) over a prosthesis may look and sound horrible, but gives a good result in correcting any deformity. The mechanical reliability of modern multipart inflatable prostheses has improved so much that failure is now more likely to be due to surgical error (Wilson et al 1996).

Conclusion

Many patients require no more than reassurance, but in the early stages it is worthwhile trying drugs, such as tamoxifen, which interfere with the laying down of fibrous tissue. Surgery is reserved for those men with a persistent deformity that makes coitus difficult. The Nesbit procedure gives good results, but in those men with a short penis it is worth considering plaque incision and inserting a vein graft. A penile prosthesis is inserted when there is a marked vasculogenic deficit.

References

Akkus E, Carner S, Rehman J, et al (1994). Is colchicine effective in Peyronie's disease: a pilot study. *Urology* **44**:291–5.

Akkus E, Carrier S, Baba K, et al (1997). Structural abnormalities in the tunica albuginea of the penis: impact of Peyronie's disease, ageing and impotence. *Br J Urol* **79**:47–53.

Alberti C (1996). The rationale of tamoxifen in the management of retroperitoneal fibrosis and Peyronie's disease. A review. *Acta Urol Ital* **10**:7–11.

Anafarta K, Beduk Y, Uluoglu O, et al (1994). The significance of histopathological changes of the normal tunica albuginea in Peyronie's disease. *Int Urol Nephrol* **26**:71–7.

Austoni E, Colombo F, Mantovani F, et al (1995). Chirurgia radicale e conservazione dell'erezione nella malattia di La Peyronie. *Arch Ital Urol* **67**:359–64.

Benson RC Jr, Knoll LD, Furlow WL (1991). Interferon-2β in the treatment of Peyronie's disease (abstract). *J Urol* **145** (suppl):1342.

Brock G, Kadioglu A, Lue TF (1993). Peyronie's disease: a modified treatment. *Urology* **42**:300–4.

Byström J, Alfthan O, Gustafson H, et al (1972a). Early and late results after excision and dermo-fat grafting for Peyronie's disease. *Prog Reprod Biol* **9**:78–84

Byström J, Johansson B, Edsmyr F, et al (1972b). Induratio penis plastica (Peyronie's disease): the results of the various forms of treatment. *Scand J Urol Nephrol* **6**:1–5.

Colletta AA, Wakefield LM, Howell FV, et al (1990). Anti-oestrogens induce the secretion of active transforming growth factor beta from human fetal fibroblasts. *Br J Cancer* **62**:405–9.

Dalkin BL, Carter MF (1991). Venogenic impotence following dermal graft repair for Peyronie's disease. *J Urol* **146**:849–51.

Devine CJ, Horton CE (1974). Surgical treatment of Peyronie's disease with a dermal graft. *J Urol* **111**:44–9.

Dominguez-Malagon HR, Alfeiran-Ruiz A, Chavanna-Xicotencatl P (1992). Clinical and cellular effects of colchicine in fibromatosis. *Cancer* **69**:2478–83.

Duncan MR, Berman B, Nseyo UO (1991). Resolution of the proliferation and biosynthetic activities of cultured human Peyronie's disease fibroblasts by interferon-alpha, -beta and -gamma. *Scand J Urol Nephrol* **25**:89–94.

Faerber GJ, Konnak JW (1993). Results of combined Nesbit penile plication with plaque incision and placement of dacron patch in patients with severe Peyronie's disease. *J Urol* **149**:1319–20.

Ganabathi K, Dinochowski R, Zimmera PE, et al (1995). Peyronie's disease: surgical treatment based on penile rigidity. *J Urol* **153**:662–6.

Gasior BL, Levine FJ, Howannesian A, et al (1990). Plaque-associated corporal veno-occlusive dysfunction in idiopathic Peyronie's disease: a pharmaco-cavernosometric and pharmacocavernosographic study. *World J Urol* **8**:90–6.

Geertsen UA, Brok KE, Andersen B, et al (1996). Peyronie curvature treated by plication of the penile fasciae. *Br J Urol* **77**:733–5.

Gelbert MK (1995). Relaxing incisions in the correction of penile deformity due to Peyronie's disease. *J Urol* **154**:1457–60.

Gelbert MK, Dorey F, James K (1990). The natural history of Peyronie's disease. *J Urol* **144**:1376–9.

Gelbert MK, Jones K, Raich P, et al (1993). Collagenase versus placebo in the treatment of Peyronie's disease: a double blind study. *J Urol* **149**:56–8.

Grainger DJ, Metcalfe JC (1996). Tamoxifen: teaching an old dog new tricks? *Nature Med* **2**:381–5.

Hall SJ, Basile G, Bertero EB, et al (1995). Extensive corporeal fibrosis after penile irradiation. *J Urol* **153**:372–7.

Iacono F, Barra S, De Rosa G, et al (1993). Microstructural disorders of tunica albuginea in patients affected by Peyronie's disease with or without erectile dysfunction. *J Urol* **150**:1806–9.

Jordan GH, Angermeier KW (1993). Preoperative evaluation of erectile function with dynamic infusion cavernosometry/cavernosography in patients undergoing surgery for Peyronie's disease: correlation with postoperative results. *J Urol* **150**:1138–42.

Judge JS, Wisniewski ZS (1997). Intralesional interferon in the treatment of Peyronie's disease: a pilot study. *Br J Urol* **79**:40–2.

Kim ED, McVary KT (1995). Long term follow-up of treatment of Peyronie's disease with plaque incision, carbon dioxide laser plaque ablation and placement of a deep dorsal vein patch graft. *J Urol* **153**:1543–6.

Kinzbrunner B, Ritter S, Domingo J, et al (1983). Remission of rapidly growing desmoid tumours after tamoxifen therapy. *Cancer* **52**:2201–4.

Klevmark B, Andersen M, Schultz A, et al (1994). Congenital and acquired curvature of the penis treated surgically by the plication of tunica albuginea. *Br J Urol* **74**:501–6.

Krishnamurti S (1995). Penile dermal flap for defect reconstruction in Peyronie's disease: operative technique and four years' experience in 17 patients. *Int J Impotence Res* **7**:195–208.

Levine LA, Merrick PF, Lee RC (1994). Intralesional verapamil injection for the treatment of Peyronie's disease. *J Urol* **151**:1522–4.

Licht MR, Lewis RW (1997). Modified Nesbit procedure for the treatment of Peyronie's disease: a comparative outcome analysis. *J Urol* **158**:460–3.

Lopez JA, Jarow JP (1993). Penile vascular evaluation of men with Peyronie's disease and erectile failure. *J Urol* **149**:53–5.

Ludwig G (1991). Evaluation of conservative therapeutic approaches to Peyronie's disease (fibrotic induration of the penis). *Urol Int* **47**:236–9.

Montorsi F, Guazzoni G, Bergamaschi F, et al (1994). Vascular abnormalities in Peyronie's disease: the role of colour doppler sonography. *J Urol* **151**:373–5.

Moriel EZ, Grinwald A, Rajfer J (1994). Vein grafting of tunical incisions combined with contralateral plication treatment of penile curvature. *Urology* **43**:697–701.

Nesbit RH (1965). Congenital curvature of the phallus: report of three cases with description of corrective operation. *J Urol* **93**:230–2.

Nooter RI, Bosch JLHR, Schröder FH (1994). Peyronie's disease and penile curvature: long-term results of operative treatment with the plication procedure. *Br J Urol* **74**:497–500.

Poulsen J, Kirkeby HJ (1995). Treatment of penile curvature – a retrospective study of 175 patients operated upon with plication of the tunica albuginea or with the Nesbit procedure. *Br J Urol* **75**:370–4.

Pryor JP (1987). Peyronie's disease. In: *Recent Advances in Urology*, Vol. 4, ed. WF Hendry, pp. 245–61. Churchill Livingstone, London.

Pryor JP, Farell CF (1983). Controlled clinical trial of Vitamin E in Peyronie's disease. *Prog Reprod Biol* **9**:41–5.

Pryor JP, Fitzpatrick JM (1979). A new approach to the correction of the penile deformity in Peyronie's disease. *J Urol* **122**:622–3.

Ralph DJ, Brooks MD, Bottazzo GF, et al (1992a). The treatment of Peyronie's disease with tamoxifen. *Br J Urol* **70**:648–51.

Ralph DJ, Hughes T, Lees WR, et al (1992b). Pre-operative assessment of Peyronie's disease using colour doppler sonography. *Br J Urol* **69**:629–32.

Ralph DJ, Al-Akraa M, Pryor JP (1995). The Nesbit operation for Peyronie's disease: 16–year experience. *J Urol* **154**:1362–3.

Rehman J, Benet A, Minsky LS, et al (1997). Results of surgical treatment for abnormal penile curvature: Peyronie's disease and congenital deviation by a modified Nesbit plication (tunica shaving and plication). *J Urol* **157**:1288–91.

Rigaud G, Berger RE (1995). Corrective procedures for penile shortening due to Peyronie's disease. *J Urol* **153**:368–70.

Rodrigues CI, Njo KH, Karim AB (1995). Results of radiotherapy and vitamin E in the treatment of Peyronie's disease. *Int J Radiat Oncol Biol Phys* **31**:571–6.

Saissine AM, Wespes E, Schulman CC (1994). Modified corporoplasty for penile curvature: 10 years experience. *Urology* **44**:419–21.

Sampaio JS, Passarinho A, Olivera AG, et al (1992). Surgical correction of severe Peyronie's disease without plaque excision. *Eur Urol* **22**:130–3.

Shah PJR, Green NA, Adib RS, et al (1983). A multicentre double-blind controlled clinical trial of potassium paraaminobenzoate (Potaba) in Peyronie's disease. *Prog Reprod Biol* **9**:47–60.

Sulaiman MN, Gingell JC (1994). Nesbit's procedure for penile curvature. *J Androl* **(Suppl)**:545–65.

Viljoen IM, Goedhals L, Dom MJ (1993). Peyronie's disease: a perspective on the disease and the long term results of radiotherapy. *South Afr Med J* **83**:19–20.

Waddel WR, Gerner RE, Reich MP (1983). Nonsteroid antiiinflammatory drugs and tamoxifen for desmoid tumours and carcinoma of the stomach. *J Surg Oncol* **22**:197–211.

Wegner HEH, Andresen R, Knipsel HH, et al (1995). Treatment of Peyronie's disease with local interferon-a2b. *Eur Urol* **28**:236–40.

Wegner HEH, Andresen R, Knipsel HH, et al (1997). Local interferon alpha 2b is not an effective treatment in early stage Peyronie's disease. *Eur Urol* **32**:190–3.

Weidner W, Schroeder-Printzen I, Weiske Wolf-H, et al (1997). Sexual dysfunction in Peyronie's disease: an analysis of 222 patients without previous local plaque therapy. *J Urol* **157**:325–8.

Williams JL, Thomas GG (1970). The natural history of Peyronie's disease. *Br J Urol* **103**:75–6.

Wilson SK, Delk JR (1994). A new treatment for Peyronie's disease: modelling the penis over an inflatable prosthesis. *J Urol* **152**:1121–3.

Wilson SK, Cleves M, Delk JR (1996). Long term results with Hydroflex and Dynaflex prostheses: device survival and comparison to multicomponent inflatables. *J Urol* **155**:1621–3.

Yachia D (1990). Modified corporoplasty for the treatment of penile curvature. *J Urol* **143**:80–2.

Index

Note: page numbers in *italics* refer to figures and tables

acetylcholine, 19, 20, 28, 256
acromegaly, 59
actin, 15, 16
Acu-Form prosthesis, *234*, 235
adenosine self-injection therapy, 174
adenylate cyclase, 166
adrenal function testing, 60
adrenaline, 18
adrenergic antagonists, premature
    ejaculation, 260
α-adrenoceptors, 99
  agonists, 115
  antagonists, 99–100, 110–12, *160*
α_1-adrenoceptors
  activation, 30, 82
  antagonism, 32
  cavernous smooth muscle, 157
  signaling, 33
  stimulation, 34
  subtypes, 99–100
α_2-adrenoceptors, penile vessels, 157
β_2-adrenoceptors, 157
adult Leydig cell failure, 39
albumin, 40–1
alcohol use, 52
alpha adrenergic receptors, 18
alpha-blockers, 263
alprostadil *see* prostaglandin E_1
American Medical Systems
  penile prostheses, *234*, 235
  three piece inflatable prosthesis, 238,
    239
  two piece inflatable prosthesis, 240, *241*
anaesthetics, topical, 259–60, 265
androgen decline in the aging man
  (ADAM), 142, 153

androgens
  age-associated decline, 39
  exogenous administration, 146, *147*
  normal male aging, 40–1
  receptors, 60
  resistance, 60
  supplemental, 145–6, *147*, 148–50
  withdrawal, 39
andropause, 141
angiography, pharmaco-penile, 92–3
angiotensin II, 159, 160
  antagonists in self-injection therapy,
    174
  secretion suppression by PGE_1, 165
anti-serotinergic inhibitors, self-
    injection therapy, 174
antiarrhythmics, 43
antibiotic prophylaxis, 245
antidepressants, 43
antihypertensives, 43
antipsychotics, 43
anxiety
  patient-related, 71
  premature ejaculation, 258
apomorphine, 28, 113, 152, 263
  central initiator, 134
  injected, 113–14
  oral, 114, 115
arginine analogs, 29
Aristotle, 2
arterial disease, 52
arterial occlusion, traumatic, 81
arterial stenosis, *88*
arteriogenic erectile dysfunction, 81
arteriogenic impotence, 60
arteriography, 62, 64
  selective, 130
arteropathies, 39
atherosclerotic vascular disease, 81